Concepts of
Epidemiology

Concepts of Epidemiology

Integrating the ideas, theories, principles and methods of epidemiology

SECOND EDITION

Raj S. Bhopal, CBE, MD, DSc (hon), MPH,

BSc (hon), MBChB, FFPH, FRCP(E)
Alexander Bruce and John Usher Professor of Public Health
and
Honorary Consultant in Public Health, NHS Lothian Board
(Head of the Division of Community Health Sciences, 2000–2003)
University of Edinburgh, Scotland
formerly
Professor and Head of the Department of Epidemiology
and Public Health
University of Newcastle Upon Tyne

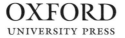

OXFORD
UNIVERSITY PRESS

OXFORD
UNIVERSITY PRESS

Great Clarendon Street, Oxford OX2 6DP

Oxford University Press is a department of the University of Oxford.
It furthers the University's objective of excellence in research, scholarship,
and education by publishing worldwide in

Oxford New York

Auckland Cape Town Dar es Salaam Hong Kong Karachi
Kuala Lumpur Madrid Melbourne Mexico City Nairobi
New Delhi Shanghai Taipei Toronto

With offices in

Argentina Austria Brazil Chile Czech Republic France Greece Guatemala
Hungary Italy Japan Poland Portugal Singapore South Korea Switzerland
Thailand Turkey Ukraine Vietnam

Oxford is a registered trade mark of Oxford University Press
in the UK and in certain other countries

Published in the United States
by Oxford University Press Inc., New York

First published 2002

Reprinted 2002 (with corrections), 2003 (twice), 2004, 2005
(twice, once with corrections), 2006, 2007 (with corrections), 2009

British Library Cataloguing in Publication Data

Data available

Library of Congress Cataloging in Publication Data

Data available

Typeset in Minion
by Cepha Imaging Pvt. Ltd., Bangalore, India.
Printed in Great Britain
on acid-free paper by
Ashford Colour Press, Gosport, Hampshire

ISBN 9780199543144 (Pbk.)

10 9 8 7 6 5 4 3 2

Foreword to the second edition

The exciting, innovative features of Raj Bhopal's book are the emphasis throughout on a conceptual approach and the systematic focus on underlying concepts and fundamental principles. This approach leads students of epidemiology, the intended readers of the book, to a logical understanding of the methods and procedures used in epidemiological research and practice. That was why I endorsed the first edition with unqualified enthusiasm.

The second edition is a thorough revision of the first. There is extensive rewriting and updating throughout the text, which remains crystal clear, easy to read, and easy to understand. The details are specified in the Preface. Students of epidemiology who use this book to enter upon their study of epidemiology have every reason to be grateful to Raj Bhopal for making their task easier and more pleasurable than it might otherwise be.

I am happy to endorse this new edition with the same unqualified enthusiasm with which I greeted the first edition.

John M Last
Emeritus Professor of Epidemiology
University of Ottawa

Foreword to the first edition

When I was learning epidemiology in the late 1950s, I was inspired by the first edition of Jerry Morris's now classic little monograph, *Uses of Epidemiology*, but there were hardly any comprehensive current textbooks to guide me. The few available books were either unreadable, unhelpful, or failed to orient my thoughts along the directions my ideas were taking. How times have changed! Now there are so many good books that it is difficult for the uninitiated to select the most suitable one to meet their needs. In 1997, Raj Bhopal reviewed twenty-five textbooks of epidemiology, discussing their approach to the subject, and their strengths and weaknesses, in a critical commentary that is helpful to teachers and learners alike. Now, from the University of Edinburgh (where I spent five happy years in the 1960s), Raj Bhopal, who holds the Usher chair of public health, has written his own introductory textbook for graduate students who are embarking upon the detailed study of epidemiology.

This is an excellent introduction. Raj Bhopal's approach is conceptual—he describes and explains the underlying concepts and methods of epidemiology with clarity and with apt examples, and simple, elegant illustrations. Frequently throughout the text he asks penetrating questions that will test the limits of his readers' intellectual capacity—an admirable feature that other authors could copy with benefit to themselves and their readers. All the essentials are here: the person–population dyad, variation, error, bias, confounding, causality, the spectrum of disease, the 'iceberg' concept, risk and its relationship to disease frequency, study design, the ethical framework within which we practise epidemiology and conduct research, the relationship of epidemiology to other scholarly pursuits, and finally, some thoughts about the way the discipline has evolved and is likely to continue to evolve in the lifetime of those now entering upon careers in this field.

If I may speak directly to students starting the study of epidemiology: you can be grateful that there is a book like this to guide you along the fascinating pathway that leads to epidemiological enlightenment and understanding. This book will enable you to comprehend the connections between individual and population health, the natural history of disease, the methods of epidemiology, the interventions that work and don't work, and the role of epidemiology as the fundamental public health science. This is a book for you to buy, to read, to study, and to enjoy.

John M. Last
Emeritus Professor of Epidemiology
University of Ottawa

Dedication to the Second Edition
I dedicate this second edition to my brothers Sohan, Kalwant (deceased), Jaswant, Surinder and Mhinder, and my sisters Harbans, Sheila and Baljinder for their love, support, example and direction.

Dedication to the First Edition
I dedicate this book to my mother Bhagwanti Kaur Bhopal for impressing on me (and my siblings) the importance of education, and encouraging us to make up for her own lack of schooling and formal education; and to my father Jhanda Singh Bhopal for setting an example of how to work hard, shoulder responsibility, and strive for self-improvement.

Preface to the Second Edition

Criticism and feedback are the life blood of the academic life. They keep academics alert, on course and on the path to improvement. Criticism can often be painful. It has been wonderful and somewhat surprising that my book has earned so much praise and so little criticism. (One critic did imply that the book did not justify its title, so I hope I have done better this time.) The pleasant problem that this left me with was this: how do I improve the book? I sought answers to this question from colleagues, reviewers, masters-level students and participants in my annual crash course in epidemiology. I hope I have justified the time people spent on giving feedback.

Readers of the second edition can expect even more emphasis on the previous interactive approach-based on questions, exercises and practical and theoretical problems arising in the breadth of epidemiological research and the application of epidemiology into public health practice. The preface to the first edition is still relevant. In addition they will see the following changes (numbers refer to book sections):

- simpler writing, particularly to meet the needs of students whose main language is not English, and those without a medical/clinical background (who might wish to start by reading the glossary)

- several new questions, answers, problems and exercises (the old ones are in an appendix for revision), including 20 questions in Chapter 9 to test students' understanding of study design

- An earlier introduction to the basic tools of rates and study design (1.7)

- a set of examination questions (used at the University of Edinburgh) with model answers so students can test themselves at the end of each chapter

- a brief, foundational introduction to the burgeoning field of genetic epidemiology (Chapters 3 and 10)

- a broader range of concepts are explained including regression to the mean and regression dilution bias (4.2.7), interaction (4.2.5), receiver operating curves (6.5), the counterfactual approach (4.2.4), birth cohort analysis in relation to cross-sectional and secular trends (9.8)

- an introduction to population impact numbers (NEPP and PIN-ER-t) (8.11 and 8.6.2)

- an introduction to the purposes and principles of reviews, systematic reviews and meta-analysis (5.4.4)

- a clearer exposition of epidemiology's relation to statistics based on the principles underpinning epidemiological analysis of data (throughout and 9.11) and introduction to correlation/regression (9.11.5)
- revision of the material in the first edition mainly to ensure it is up to date, and technically correct, including expansion such as on epidemological variables and changes of emphasis, e.g. on data privacy (e.g. Chapter 10)
- 10 tips on how to write for students (appendix, chapter 9)
- †or course teachers, suggestions for the curriculum content for undergraduates, postgraduates, and for continuing education for policy-makers and managers (Appendix at the end of the book)
- updated bibliography (References, websites etc.), and
- a selection of important internet portals (References, websites etc.).

The adage, 'If you like what you see, tell others, if you don't like it tell me', applies here. Please let me know if you have any ideas on improving this book. Write to me at raj.bhopal@ed.ac.uk

Raj Bhopal
29 February 2008

Preface to the First Edition

The purpose of this book is to explain and illustrate the key concepts which underpin the science of epidemiology and its applications to research, policy making, health service planning and health promotion. The book emphasizes theory, ideas, and epidemiological axioms. In doing this I hope to counter the mounting criticism that epidemiology is an atheoretical discipline.

A concept is an idea, but the word is usually reserved for complex, or interrelated, ideas. A concept is the idea behind the word or phrase we use to describe something. This book, then, aims to explain the ideas underlying the language, principles, and basic methods in epidemiology. For example, the attributable risk and odds ratios are not considered merely as arithmetical equations or tools, but also in terms of the ideas underlying their calculation, applications, strengths, and limitations.

This book is primarily written for postgraduates beginning courses on epidemiology anywhere in the world, for the concepts are the same everywhere. Only the examples will differ. The book may be of interest to public health and other epidemiological practitioners interested in revisiting the fundamental ideas of their discipline. Undergraduates who are keen on epidemiology may find it helpful in deepening their understanding generally, or while studying some topics in a little depth. Health professionals (including busy doctors) may find this material an interesting adjunct to their use of epidemiological techniques or data. Finally, health service managers and policy-makers may find this book a source of insights into the world of epidemiology.

There are 10 chapters. Many introductory courses are designed around 10–15 or so sessions. I envisage that the core of this book could be grasped in 10 days of committed study, preferably in the context of a taught course, but also independently.

The book is written in plain language but a basic understanding of biology is needed, as is some familiarity with illness and disease. However, medical terminology is explained and defined in a glossary. The learning objectives are expressed in terms of the reader acquiring understanding. I believe that achieving understanding is the highest form of learning; from that may flow a lasting and usable knowledge base, change of attitude, and the achievement of skills. There are exercises to help readers to deepen their understanding. Each chapter ends with a summary.

The motivation to write this book came from two directions, one in academia, the other in public health practice. As an examiner of both undergraduate and postgraduate students I was surprised, and crestfallen, to see how many students could not clearly explain basic ideas such as the difference between a case–control and cohort study, some-times even after a year of study. In my duties in the health service I participated in many discussions on why service demands exceeded supply even after new investments were made. Not once did anyone invoke the crucial concept of the iceberg of disease and symptoms to explain this phenomenon, and clearly even those who knew of it did not make the leap from the classroom to the boardroom. This book is deliberately discursive, not simply descriptive, to help readers to achieve a deeper understanding and to help bridge the world of theory to that of practice.

Students rapidly grasp the importance and worth of studying concepts, and demand more. The depth of understanding of concepts gained from most books and courses is insufficient to permit students to apply what they have learned to the problems they are to solve. The acid test of this book is whether readers find themselves using epidemiological concepts in their everyday work, not seeing them merely as theoretical constructs for the classroom and examination hall.

The conceptual frameworks within which the practice of epidemiology operates take a slightly different perspective from those of the science of epidemiology. The nature of research questions, the relative value of the various methods, and the approach to data analysis, presentation, and interpretation differ. This book demonstrates these differences and makes the implications explicit.

The book places heavy emphasis on integrating the ideas of epidemiology. The interdependence of epidemiological studies and their essential unity is an important theme of this text. It is, therefore, designed to be read as a whole, either as a foundation text or as a refresher. Each chapter, however, can be read independently if necessary, with cross-references to other chapters for required definitions.

This book differs in many ways from alternatives, for example:

- The concepts of epidemiology are discussed in detail, and in an integrated way.

- The concepts are dominant whereas in other books the methods dominate.

- The epidemiological idea of population is explicitly the foundation of the whole book. In most other books the population idea is implicit and in some it is neglected.

- The practical applications of each concept are considered, and illustrated with examples drawn from contemporary research and public health practice, including health care policy and planning. The idea is that the reader will acquire the depth of knowledge to use the concepts and not merely be aware of them.

- The work is rooted in the basic ideas of the science of epidemiology, which are wholly applicable worldwide, not just in Europe or North America.

- The emphasis is on gaining understanding, and not on calculations, except where this is essential to understanding.

- Most of the exercises require reflection not calculation.

In short this textbook focuses on a theme which is the most important in any science, is too often overlooked, and which students demand more of: concepts.

R.S.B.
Written 2001

Acknowledgements for the Second Edition

My debts as recorded in the first edition, reprinted here, are still outstanding and can never be repaid. I am grateful to the many people who spontaneously provided feedback on the first edition and those who wrote reviews for publication in journals and websites. OUP has proven itself a most supportive publisher with many highly professional colleagues – I thank especially Helen Liepman, Georgia Pinteau, Rosemary Bailey and Claire Caruana for their feedback, encouragement and help over the years that has spurred me to prepare this edition.

Permissions for reproducing material are noted separately, but I record my gratitude to publishers here.

Professor John Last's support has been constant and reflected in his splendid second foreword for me. Dr Colin Fischbacher's comments on all the new sections were invaluable for he has a keen and critical eye. My postdoctoral colleague Dr Charles Agyemang gave prompt, enthusiastic and able feedback on the new material. Professor Harry Campbell offered expert guidance on my introduction to genetics. Professor Richard Heller provided excellent material on population impact numbers, so if my distillation has impurities, this is my responsibility. Dr Sarah Wild helped me think about the section on interaction.

I could not have coped with a task like this revision without my secretary, Anne Houghton. The support of my academic colleagues in Edinburgh University is worth noting for they, surely, must have been patient as their own priorities awaited my more than usually distracted attention.

The support of one's institution is vital to a project like this. The University of Edinburgh is a research-intensive university, and writing textbooks is a little wayward, especially in the College of Medicine. I thank my institution for allowing me to go slightly astray.

Students are the teachers' teachers. I have learned a great deal from my undergraduate, postgraduate and postdoctoral colleagues and this book hopes to repay them.

My family is now used to me and my scribbles. I thank my children Sunil, Vijay, Anand and Rajan for the joy and fulfilment they give me. Without the tolerance and love of my wife, Roma, I would not have had the peace of mind, focus and drive to pursue my academic passions. In trying to thank her I am, for once, lost for words!

February 2008

Acknowledgements for the First Edition

My foremost debt is to the innumerable people who have taught me, whether in the classroom, seminar, and conference, or by their writings. One absorbs ideas and facts from others and over time synthesizes them with one's own thoughts and experiences. Eventually, it is impossible to distinguish one's own ideas from those of others. If my readers recognize their own ideas, and think they are incompletely acknowledged, then please accept my thanks and let me know.

Needless to say, I am responsible for all remaining errors of fact or interpretation—readers would do me a great favour by alerting me to any they discover (E-mail raj.bhopal@ed.ac.uk).

Many people have helped me by giving encouragement, information, constructive criticism, and by helping to prepare the manuscript. I can list only a few here; the others are not forgotten.

Marcus Steiner, an MSc (Epidemiology) student and graduate at Edinburgh University, was my postgraduate reader-critic and helper. His advice and help, particularly with the technical preparation and development of the figures, was immensely useful. His comment after reading an early draft, 'I wish I knew all this before', was highly motivating to me at times of difficulty.

Dr Sonja Hunt stimulated me to think about Figure 10.1. Dr Colin Fischbacher helped me proof-read the manuscript and made several thoughtful observations. Professor John Last enthusiastically agreed to write the foreword.

Others who provided academic advice on one or more specific chapters include: Professor Carl Shy, Dr David Chappel, Dr Eileen Kaner, and four anonymous referees who commented on the book proposal and chapter outlines.

I thank Dr Mike Lavender for permission to use extracts from our joint unpublished paper on the role of epidemiology in priority setting, and co-authors on various publications that I have drawn on (these are referenced). I have drawn heavily on my publications to prepare Chapter 10 and acknowledgements are given below.

Helen Liepman, Commissioning Editor at Oxford University Press, deserves thanks for her enthusiasm, expert support, and patience.

I conceived this book while in my post as Professor of Epidemiology and Public Health at the University of Newcastle upon Tyne, England. The embryonic and fetal growth stages of the idea were nourished during my sabbatical at the Department of Epidemiology of the School of Public Health at the University of North Carolina at Chapel Hill, and on my return to Newcastle. The birthplace of the book, however, was in Edinburgh, during my tenure as Alexander Bruce and John Usher Professor of Public

Health in the Section of Public Health, Department of Community Health Sciences, Edinburgh University. I thank these departments and institutions, and my colleagues within them.

Secretarial support was provided chiefly by Lorna Hutchison, Carole Frazer (both Newcastle University), Betsy Seagroves (University of North Carolina), Janet Logan, and Hazel King (both Edinburgh University). Hazel bore the dual challenge of making sense of the styles of many other secretaries, and finishing the job.

It is customary to thank one's family, for many sacrifices including forsaking the dining room which is taken over by the author as a writing den. In my case I offer grateful thanks to my wife Roma for encouraging me to finish the project, for accepting the sleep disruption caused by early morning shuffling as I slipped out of bed and into the study, and for my lack of enthusiasm for late night revelries. She also allowed me to use the dining room as the second study in the last month of the project! I have four sons, Sunil, Vijay, Anand, and Rajan, and I ask their forgiveness for sometimes being too busy and distracted to give them and their passions the attention they deserved.

R.S.B.
Written 2001

Permissions

Permission to use material published elsewhere and due acknowledgements

I have drawn upon *A Dictionary of Epidemiology (4th Ed)* by J. Last, throughout the book and, especially, the glossary (with the permission of the author). Direct quotations are attributed but readers will recognize the general debt I owe. I have reutilized my own published work, albeit in new contexts and with heavy editing, mostly as acknowledged and with permissions.

Chapter 2

Figure 2.2 is adapted from Figure 2 in G. Rose (1985) *International Journal of Epidemiology*, **14**, 32–38 (with permission).

Chapter 3

Figures 3.1, 3.2, 3.3, and Table 3.4 are based on the concepts in R. Bhopal (1991) *Journal of Public Health Medicine*, **13**, 281–9 (published with permission).

The artwork for Figs 3.4–3.7 was originally done by the Newcastle Medical School's Medical Illustration Unit under my direction.

Figure 3.7 and Tables 3.5 and 3.6 were first published in R. Bhopal *et al.* (1992) *British Medical Journal*, **304**, 1022–7 (Figure 1 and Tables 2 and 3). They are published here with permission.

Figure 3.8 was first published in Bhopal *et al.* (1991) *British Medical Journal*, **302**, 378–83, and Table 3.7 is an extract from the same paper (Table 2). They are published here with permission.

Chapter 4

The abstract in Box 4.6 is similar to the one published in Bhopal *et al.* (1998) *Occupational and Environmental Medicine*, **55**, 812–22 (published with permission from the BMJ Publishing Group).

The data in Table 4.2 were first published by the Health Education Authority, a body that no longer exists. The source is acknowledged.

Chapter 5

The statistics for Table 5.1 are extracts from I. Semmelweiss's book *The etiology, concept, and prophylaxis of childbed fever,* republished in C. Buck *et al.* (1988) *The challenge of epidemiology.* PAHO, Washington.

The drawings of the triangle (Fig. 5.4) and wheel of causation (Fig. 5.7), now in widespread use, were inspired by those published in Mausner and Kramer (1985) *Epidemiology*, 2nd edn. Saunders, Philadelphia.

The model of the component causes (Fig. 5.11) is based on the ideas and diagrams in K. Rothman and S. Greenland (1998) *Modern Epidemiology*. Lippincott, Philadelphia.

Chapter 6

Figure 6.8 is based on Figure 9.6 in Mausner and Kramer (1985) *Epidemiology*, 2nd edn. Saunders, Philadelphia. It is published with permission. Mausner and Kramer, in turn, based it on data from T. J. Vecchio (1966) *New England Journal of Medicine*, 274, 1171 (with permission).

Table 6.2 is prepared from text published in W. Holland and S. Stewart (1990) *Screening in health care*, pp. 12–13. Nuffield Provincial Hospitals Trust with permission.

Figure 6.10 is from Raffle, A.E. (2000) Honesty about screening programmes is best policy. *British Medical Journal*, **320**, 872 (with permission from the BMJ Publishing Group).

Chapter 7

Figure 7.3 is from unpublished work by R. Williams and based on data reported in an abstract (Bodansky, H. J., Airey, C. M., Chell, S. M., Unwin, N. and Williams, D.R.R. (1997) The incidence of lower limb amputation in Leeds, UK: setting a baseline for St Vincent. International Diabetes Federation Meeting. *Diabetologia*, A1850. The figure is published here with permission of the senior authors D.R.R. Williams and N. Unwin.

The bath model (Fig. 7.6) develops a diagram given to me by Ms Denise Howel: thanks are recorded.

The codes in Table 7.6 are extracted, with acknowledgement, from WHO's ICD-10 (International statistical classification of diseases and related health problems. World Health Organisation, Geneva, 1992).

Chapter 8

Table 8.1 is a small extract from a large table published in M. Marmot *et al.* (1984) *Immigrant mortality in England and Wales*. HMSO, London. The source is acknowledged. Table 8.2 is a small extract of a table published in T. Pless-Mulloli *et al.* (1998) *Environmental Health Perspectives*, **106**, 189–96. The source is acknowledged.

Table 8.12 extracts data from R. Doll and A. Bradford Hill (1956) *BMJ*, 2,1071–81 as summarized by Mausner and Bahn in *Epidemiology*, Table 7.4. Table 8.12 adapts this table (with permission from the BMJ and Elsevier).

Table 8.14 is based on that published on p. 29 in J. Mackintosh *et al.* (1998) *Step by step guide to epidemiological health needs assessment*. Newcastle University, Newcastle upon Tyne (there is no copyright, and R. Bhopal is the second author).

Table 8.15 is based on that published in *BMJ* (1994) **309**, 327–30 and is published here with permission.

Tables 8.17, 8.18, and 8.19 are based on work reported in Lee (1998) *International Journal of Epidemiology*, **27**, 1053–6 (with permission of the author and the editor).

Chapter 9

The data in Table 9.3 are extracted from a large table in R. Bhopal *et al.* (1998) *Occupational and Environmental Medicine*, **55**, 812–22 (with permission).

Table 9.6 is adapted from Table 1, in Frost W. H. The age selection of mortality from tuberculosis in successive decades. *American Journal of Hygiene* 1939, **30**, 91–96.

Chapter 10

Table 10.1 was first published by R. Bhopal in: S. Rawaf, V. Bahl (ed.) (1998) *Health needs assessment in ethnic minority groups.* Royal College of Physicians, London (used with permission).

Table 10.2 is adapted from a joint unpublished work with M. Lavender (published with permission of the co-author).

The text in Chapter 10 combines new and edited published writings. The edited material is as follows:

Discussion on paradigms, e.g. some of 10.1 and 10.5 draws on Bhopal, R. S. (1999) Paradigms in epidemiology textbooks: In the footsteps of Thomas Kuhn. *American Journal of Public Health*, **89**, 1162–5. Copyright 1999 by the American Public Health Association (with permission).

Section 10.3 draws on an unpublished paper with M. Lavender (with permission of the co-author).

Discussion on the US and UK context, e.g. Section 10.8 draws on Bhopal, R. S. (1998) The context and role of the American School of Public Health: Implications for the UK. *Journal of Public Health Medicine*, 20, 144–8 (with permission).

Sections 10.10.1 and 10.11 on tobacco draw on Edwards, R., Bhopal, R. (1999) The covert influence of the tobacco industry on research and publication: a call to arms. *Journal of Epidemiology and Community Health*, **53**, 261–2 (with permission from the BMJ Publishing Group).

Section 10.10.2 draws on Bhopal, R. S., Rankin, J., McColl, E., Thomas, L., Kaner, E., Stacy, R., Pearson, P., Vernon, B. and Rodgers, H. (1997) The vexed question of authorship: views of researchers in a British medical faculty. *British Medical Journal*, **314**, 1009–12, and other work with these colleagues. This help is acknowledged.

Section 10.10.3 and other discussions on race, ethnicity, and health draw upon Bhopal, R. (1997) Is research into ethnicity and health racist, unsound, or important science? *British Medical Journal*, **314**, 1751–6 (with permission from the BMJ Publishing Group).

Sections 10.14 and 10.15 draw on Bhopal, R. (2001) *Generating health from the pattern of disease.* Royal College of Physicians, London **31**, 293–8 (with permission).

The Section 10.12 draws heavily on P. Skrabanek (both deceased) and J. McCormick's book *Follies and fallacies in medicine* (with permission of the Trinity College Dublin).

Contents

Glossary, including many of the concepts considered in this book

Acute An adjective commonly applied to diseases that have a short time course.

Adenocarcinoma A cancer of musosal cells.

Aetiology/aetiological Causation/about causation.

AIDS Acquired immune deficiency syndrome is the serious multisystem disease resulting from infection by the human immodeficiency virus (HIV).

Allele See **gene**.

Anorexia Impaired appetite for food which can lead to serious illness; when caused by psychological factors it is called anorexia nervosa.

Angina See **Rose angina**.

Aristotle Greek philosopher, scientist and general scholar living 384–322 BC.

Arrhythmia An abnormal rhythm—usually applied to the heart, e.g. atrial fibrillation.

Association A link, connection, or relationship, between risk factors, diseases, and most usually between risk factors and diseases.

Asthma A respiratory disease characterized by difficulty in breathing caused by narrowing of the airways (which is reversible).

Atherosclerosis/atherosclerotic The process of deposition of lipids and other materials in the walls of arteries leads to their narrowing and to inflammation. Such an artery is atherosclerotic (also known as arteriosclerosis/arterosclerotic)

Atrial fibrillation An irregular heart beat resulting from very rapid and irregular contractions of the atrium (one of the chambers of the heart).

Attenuation Reduction of the effect of a cause. Used in microbiology where the virulence of microbes may be reduced through process that attenuate the effects, e.g. in the production of vaccines.

Autopsy See **necropsy**.

Autosomal A genetic disorder relating to any chromosome except the sex chromosomes.

Berkson, Joseph (1899–1982) and **Berkson's Bias** The bias, explained in the text, was first described by this American statistician.

Blood pressure Usually refers to the pressure in the systemic arteries (not veins and pulmonary arteries), as measured by sphygmomanometer (see below).

Bradford Hill (Austin) Statistician, 1897–1991, renowned for his work on smoking and cancer, and clinical trials, and for guidance on causal interpretation of data.

Brucellosis An infection caused by Brucella microorganisms, characterized by recurrent fevers.

Capture–recapture methods A technique whereby two or more incomplete data sets are used to estimate the true size of the population of interest. Usually, the method is applied to elusive populations, e.g. the homeless.

Carcinogen(ic) A substance that increases the risk of developing a cancer (an adjective describing such a substance).

Case A person with the disease or problem under investigation.

Caseous An adjective applied to cheese-like lesions produced in response to inflammation, e.g. in tuberculosis.

Cataract An opacity in the lens of the eye.

Causation The term is commonly used in medicine as an alternative to aetiology.

Cause Something which has an effect, in the case of epidemiology, this effect being (primarily) a change in the frequency of risk factors or adverse health outcomes in populations.

CAD or **Coronary artery disease** See **Coronary heart disease**.

Cholesterol A lipid (fatty substance) that is essential to many bodily functions that is transported in the blood via lipoproteins. Cholesterol and other lipids carried by low/very low-density lipoproteins (LDL/VLDL) are a risk factor for coronary heart disease (and like vascular diseases), while those carried by high-density lipoproteins (HDL) seem to be protective.

Chromosome See **gene**.

Chronic An adjective commonly applied to diseases that have a long-lasting time course, and usually applied to non-toxic and non-infectious diseases.

Chronic bronchitis A lung disease characterized by production of excess sputum, wheezing, shortness of breath and eventual respiratory failure.

Circadian A rhythm with a cycle lasting about 24 hours, corresponding to each day.

Competing causes A concept where alternative causes of disease, or more usually causes of death, are in competition with each other; for example, in African Caribbean populations one explanation of the comparatively low CHD rates is that the atherosclerotic process kills people from stroke. If stroke were to be controlled, it may be that CHD would become more common.

Confidence interval The interval, with a given probability, within which is contained the population value of a summary measure from a sample such as a mean, or odds ratio.

Confounding The distortion of the measure of an association by other (confounding) factors that influence both the outcome and risk factor under study.

Contagion/contagious The infectious diseases that may be transmitted from person to person.

Congenital A health problem present at birth.

Cooling tower A term that describes a structure (sometimes including evaporative condensers, designed to extract heat from a liquid—usually water—before its recirculation).

Coronary heart disease/coronary artery disease A group of diseases resulting from reduced blood supply to the heart, most often caused by narrowing or blockage of the coronary arteries that provide the blood supply to the heart.

Correlation analysis The extent that variables are associated with each other. The word is usually applied to continuous variables. The association can be measured by a statistical technique giving the correlation coefficient (which varies from −1 (inverse correlation) to +1, positive correlation).

Cot death A synonym for the sudden infant death syndrome, which is unexplained death in infancy (full definition in text).

Crick (Francis) 1916–2004 One of three scientists receiving the Nobel prize for discovering the structure of DNA in 1953.

Crohn's disease A disorder usually of the lower part of the small intestine, characterized by inflammation.

Cutaneous Associated with the skin.

Davey Smith (George) Epidemiologist, 1959–, working primarily in life-course epidemiology and inequalities in health.

Deep vein thrombosis Clotting of blood in the deep veins usually of the calves, thigh, and pelvis. The clots may lead to a pulmonary embolus.

Degenerative An adjective applied to disease thought to be resulting from deterioration of tissues over time, i.e. with age.

Demographic transition The change in the age structure of the population when death rates and fertility declines, with a comparatively older population being the result.

Demography The scientific study of population, particularly the factors that determine its size and shape, including birth and death. A cousin of epidemiology.

Depression A serious clinical illness with a characteristic set of symptoms and behaviours that, in its most severe form, may lead to suicide.

Diabetes (mellitus) A disease characterized by high levels of glucose in the blood caused by either lack or ineffectiveness of the hormone insulin.

Diethylstilboestrol A medication containing the hormone oestrogen.

Differential diagnosis A preliminary list of the most likely diseases in a patient, to be confirmed by further investigation.

Disease A bodily dysfunction, usually one that can be described by a diagnostic label. (For simplicity, this book concentrates on discussing diseases and uses this word when other words describing other health problems would also be appropriate, e.g. death, disability, illness, sickness, etc.)

Distribution The frequency with which each value (or category) occurs in the study population. The distribution of many variables takes on a characteristic shape. (See **normal distribution**.)

Dizygotic Usually refers to non-identical twins who have shared the womb, but result from two fertilized eggs (see monozygotic).

Down's syndrome A congenital genetic disorder, leading to mental retardation and a characteristic face caused by the presence of three chromosomes instead of two at the site of the 21st chromosome.

Durkheim (Emile) 1858–1917, French social theorist and eminent sociologist.

Effect modifier The concept is explained in the text, but briefly a factor that alters the causal impact of another factor, the classical example being that smoking cigarettes greatly increases the risk of lung cancer after exposure to asbestos and vice versa.

Einstein (Albert) Physicist, 1879–1955, most famous for the theory of relativity.

Elective In health care, a procedure done at a time chosen for its convenience, as opposed to being dictated by an emergency, e.g elective surgery.

Electrocardiogram (ECG) A recording of the electrical activity of the heart made by an instrument called an electrocardiograph.

Emphysema When applied to the lungs (pulmonary emphysema) a condition caused by destruction of lung tissue with gaseous distension.

Environment A broad concept in epidemiology, sometimes meaning everything except genetic and biological factors, and sometimes more qualified and narrow, e.g. physical environment.

Epidemiological transition The change in disease patterns that accompanies the demographic transition, with both usually following economic, educational or social improvements. See text for details.

Epidemiology See text, but in short, the study of the pattern of diseases and their causes in populations.

Epilepsy A complex disease of the brain characterized by temporary, involuntary, altered states of consciousness, including fits (convulsions).

Equity/inequity An equality that is required by our rules on fairness and justice. An inequality that is unfair or unjust is called an inequity. So inequity is a subset of inequality, as not all inequalities are unfair.

Ethnicity The group you belong to, or are perceived to belong to, or a mix of both, as a result of cultural factors such as dress, religion, diet, name, and physical appearance, the latter a result of ancestry, e.g. skin colour.

Evans (Alfred) Epidemiologist, 1917–1996, who developed ways of assessing causality, based on the Henle–Koch postulates.

Exposure A general term to indicate contact with the postulated causal factors (or agents of disease) used in a way similar to risk factor.

Fetal origins of disease hypothesis The phrase encapsulating the idea that early life circumstances, particularly *in utero*, have an important and lasting effect in determining health and disease in later life.

Galton (Francis) 1822–1911 A British scientist who made numerous contributions including to biology (genetics) and statistics. Founder of eugenics, the science of good breeding, that was widely abused by governments across the world, including Nazi Germany.

Gaussian (see **normal distribution**)

Gene The discrete basic unit (made of DNA or deoxyribonucleic acid) of the chromosome, which itself consists of numerous genes and other DNA material. Genes carry information coding for specific functions, e.g. making proteins. There are two copies of each gene, one on each of the pair of chromosomes. The two copies of the gene at a particular location on the pair of chromosomes are called alleles. There are 23 pairs of chromosomes in each cell in human beings (46 in total), and the number of genes is variously estimated as 25–30,000 (until recently 50–100,000).

Generalisation Drawing principles or conclusions that go beyond the data at hand and, often in epidemiology, the population studied. In sciences, epidemiology being no exception, generalizability is a much coveted property.

Genetic drift Genetic evolution, characteristically observable in small populations, arising from random variations in gene frequency.

Gestational diabetes High levels of blood glucose in association with pregnancy (see diabetes).

Goldberger (Joseph) 1874–1927 American public health doctor and epidemiologist famed for his work demonstrating the nutritional basis of pellagra.

Gonorrhoea Sexually transmitted infection caused by the bacterium *Neisseria gonorrhoeae.*

Gregg (Norman) 1892–1966 Australian opththalmologist famed for his hypothesis that rubella (German measles) in the mother could lead to congenital abnormalities in the fetus (Rubella syndrome).

Henle (Jacob) 1805–1885 German pathologist who provided three of the four (Henle–Koch) postulates that underpin analysis of whether a microbe causes disease.

HDL See **cholesterol**.

Heaf test A skin test similar to the Mantoux test (see below).

Health A desired ideal, which includes being alive and free of disease, disability, and infirmity, characterized by well-being and efficient functioning in society.

Helicobacter pylori A bacterium that lives in the human stomach, and in some circumstances causes gastritis, ulcers, and stomach cancer.

Herd immunity The resistance of an entire community to spread of infection arising from immunity to the infection in a high proportion of the population preventing easy spread of disease.

Herpes Infection with the herpes simplex virus, characterized by small blisters, usually in and around the mouth (type I virus) and on and around the genitals (type II virus).

Hippocrates (460–377 BC) approximately Influential teacher and leader of a school of medical thought that continues to be influential, and not only in relation to the Hippocratic Oath.

Histology The examination of tissues microscopically (and the results thereof).

Human papillomavirus (HPV) A viral microorganism that causes, among other problems, cervical cancer.

Hume (David) Scottish philosopher and historian living 1711–1776.

Hypersensitivity reaction An abnormally powerful reaction by the immune system to exposure to some substances (allergens) such as peanuts, fur or pollen.

Hypertension A condition of having blood pressure above an arbitrarily defined level (presently 140/90). Hypertension is associated with many adverse outcomes, particularly atherosclerotic diseases.

Hypertrophy Unnatural enlargement of the tissues or structures.

Hypothesis A proposition that is amenable to test by scientific methods. (See **null hypothesis**.)

Illness The state of being unwell, usually due to disease.

Impaired glucose tolerance An abnormality of glucose metabolism detected after glucose measurements following a fast and the ingestion of a standard glucose load. It predicts a higher risk of CHD and of diabetes.

Inequity See **equity**.

Jenner (Edward) 1749–1823 British medical practitioner who tested a hypothesis that exposure to cowpox protects against smallpox. This laid the scientific foundation for the eradication of smallpox and immunization.

Kaposi's sarcoma A cancer of cells (called reticuloendothelial cells) that is characterized by brown/purple patches on the skin.

Koch, Robert (1843–1910), a German bacteriologist who established the bacterial cause of many infectious diseases, including anthrax (1876), tuberculosis (1882), conjunctivitis (1883), and cholera (1884).

Kuhn (Thomas) Science philosopher, 1922–1996, who is renowned for his work on the nature of scientific revolutions.

LDL/VLDL See **cholesterol**.

Lead-time The extra time gained by earlier than usual detection of disease, as in screening.

Legionnaires' disease A pneumonia usually caused by the bacterium *Legionella pneumophila* (so-called because of the major outbreak among the US Legionnaires attending a convention in Philadelphia in 1976).

Leprosy A multisystem infection caused by the bacterium *Mycobacterium leprae.*

Leukaemia A group of cancers of blood cells, with various types, e.g., chronic myeloid leukaemia, acute leukaemia, etc.

Life-grid approach A technique of data collection from the past where the information of interest, say, smoking habits, is linked to key life events, e.g. date of marriage, change of job, etc.

Lind (James) 1716–1794 British naval physician who did a controlled trial (one of the first on record) of treatments for scurvy, finding that oranges and lemons were curative.

Logistic regression See **multiple regression**.

Lyme disease An infection caused by the microorganism *Borrelia burgdorferi*, characterized by skin rash and arthritis.

Lymph glands or nodes The fluid from the spaces between cells drains into the lymphatic system, a network of tubes. The lymph glands/nodes are lymphatic organs connecting into the lymphatic system, and are important in the immune system.

Mantoux test A skin test to assess the level of immune response to tuberculosis, using a protein derived from the tubercle bacillus.

Mean A statistical measure of the average, where the values for all the members of a group are added up, and the total is divided by the number of members.

Median A statistical measure of the average; the value that divides a group into two equal parts, those below and those above the median.

Melanoma A skin cancer of the pigment producing cells of the skin or eye.

Mendel (Gregor) 1822–1884 He published in 1866 his research on the laws of heredity based on his observations and experiments on garden peas. This was the beginning of the science of genetics.

Meningitis/meningococcal meningitis An inflammation of the lining around the brain (meninges), as, for example, caused by infection by the meningococcus bacterium.

Miasma An impurity in air capable of causing diseases, the impurity arising from a number of sources including decaying matter and from cases of disease. Cholera was long thought to be caused by miasma.

Microorganism A term to refer to unicellular organisms including viruses, bacteria, protozoa, and algae.

Mm Hg Pressure recorded as millimetres of mercury (Hg) because traditionally mercury has been used in the sphygmomanometer.

Mode A statistical measure of the average; simply the most commonly occurring value.

Monozygotic Refers to identical twins born from one fertilized egg. Twin studies are important in epidemiology to help judge the relative importance of environment and genes.

Multiple (logistic) regression In regression analysis a mathematical model is constructed to describe the relation between one variable X (say, height), and another Y (say weight). The method then predicts Y, knowing X (the independent variable). Multiple regression permits the simultaneous assessment of the relation between several variables (X1, X2, etc.) and Y The multiple logistic model is a variant where the predicted variable (Y) is the probability of an event and hence is of particular interest in epidemiology. Regression is discussed in the text.

Mutagen A substance such as radiation that damages the structure of DNA (or RNA) through mutations i.e. permanent alterations in the chemical structure of DNA.

Myocardial infarction The death of heart muscle from insufficient blood supply to the heart, usually caused by blockage of the coronary arteries (see **atherosclerosis and coronary heart disease**).

Natural history of disease The course of disease from inception to resolution (or death).

Necropsy An autopsy, i.e. an examination of the dead body by a pathologist usually to find the cause of death or to find evidence in the case of crime. This is a very important way of judging the accuracy of death statistics.

Neoplasm/neoplastic A new growth, usually applied to a cancer/an adjective usually used to describe something that is cancerous.

Normal distribution A distribution that describes well a great many biological variables. The mean, median and mode values are identical, the distribution is symmetrical around this value, and one standard deviation includes 68 per cent of the population.

Null hypothesis A testable hypothesis stated in a way that implies that there is no difference between comparisons, other than that which could occur by chance alone.

Osteoporosis Loss of bone density caused by loss of calcium and phosphorous from bone.

Parasuicide A suicide attempt that does not lead to death.

Participant The word that is replacing subject, as in study participant.

Pathogen An organism (usually reserved for microorganisms) that causes disease.

Pathogenesis The mechanisms and processes by which disease occurs.

Pathology The study of the processes leading to, during and following disease. Pathology is a vital partner to epidemiology.

Pellagra A nutritional deficiency disease caused by lack of the vitamin niacin with problems including dermatitis, diarrhoea, and neurological disorders.

Person-to-person spread Direct transmission of disease, usually infections, resulting from close proximity of persons.

Phenylketonuria A genetic disorder in which the amino acid phenylalanine cannot be metabolized properly, leading to mental deficiency.

Placebo An inactive substance or procedure used as a therapeutic intervention for psychological effect; and commonly used in the control group in a trial.

Popper (Karl) Philosopher, 1902–1994, who contributed to science by promoting the key idea of falsifying rather than proving hypotheses.

Population A complex concept with multitude meanings in epidemiology, but crucially, the group of people in whom the problem under study occurs, and in whom the results of the research are to be applied. The concept is discussed extensively in the text.

Post-mortem See **necropsy**. Also used more loosely to mean an investigation after some problem has arisen.

Probability The chance that an event will occur expressed between the values of 0 (no chance) and 1 (100% chance). The (cumulative) incidence rate is the epidemiological measure of probability.

Prognosis Forecast of the outcome of a disease or other health problem with appropriate management (cf. **natural history**, which is without such management).

Proportional mortality (or morbidity) ratio (PMR) A summary measure of the proportion of deaths/disease due to a specific cause in the study population compared to either all causes or another cause.

Prostate A gland at the base of the male bladder.

Psychotic A term used for some serious mental health problems e.g. schizophrenia.

Public health (medicine) An activity to which many contribute, most usually defined as the science and art of prolonging life, preventing disease and promoting health through the organized efforts of society. Public health medicine is one of the many names given to the specialty of medical doctors who focus on public health.

Pulmonary Associated with the lungs.

Pulmonary embolus A blood clot lodged in the artery structure of the lungs.

Race The social group you belong to, or are perceived (or assigned) by others as belonging to, on the basis of a limited set of physical characteristics, particularly skin colour, hair and facial features. Race has been seriously discredited as a useful scientific construct and is being superseded by ethnicity.

Ramanujan (Srinivasan) Mathematician, 1887–1920, renowned for his intuition that led him to enunciate complex formulae that are still being proved.

Regression See **Multiple regression**.

Risk factor A factor associated with an increased probability of an adverse outcome, but not necessarily a causal factor.

Rose angina Angina is the characteristic chest pain arising from a shortage of oxygen to the heart muscle. Rose angina is the measure of whether chest pain is angina using the Rose angina questionnaire (also known as the London School of Hygiene and Tropical Medicine questionnaire).

Rothman (Kenneth) Epidemiologist, 1945 to 19–, known for conceptual and technical advances, and for his text *Modern Epidemiology*. (See References.)

Rubella syndrome A complex set of congenital malformations caused by infection of the mother by German measles (rubella) and transmitted to the fetus.

Sampling The approach to selection of people to participate in studies. In epidemiology, the sampling methods are chosen to minimize selection biases, given other restraints.

Sarcoidosis A disease of unknown cause, where the histology resembles tuberculosis. Most commonly affects the lungs, liver, eyes, and skin.

Scurvy A disease caused by vitamin C deficiency, characterized by symptoms/signs including bruising and bleeding readily.

Senile dementia Brain disease characterized by loss of intellect, usually irreversible and caused by degenerative processes associated with old age.

Sexually transmitted diseases (STDs) The group of diseases mainly transmitted during sexual behaviour, e.g. syphilis. Some STDs may be transmitted in other ways too, e.g. AIDS.

Sickle cell disease/anaemia A genetic disorder, whereby the haemoglobin, the oxygen-carrying molecule in red blood cells, crystallizes and distorts the blood cell into a sickle shape when oxygen in the cell is low.

Sickness The state of being unwell or dysfunctional, usually as a result of disease.

Significance Usually shorthand for the much preferred phrase statistical significance, as given by the *P*-value (see **Significance test**).

Significance test A shorthand for tests of statistical significance whereby the *P*-value indicates the probability that the observed difference could have been obtained by chance alone.

Skrabanek (Petr) Epidemiologist living 1940–1994, known for his capacity for critical appraisal.

Smallpox A severe viral disease, now extinct, characterized by skin blistering.

Snow (John) 1813–1858 Pioneer in both epidemiology and anaesthetics. His investigations of cholera was pivotal in the development of epidemiology.

Sphygmomanometer A device for measuring arterial blood pressure using an inflatable cuff (usually applied to the upper arm). The cuff is inflated until blood flow stops, then deflated until blood flow begins (systolic blood pressure) and then occurs freely (diastolic blood pressure).

Standard deviation A measure of variation around the mean, measured as the square root of the variance (see below).

Standardized mortality (or morbidity) ratio (SMR) A summary measure of the rate of death/disease in a population adjusted for one or more confounding factors (usually age or sex or both) using the indirect method. The ratio is of deaths observed/deaths expected if the rates in the standard population had applied in the study population. This is discussed in detail in the text.

Statistical significance See **significance**.

Stratified sample The people selected for (or participating in) a study where the sampling frame is organized by subgroups, e.g. men and women, or age groups. Then random samples are chosen within each subgroup.

Streptococcus/cocci One of a number of species of bacteria, some of which cause serious human diseases.

Subject A person who is studied, i.e. a member of the population under study (see participant).

Suicide Purposive action that leads to one's own death.

Target population The population about which inferences or generalizations are to be made or interventions designed for.

Tesh (Sylvia) Public health scholar (1937–) and author of a wide-ranging and controversial book on public health—*Hidden arguments*.

Theory A system of ideas offered to explain and connect observed factors or conjectures. A statement of general principles or laws underlying a subject.

Trisomy 21 See **Down's syndrome**.

Tuberculosis A multisystem infection caused by the bacteria *Mycobacterium tuberculosis*.

Variance A measure of the variation in a set of observations, defined as the sum of the square of the deviation of each value from the mean (in other words, each value is subtracted from the mean value and squared (always a positive number)), divided by the degrees of freedom (often the number of observations minus 1).

Watson (James) 1928 – American scientist who in 1953 co-discovered the structure of DNA, winning the Nobel Prize in 1962 (see also **Crick**).

Zoonoses Diseases transmitted from animals to humans.

Chapter 1

What is epidemiology?
The nature and scope of a biological, clinical, social, and ecological science and of its variables

Objectives

After reading this chapter you should understand:

- that the prime focus of epidemiology is on the pattern of disease and ill-health in the population;
- that epidemiology combines elements of clinical, biological, social and ecological sciences;
- that epidemiology is dependent on clinical practice and the clinical sciences to make a diagnosis, which is essential to most epidemiological work;
- that the central goal of epidemiology as a science is to understand the causes of disease variation and use this knowledge to better the health of populations and individuals;
- that the central goal of epidemiology as a practice is preventing and controlling disease in populations, guiding health and health-care policy, and planning and improving health care in individuals;
- that useful epidemiological variables should meet the purposes of epidemiology;
- that both research and practice in epidemiology is based on theories though these may not be made explicit.

1.1 The individual and the population

Humans cherish the fact that they are unique, not only in their physique but also in their character, personality and behaviour (identical twins excepted). The health of an individual is also unique, and only the facts of birth and death are universally shared.

Some people who smoke develop lung cancer and others do not. Some people drink alcohol and become aggressive, while others become passive. These outcomes are not easily predictable at the individual level. Such prediction remains an elusive key goal of science. It is self-evident, nonetheless, that the characteristics of individuals play a part in causing their diseases. According to Hippocrates, writing more than 2000 years ago, medicine should consider the health of the inhabitants of a place, for example, 'are they heavy drinkers and eaters and consequently unable to stand fatigue or, being fond of work and exercise, eat wisely but drink sparely?' Hippocrates also wrote about the role of the environment on disease, particularly the seasons, the winds and water (see Chadwick and Mann 1950).

It is less intuitive but true that as with individuals, population groups have distinctive patterns of disease. Before reading on reflect on why this is so, considering the role of individual behaviour, social interaction, genetic factors and the environment.

This distinctive pattern is a result of varying exposure of populations to the causes of disease. If different populations were exposed equally to the causes they would have much the same patterns of disease. Some variation would remain due to genetic differences, which are small between populations (but these too are mainly due to the effects of environmental differences over evolutionary periods).

The population pattern of disease is dependent on the characteristics of individuals and the interaction between individuals with each other and the environment. Population patterns of diseases may arise from difference in the interaction of individuals. For example, sexually transmitted diseases arise only when having more than one sexual partner is common in society. If a few non-diseased people had multiple sexual partners in a society where a single sexual partner was the norm for others, this would not raise their own risk of sexually transmitted disease (nor that of others in the society). Herd immunity is the protection given to children who are not immunized by the immunization of other children in the society. The population's pattern of disease arises from its intrinsic social characteristics. If society changed, the individual's risk of disease would also change, even when the individual does not change—as reflected in the examples of sexually transmitted disease and immunization. Patterns of diseases in populations, therefore, result from the characteristics of individuals, societies and the environment (as discussed in detail in Chapter 2). The science and practice of epidemiology seeks to describe, understand and utilize these population patterns to improve health.

1.2 Definition of epidemiology and a statement of its central paradigm

The identity of the person who coined the term epidemiology is unknown but it is derived from the Greek words meaning study upon populations (*epi* = upon, *demos* = people, *ology* = study). This derivation does not convey what is studied or the nature of that study and is effectively the same as demography, which is the study of the characteristics of populations, such as size, growth, density, distribution and vital statistics. Epidemiology is concerned primarily with disease, and how disease detracts from health. A more descriptive word would be epidemiopathology (pathos is the Greek word for suffering and disease) but it is too clumsy to recommend.

The word epidemic was used by Hippocrates, but his writings were mainly compilations of the case histories of affected people and not a study of the causes or the pattern of the epidemic in the population. The early applications of epidemiology were in the study of infectious disease epidemics, environmental hazards, and social and nutritional problems. Most epidemiology is on human populations but veterinary epidemiology is important also, both in its own right and in the study of the interaction of humans and animals causing the diseases known as the zoonoses.

Last's (2001) dictionary gives a definition of epidemiology that includes 'The study of the distribution and determinants of health-related states or events in specified populations, and the application of this study to control of health problems' (see glossary.)

Based on what it has done in the last 150 years, epidemiology is the science and practice which describes and explains disease patterns in populations, and uses this knowledge to prevent and control disease and improve health. Thomas Kuhn's (1996) influential concept of scientific paradigms is helpful (Chapter 10). The central paradigm of epidemiology is that patterns of ill health and disease in populations may be analysed systematically to understand their causes and to improve health. The key strategy of epidemiology is to seek differences and similarities ('compare and contrast') in the disease patterns of populations to gain new knowledge. Most epidemiologists are interested in health but study it indirectly through disease, partly because of the difficulty of measuring health directly. Nearly all the examples in textbooks and in collections of great epidemiological papers are based on this paradigm. Epidemiology is, however, evolving new paradigms, as discussed in the next section and again in Chapter 10.

The valid measurement of the frequency of disease, and factors that may influence disease and are therefore potential explanations for the observed patterns, is crucial (Chapters 3, 4, 7, and 8). Measurement, however, is a means to an end. Excellence in measurement will not, in itself, yield excellence in epidemiology. The quality of epidemiology must be judged by its contributions to its goals. The same applies to the design of epidemiological studies (Chapter 9).

1.3 Directions in epidemiology and its uses

A great expansion in the scope of epidemiology is underway. The ideas which have proven themselves in the study of disease are used increasingly to study health and health care. Epidemiology is useful in the laboratory, both in contributing to ideas to help understand biological processes and in pragmatic ways such as defining ranges for the normal values of biological measures. Normal values are usually derived by demonstrating the distribution of the values in healthy populations or, better, by demonstrating the health problems associated with particular values. Epidemiology is central in the practice of clinical medicine, and though its uses have been insufficiently demonstrated, its potential for the professions allied to medicine, such as nursing and physiotherapy, is promising.

The standard definitions of epidemiology, such as the science of the distribution and determinants of disease, or the occurrence of disease in populations, do not capture the essence of applied epidemiology in health care settings, though they do describe well the tradition of the science. Morris's (1964) classic book, *The Uses of Epidemiology*, fully recognized the huge contribution of epidemiology to health care, opening the chapter on community diagnosis with the words 'Epidemiology provides "intelligence" for the health services' (1964, 2nd edition). Modern epidemiology is more than a science: it is a craft, vocation and profession—in this sense it is a partner of public health and clinical care, not just a science of these disciplines. Currently, epidemiology is seen as useful in:

- yielding understanding of what causes or sustains disease in populations;
- preventing and controlling disease in populations;
- guiding health and health-care policy and planning;
- assisting in the maintenance of health and management of disease in individuals.

1.4 Epidemiology as a science, practice, and craft

Nearly all definitions of epidemiology say it is a science, and there are claims for it to be the underlying science of public health (Chapter 10). Some critics have claimed epidemiology is not a science but just a toolkit of methods for other sciences and professions to use. An understanding of whether epidemiology is a science is important in an era when the label 'science' is vital to the credibility of both research and professional practice. Try the exercise in Box 1.1 before reading on.

Science is about knowledge, for the word is derived from the Latin *scientia* meaning knowledge and the French *scíre*, to know. Dictionary definitions of science tend to be complex, for example:

1 the observation, identification, description, experimental investigation, and theoretical explanation of phenomena

2 such activities restricted to a class of natural phenomena

3 any branch of knowledge based on systematic observations of facts and seeking to formulate general explanatory laws and hypotheses that could be verified empirically.

Clearly, not all systematic study is science; for example, literature, art, philosophy and religion are not sciences, though they may be rigorous and systematic, and even emulate the methods and measurement techniques of science. Science is the systematic study of natural phenomena. Furthermore, science is not just about the methods and techniques, which can be applied in many non-scientific circumstances (for example political polling), but the mode of thought. The mode of thought of sciences pursues new knowledge based on theory and verified by direct, research-based observation.

Box 1.1 The nature of science in relation to epidemiology

- What are the characteristics of a science?
- Name some disciplines that are sciences and some that are not.
- Compare the disciplines that are sciences to those that are not.
- Is public health a science? Is medicine a science?
- Is epidemiology a science?
- Is epidemiology also a practice?

Box 1.2 The question as the basis of science

That is the essence of science: ask an impertinent question, and you are on the way to a pertinent answer.

Jacob Bronowski (1908–74), British scientist, author of *The ascent of man* (1973) chapter 4

Scientists are engaged in extending or consolidating the knowledge base, sometimes through deliberate repetition of research. Science is a creative endeavour that relies as much on questioning, imagination and exploration as art, but the difference is that science tests out its ideas by seeking empirical evidence rooted in the natural world.

The idea to be tested is often stated as a question. The question may be expressed in a way that lends itself to systematic test. If so, it is called a hypothesis. Reflect on the importance of the testable question as emphasized in Box 1.2.

The idea, the question, the testable hypothesis, the research test, and the interpretation of the research data to advance understanding of natural phenomena, together comprise science. Epidemiology studies the nature of diseases and their causes, and it uses systematic methods of measurement to test ideas, questions and hypotheses, and hence it is a bioscience, serving medicine and public health just as medical sciences such as pathology and microbiology do. Epidemiology has been particularly relevant to medicine rather than laboratory science, but the increasing collaboration between geneticists and epidemiologists is changing the balance.

Epidemiology is, however, primarily concerned with disease and health hazards in populations. Human populations live in societies, where behaviour and attitudes are shaped by interaction among people, which create the conventions and laws of the society. Epidemiology, therefore, studies disease within a sociocultural context. Epidemiology is, therefore, not only a bioscience but also a social science. Populations exist in a physical environment, which is dominant in determining health. The study of life in relation to the environment is ecology (the word derives from the Greek for house), so epidemiology is, in addition, the science of the ecology of disease.

The science of epidemiology, therefore, combines elements of biology, social sciences and ecology: a biosocial–environmental science focusing on disease in populations. By its nature, epidemiology is multidisciplinary. The closest partner of the epidemiologist is the statistician, for reasons that will become apparent.

Epidemiological science is easily applied. Understanding the causes of diseases, more than any other information, transforms the practice of clinical care and public health. For example, the epidemiological work showing that smokers have a much higher risk of a multiplicity of diseases than non-smokers has transformed health care, public health and health politics. Epidemiological data has value for creating health policy for the nation or for a plan to meet the needs of patients with cancer or risk of cancer.

While many epidemiologists are simultaneously engaged in both research and practice, some only apply available knowledge. Their applied work is not science, though it draws upon science. In this regard, epidemiology is no different to, for example, medicine, nursing, geology and chemistry, where there are scientists and practitioners, and often the two roles are combined. Scientific research and practice in epidemiology are symbiotic, but not identical, activities. Recent criticisms of epidemiology may partly arise from a failure to separate the roles of epidemiology as a science and as a craft or practice (see Chapter 10). Analogously, there are criticisms of physics for discoveries that have underpinned poor energy policy (disasters in nuclear energy power plants, for example) and criticisms of biology for unethical and erroneous interpretation of data on intelligence (for example, the Immigration Bill of 1924 in the USA kept Jews from migrating to America on the basis of their supposedly low intelligence). Criticisms of the research need to be separated from those of its application.

The practice of epidemiology operates somewhat differently from the science of epidemiology. The research questions, the value of the various methods, data analysis, presentation and interpretation may differ; something which needs to be appreciated. These differences and their implications will be emphasized throughout the text.

1.5 **The nature of epidemiological variables**

The word variable is in common use in research including epidemiology, but its meaning is seldom defined. Most people have used the word variable. Before reading on you should reflect on its meaning—what is it?

A variable is anything which varies and has different values. Clearly, this applies to most phenomena, but only a few are chosen for study. Variation in disease pattern is the foundation of epidemiology, but in epidemiology the word variable is seldom applied to diseases, which may be referred to as outcome variables or, more commonly and simply, outcomes. It is usually applied to factors which help to describe and understand disease pattern. These are called exposure variables or risk factors (see Chapter 7).

Epidemiological variables aid in the description, analysis and interpretation of disease patterns. Analysis of disease by age, sex, economic status, social class, occupation, country of residence, country of birth, region of residence and racial or ethnic classification are powerful ways of showing and interpreting variations in diseases and health states.

Many variables used in epidemiology are markers for complex underlying phenomena which cannot be measured easily, if at all. For example, social class is an indirect indicator of various differences between populations in factors such as occupation, income, education and styles of consumption. Sex is a proxy for genetic, hormonal, psychological, or social status in different studies. It is important, therefore, that we can disentangle and study separately the component influences of such epidemiological variables.

Before reading on do the exercise in Box 1.3.

A good epidemiological variable should:

- have an impact on health status in individuals and populations;
- be measurable accurately;

Box 1.3 The epidemiological exposure variable

- What qualities should an exposure variable have to make it important and useful in epidemiology?
- How do the purposes and uses of epidemiology help to assess the potential value of an exposure variable?

- differentiate populations in terms of patterns of disease or health status;
- differentiate populations in some underlying characteristic relevant to health e.g. income, childhood circumstance, hormonal status, genetic inheritance, or behaviour relevant to health;
- generate testable causal hypotheses, and/or
  - help to develop health policy, and/or
  - help to plan and deliver health care, and/or
  - help to prevent and control disease.

These characteristics, which are closely tied in to the purposes of epidemiology, can help to evaluate exposure variables (risk factors). In Chapter 10, and other parts of the book, they will be used to illustrate the strengths and weaknesses of epidemiological variables, particularly in the context of the controversies around race and ethnicity (see section 10.10.3).

Table 1.1 summarizes the concepts here in the context of age, the most influential and important of all epidemiological variables. Before reading on, however, try the exercise in Box 1.4.

Biological changes related to ageing have a profound influence on susceptibility to many diseases. For example, disorders of growth and development occur in the young; degenerative diseases such as osteoporosis or senile dementia mostly in the old. So, age is associated with and impacts on health of populations.

In most populations age is accurately measured by asking people. Alternatively, age can be obtained from birth registration data. In some populations, mainly in developing countries, where registration at birth is not operative or effective, age may not be

---

Box 1.4 Thinking about age as an epidemiological variable

- Is age easily and accurately measured?
- Is age good at showing population differences in disease experience?
- What underlying differences between people does age reflect?
- How can these differences be used to advance understanding of disease causation, or health policy or health-care planning?

Table 1.1 Age as an epidemiological exposure variable

Characteristics of a good epidemiological variable	Characteristics in relation to age
Impacts on health in individuals and population	Age is a powerful influence on health
Be measurable accurately	In most populations age is measurable to the day, but in some it has to be guessed and may deliberately be reported wrongly
Differentiates populations in their experience of disease or health	Huge differences by age are seen for virtually every disease, health problem, and for factors which cause health problems
Differentiates populations in some underlying characteristic relevant to health e.g. income, childhood circumstance, hormonal status, genetic inheritance, or behaviour relevant to health	Differences in disease patterns in different age groups reflect a mix of environmental factors and may reflect population changes in genetic factors, particularly in populations where migration has been high
Generates testable causal hypotheses, and/or	It is hard to test hypotheses because there are so many underlying differences between populations of different ages
helps in developing health policy, and/or	Age differences in disease patterns profoundly affect health policy decisions
helps to plan and deliver health care and/or	Knowing the age structure of a population is critical to good decision-making in health care
help to prevent and control disease	By understanding the age at which diseases start, preventive and control programmes can be targeted at appropriate age groups

known accurately. In some societies, for social reasons, there is a tendency to exaggerate age on self-report, in others to understate it.

Age is superb at showing variations in most diseases, so differentiating populations (see Table 8.17, Chapter 8). Variations by age seldom yield easy explanation, for their causes are a complex mix of social, environmental and biological factors. Causal hypotheses about age and disease are not easily tested. Generally, the more complex the variable, the harder it is to explain the underlying reason for the associated variation in disease experience. This is why it is imperative to understand the underlying concept behind the variable, for in causal studies additional data will be needed and these will be dependent on such understanding. The epidemiological concept of ageing is a mix of biological and environmental components. As the body grows older the biology changes, but at the same time the body absorbs a barrage of environmental insults. The combined effects lead to differences in disease patterns in different age groups and in different generations (see section 9.8 on cohort effect). Furthermore, the social circumstances, and particularly social support networks, of people change at different ages and these affect health. Age differentiates populations in characteristics relevant to health. The differences in disease experience at different ages are profoundly important to clinical care, preventing and controlling disease, making sound health policy, and for effective health-care planning.

Box 1.5 Categorizing the differences between sexes

List the differences between women and men which could explain their different patterns of disease. (You may wish to focus your thinking using heart disease which is more common in men than women.) Can you put these differences into categories?

The epidemiological concept of sex is also a mix of biological and social. Try the exercise in Box 1.5 before reading on.

To begin to understand the sex variation in the occurrence of coronary heart disease, the investigator needs to know what differences there are between men and women in the population studied. Table 1.2 categorizes some of the differences as biological, coexisting disease (or comorbidity), behavioural, social, occupational, economic and health care. There are complex differences between men and women, so using this variation to explain the different patterns of heart disease is immensely difficult. To ascribe differences solely to genetic factors would be a serious though tempting error. By contrast, differences between men and women in the risk of breast cancer are likely to be

Table 1.2 Categorizing and analysing the factors which may underlie an epidemiological variable: the example of male/female differences in heart disease

Category of underlying difference	Example of possible specific differences by sex	Implications for science of epidemiology
Biological	Hormonal, e.g. oestrogen levels	Collect biological data
Coexisting diseases	Women may have less of the other diseases which raise the risk of heart disease e.g. diabetes	Collect clinical data
Behavioural	Women eat more fruits, vegetables and salads than men, and generally smoke less	Collect data on behaviours relating to health
Social	Women spend more time with friends and family	Collect psychosocial data as potential explanations
Occupational	The pattern of working, including likelihood of employment, the hours worked and the type of occupation is substantially different	Collect data on employment histories
Economic	Women earn less money than men	Collect data on differences and their effect on lifestyles and stress levels
Health care	Women with heart disease are treated differently than men by health-care professionals	Collect data on level and timing of interventions

biological and for cervical cancer are, of course, wholly biological because men don't have a cervix. The depth of the analysis will, therefore, be disease- and context-specific. Differences in health care between men and women as explanations for disease variations arouse great controversy, because inequitable health care is unethical.

Scientific understanding of the reasons for the variation by sex is extremely helpful in designing preventive interventions, but in its absence the variations can be used to set priorities and target resources.

For the science of epidemiology, concerned to advance causal knowledge, variables which highlight variations between and within populations in diseases of unknown aetiology are *potentially* of great value. If disease variation has not previously been demonstrated it is of particular value. The repetitious demonstration of variations is, however, seldom of scientific value.

For example, huge variations between countries in the incidence of cancer have been demonstrated, and these conclusively demonstrate that population variation in cancer is largely determined by environmental factors. New observations on such variations would be of scientific value only if they refuted rather than confirmed this interpretation. A great deal of effort is presently underway to show racial and ethnic variations in cancer. These mainly reconfirm the insights from international studies. Their additional value in aetiological research needs to be questioned. In his analysis of epidemiology as a science Skrabanek (1994) argued that epidemiologists must advance understanding of the causes of the associations between epidemiological variables and diseases. He cited a review of 35 case–control studies of coffee drinking and bladder cancer, which failed to provide important information on whether coffee causes bladder cancer. He likened such research to repetitively punching a pillow. A dimple forms and refills. The totality of the blows is no more than the first. He called this 'black box' epidemiology, and another epidemiologist, Kuller (1999), has criticized a similar phenomenon that he called circular epidemiology.

As the above discussion shows, epidemiological variables are of many types and with different qualities. These qualities can be summarized as follows:

♦ Categorical variables, where the individual is put into one or two or more agreed categories, or groups. Sex is an example, i.e. male or female. Another is dead or alive. Categories may be in some order, e.g. social class, where there is an expectation that as we move through the classes, say from 1 to 5, there is a step change, for example in access to resources, or likelihood of smoking. Categorical variables are of great importance in epidemiology as risk factors (exposures), confounding factors and outcomes. (Categorical variables are also called qualitative data, but this risks confusion with qualitative research.)

♦ Numerical or quantitative variables, where there is no prior grouping, and the values rise from zero onwards, with no imposed upper limit. The variables can be whole numbers, e.g. the number of episodes of asthma a person had over the last year, or the number of times a person took exercise in the last month. Such variables can also be continuous, e.g. age (measurable in seconds, days, years etc.) or amount of alcohol consumed (litres, mls etc.). Continuous measures are often converted to whole numbers such as age in years, or alcohol consumption to the nearest unit. It is also common, but often not advisable as it reduces precision, to convert quantitative variables into categorical ones e.g. age into young/middle aged/old or into 5-year or 10-year groupings.

Quantitative variables are commonly risk factors and confounding factors, but less commonly outcome variables in epidemiology, simply because death, disease and illnesses are the outcomes of greatest interest and these are categorical variables. States that are intermediate between health and disease are often measured quantitatively, e.g. blood pressure, or weight in relation to height. These are usually called intermediate traits.

1.6 Definition and diagnosis of disease: an illustration of the interdependence of clinical medicine and epidemiology

Investigating the causes and mechanisms of health problems is the essence of the science of epidemiology. Taking steps to prevent and control the problem, including providing the appropriate health services, is the essence of public health. The craft of epidemiology is in presenting the scientific evidence in ways which lead to effective public health and clinical action. Epidemiology cannot work until some basic clinical and pathological issues have been resolved, for example, on the definition of the disease. The science of epidemiology, therefore, functions in close partnership with clinical medicine and its sciences, particularly pathology. Read Box 1.6 and try the questions before reading on.

Sickness X (Box 1.6) illustrates why epidemiology requires clinical collaboration. Because the cause is unknown the disease must be defined on the clinical picture, or laboratory tests. If a definition cannot be agreed or is inaccurate, cases cannot be diagnosed accurately and epidemiology is paralysed, or led to error. The first question in epidemiology is the nature and validity of the definition of the disease or other health problem under investigation. Clinicians need to study cases and agree on a definition which will permit the classification of sick people into one of two groups: probably suffering from the disease or probably not. Diagnoses are statements of probability, and their accuracy will depend on the clarity of their definition. A definition of sickness X which accepted only patients with a rash as cases would miss those without a rash. To accept cases of disease without a rash means that more people suffering from other disorders will be wrongly diagnosed with sickness X.

Pragmatic choices need to be made. For scientific investigation, a definition which includes people with a high probability of disease is likely to be better than one which includes many people without disease. For public health a strict definition may be inadequate, for it underestimates the size of the problem and misses the people most likely to benefit: those with early symptoms and few signs. A possible definition would be that a case of sickness X is, for the purpose of epidemiological research:

+ an illness diagnosed by a physician;
+ one of a cluster or outbreak of cases;

Box 1.6 A puzzle for medicine and a challenge for epidemiology: sickness X

A sickness of unknown type, which appears as outbreaks, sometimes affecting whole communities, is spreading across a large part of continental Europe. Years later it will emerge in the USA. It will be shown to be present in many countries, though it may remain unrecognized in normal medical practice, for it may occur as solitary cases or in small numbers and not outbreaks. Sick people have a wide range of symptoms and signs on examination. Their many symptoms include simply feeling unwell, with loss of appetite and abdominal pain, disturbances of the gastrointestinal tract including diarrhoea, a skin rash on parts of the body exposed to the sun, and mental disturbances.

Sickness leads to progressive physical and mental deterioration. People who contract the sickness are likely to die, with the mortality rate as high as 60 per cent in some outbreaks. If a sufferer recovers the sickness can recur.

The sickness clusters in families, and it affects poor people living in rural areas more than any other group. Growing corn is common in areas where the disease occurs. The problem is greatest in spring, though the early symptoms occur in winter. The sickness is common in prisoners and patients in asylums. It does not affect staff in these institutions.

Physicians cannot agree on the cause of the sickness and the many 'cures' tried by physicians give variable results.

Questions

- Can you form a definition of this sickness X?
- If not, how would physicians make a diagnosis? How could the number of cases of the sickness be counted for epidemiological purposes?
- If you can define sickness how would you do it? What would be the components of your definition?

- one that occurs in an ill person who has at least two out of these three problems:
  - gastrointestinal disturbance
  - skin rash
  - mental disturbance
- one with no other clear diagnosis.

Using this pragmatic definition physicians can be asked to inform the researchers of the occurrence of cases, which can be counted and studied. The effect of error in the definition on the estimated frequency of the disease may be huge. The comparison of different populations is likely to be misleading, as will be discussed in Chapter 3, but a pragmatic definition is still essential.

Box 1.7 The nature and possible causes of sickness X

- What thoughts come into your mind about the nature of the sickness?
- What kind of sickness/disease is it? Is it, for example, genetic, congenital (present at birth), degenerative (wear and tear of age), cancer, injury, infection, toxic, nutritional, or immune disorder?
- What kind of sickness/disease is it not?
- What sort of factors could cause a sickness such as this? Think of these factors at the level of individual, family, community and national society.

Consider, for comparison, the definition used by Fraser and colleagues (1977) in their investigation of the 1976 Legionnaires' disease outbreak in Philadelphia: a case had *a fever of atleast 102 degrees and a cough, or a fever allied to chest X-ray evidence of pneumonia, plus some association with the Legion convention.* The definition was designed to separate those who were probably linked to the outbreak from those who probably were not. Later, when the importance of the Bellevue Stratford Hotel in Philadelphia as the source of exposure became clearer, the definition was revised to include only people who were American Legion conventioneers or who had entered the Bellevue Stratford Hotel after 1 July 1976. The change in definition caused confusion in the minds of the public and the media, and changed the numbers of cases involved and dead. Similarly, a change in the definition of AIDS some years ago led to changes in the numbers of cases. Changes in case definition are common, reflecting the fact that diagnosis is often pragmatic, and influenced by advancing knowledge and new techniques.

Even at this stage, some possibilities in the causation of sickness X can be ruled out using general clinical and pathological principles about the nature of disease. Try the exercise in Box 1.7 before looking at Table 1.3.

Table 1.3 summarizes some reasoning on the nature of sickness X. This disease is not a chromosomal or gene defect, congenital, an immune disorder, a result of injury, a degeneration of age, or a result of uncontrolled cell division (cancer). It may be a result of infection, exposure to toxins, or a deficiency of some essential substance. This reasoning is based on epidemiological descriptions, and draws upon the other relevant sciences. Population studies may be used by the clinician in managing the individual patient. Therapeutic ideas may be sparked off by understanding of causation and then tested on populations of patients. The results derived from populations will then be applied to individuals.

1.7 The basic tools of epidemiology: measuring disease frequency and study design

The toolbox of epidemiology is powerful, growing and changing, and it needs to be applied with great care. As with any tool wrongly applied, it can be damaging and

Table 1.3 Types of disease and some preliminary reasoning on causes of sickness/disease X

Type of disease	Reasoning for and against sickness X being this kind of disease
Genetic	Genetic diseases do not vary in their frequency over short periods of time, and do not selectively avoid certain populations, e.g. staff in institutions
Congenital	Congenital problems are present at birth, are usually diagnosed in the young and are usually permanent
Degenerative	As above. They do not tend to affect the young
Cancers	As above. They do not exhibit marked seasonal variation
Injuries	The cause of injuries is usually apparent
Infections	The picture fits, though the reason for some populations being immune is a puzzle
Toxins	The picture fits
Nutritional deficiency	The picture fits
Immune disorders	These do not present as epidemics

even dangerous. The tools are best applied with a proper understanding of the purposes, theories, principles and pitfalls of epidemiology. It is for this reason that the main tools are discussed late in this book—Chapters 7–9.

Some readers may, nonetheless, wish to read about the tools in advance of the more general material in Chapters 2–6. Others may content themselves with the brief introduction given in this section.

The fraction or ratio of the number of outcomes of interest (usually diseases or like problems) in relation to the population under study provides the core measurement tool. The most important of these measures are incidence and prevalence, and from these building blocks a multiplicity of specific disease measures arise.

Table 1.4 outlines these two measures. The study types that are mostly used in epidemiology are in Table 1.5. As we will see in Chapter 9, there is much conceptual and

Table 1.4 Introduction to incidence and prevalence rates

Measure	Key features	Type of study	Formulae
Incidence	Count of new cases over a period of time in a population of known size defined by characteristics (age, sex, etc.), and place and time boundaries	Disease register Cohort Trial	New cases ÷ population-at-risk or New cases ÷ time spent by the study population at risk
Prevalence	Count of cases (new and old) at a point in time in a population of known size defined by characteristics (age, sex, etc.) and place	Cross-sectional Disease register	All cases ÷ population at risk

Table 1.5 Epidemiological designs and applications: an overview

Study design	Essential idea	Some research purposes
1. Case series and population case series	Count cases (numerator) and relate to population data (denominator) to produce rates and analyse patterns Look at characteristics of cases for causal hypotheses	Study signs and symptoms, and create disease definitions Surveillance of mortality/morbidity rates Seek associations Generate/test hypotheses Source of cases or foundation for other studies
2. Cross-sectional	Study health and disease states in a population at a defined place and time Measure burden of disease and its causes	Measure prevalence (very rarely incidence) of disease and related factors Seek associations between disease and related factors Generate/test hypotheses Repeat studies (on different samples) to measure change and evaluate interventions
3. Case–control	Look for differences and similarities between a series of cases and a control group	Seek associations Generate/test hypotheses Assess strength of association (odds ratio)
4. Cohort	Follow up populations, relating information on risk factor patterns and health states at baseline, to the outcomes of interest	Study natural history of disease Measure incidence of disease Link disease outcomes to possible disease causes, i.e. seek associations Generate/test hypotheses
5. Trial	Intervene with some measure designed to improve health, then follow up people to see the effect*	Test understanding of causes Study how to influence natural history of disease Evaluate the effects (side-effects and benefits) and costs of interventions

* Measures designed to worsen health or to make no difference would be ethically unacceptable, though this may be done (with ethical or regulatory approval) on animals.

methodological overlap between these study designs. Moreover, each study design is capable of generating many different kinds of measure.

1.8 Seeking the theoretical foundations of epidemiology

A theory is a statement that provides an explanation or coherent account of a group of ideas, facts, or observed phenomena, like the theory of evolution does. Epidemiology has been criticized as an atheoretical discipline, comprising a mixed bag of tools, useful for solving particular problems but neither adding up to a science, nor providing a theoretical basis to the study of health and disease. Epidemiology, however, both draws upon and contributes to theories of health and disease. It may be that epidemiologists spend little time reflecting on the theories underpinning their work, but the same criticism would probably apply to other sciences. In most disciplines theories are at the core of thinking and practice. Priscilla Alderson (1998) has argued that it is not possible to think about health care without theory even though it may be implicit rather than explicit. Before reading on do the exercise in Box 1.8.

Box 1.8 Spotting theories and principles underlying epidemiology

Can you discern any theories which have guided this chapter so far? What general principles follow from these theories?

The main epidemiological theories and principles that have guided this chapter include these:

- Disease in populations is more than the sum of disease in individuals.
- Populations differ in their disease experience.
- Disease experiences within populations differ in subgroups of the population.

Principles arising:

- Disease variations can be described, and their causes explored, by assessing whether exposure variables are associated with disease patterns.
- Knowledge about health and disease in human populations can be applied to individuals and vice versa.
- Health policies and plans and clinical care can be enriched by understanding of disease patterns in populations.

Methods and techniques in epidemiology are designed to achieve the promise inherent in these theories. In turn, new methods and techniques lead to new or refined theoretical understanding. Epidemiology's contribution to the theory of health and disease will be a recurrent theme of the book, and will be summarized and developed in Chapter 10 (section 10.1).

Summary

Populations, as with individuals, have unique patterns of disease. Populations' disease patterns derive from differences in the type of individuals they comprise, in the mode of interaction of individuals, and in the environment. The science of epidemiology, which straddles biology, clinical medicine, social sciences and ecology, seeks to describe, understand and utilize these patterns to improve population health. As a science, epidemiology's central paradigm is that analysis of population patterns of disease, particularly by linking these to exposure variables (risk factors), provides understanding of the causes of disease. Epidemiology is useful in other ways, too, including preventing and controlling disease in populations and guiding health and health-care policy and planning. Causal understanding is not always essential in these latter applications. Epidemiology also helps to manage the health care of individuals.

A useful epidemiological exposure variable reflects the purposes of epidemiology and is: measurable accurately; differentiates populations in their experience of disease or health; and generates testable aetiological hypotheses, and/or helps in developing health policy and health-care plans and/ or to prevent and control disease. For advancing causal knowledge, variables which highlight differences between and within subgroups of populations in diseases of unknown aetiology are *potentially* of great value. The more complex the concept captured by the variable the harder it is to understand the reasons for the associated variation in disease experience. For health policy and planning, variables which show variations in diseases for which effective interventions are available are particularly valuable.

Understanding the epidemiology of the disease demands clinical collaboration. Clinicians need to agree on a definition that will permit screening or diagnosis. The first question for the epidemiologist, in any investigation, is the nature and validity of the definition of the disease or other problem under investigation. Then follow decisions on which populations are to be studied and the methods for making accurate measurement of the frequency and pattern of disease and the postulated risk factors. In turn, epidemiological knowledge is used by clinicians to help make diagnoses in individuals, to prescribe effective treatments, and to offer patients information on the natural history and prognosis of their diseases.

Epidemiology has evolved a large toolbox. At its core lies the measurement of the prevalence and incidence of risk factors and outcomes. These measurements are generated by study types (designs) that serve the various purposes of epidemiology.

Epidemiology is both founded on, and contributes to, theories of health and disease, though these are seldom made explicit.

Sample examination questions

Give yourself 10 minutes for every 25% of marks.

Question 1 The phrase 'outcome variable' is often used in epidemiology. Explain the meaning of this phrase, and indicate how it differs from exposure variable. (25%)
Answer The outcome variable usually refers to the disease, illness, death or preceding processes leading to these, e.g. hypertension, or obesity/overweight. The outcome variable is the variable that the study is trying to understand or explain the causes of. The potential explanations are usually referred to as exposure variable, or even more commonly, risk factors. There is an overlap in these two types of variable because sometimes epidemiologists study the effect of one disease on another (outcome variable), and sometimes of one exposure on another (outcome variable).

Question 2 Define epidemiology and briefly outline its principal strategies. (25%)
Answer Epidemiology is the study of the patterns of health, and disease, in populations. It focuses on describing and understanding these patterns, thereby shedding light on the causes of ill-health and disease. Its central strategy is to compare and contrast populations over time and between places, and using differences and similarities in risk factors and disease outcomes to aid understanding. Epidemiology uses several designs to gather data and frameworks for causal reasoning to interpret it.

Question 3 In what respects is epidemiology a science? In what respects is it not a science?

Answer Epidemiology is a science in that it studies a natural phenomenon—the causes of health and disease in populations—using systematic approaches to developing hypotheses, implementing methods, and interpreting data. It uses and develops theories of health and disease. It is a science that has elements of biological, social and ecological sciences.

Epidemiology also measures the burden and distribution of disease for applied purposes, e.g. health-care planning and setting public health priorities. In this context epidemiology is not studying causes or exploring hypotheses and theories. It is, in this context, a practice or craft, rather than a science.

Chapter 2

The epidemiological concept of population

Objectives

On completion of your reading you should understand:

♦ the meaning and applications of the idea that epidemiology is a population science;

♦ the profound influence of the characteristics of a population on its disease patterns;

♦ the potential and limitations of epidemiology in the absence of demographic population data;

♦ the expansion of possibilities in epidemiology which occurs when demographic population data are available;

♦ the impact of change in population size and characteristics on health.

2.1 The individual and the population

Epidemiology is defined as a population science. It is primarily concerned with understanding the distribution and causes of disease through the comparison of the pattern of disease in populations over time, between places and in different types of people, as symbolized in Fig. 2.1.

Populations, of course, comprise unique individuals. Humans, however, are social animals who thrive in families, groups and communities, and it is extremely rare for people to live in isolation. (Solitary confinement is one of the severest penalties in society.) The family is the basic unit of the group or community but nearly all humans live in much larger populations. The study of human groups is, without doubt, the keystone of epidemiology. No epidemiological study can be done on one person, but other medical sciences such as pathology and physiology may study one person, or even parts of a person. Even therapeutic trials can be designed for one individual.

To compare and contrast health status and disease patterns, the basis of epidemiology, you need several individuals. While epidemiology may be on very large groups—sometimes millions of people but nearly always hundreds or thousands—it can be also done on very small groups. The classic experiment of Lind in 1747 was on 12 persons, divided into six pairs of two, with each pair receiving a different nutritional supplement to try to prevent scurvy (Lind 1753). A definitive study of adenocarcinoma of the vagina by Herbst and colleagues (1971) was based on 8 cases and 32 people without disease as controls.

- Populations comprise individuals, families, groups and communities
- Epidemiology seeks variations in disease patterns over time, between subgroups and between places
- Understanding such variation yields knowledge on causation and prevention of disease

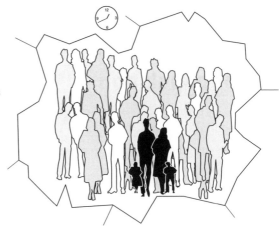

Fig. 2.1 The individual and population: the triad of time, place, and person.

Epidemiology aggregates the health experiences of individuals and tries to generalize the findings to the population from which the individuals have come, and beyond. These aggregate experiences are analysed in terms of the questions summarized in Box 2.1 to seek patterns over time, between places and between subpopulations with different characteristics. This is known as the epidemiological triad of time, place, and person. Time, place, and person can be thought of as broad exposure variables. We examine how time, place, and personal characteristics are associated with disease patterns. The strategy of epidemiology, as we saw in Chapter 1, is to discover the causes of these patterns, and ultimately the causes of disease. (A theme developed in later chapters, particularly Chapter 5.)

Answer the questions in Box 2.2 on disease X (described in Chapter 1, Box 1.6), before reading the answers in Table 2.1.

As the analysis in Table 2.1 shows, epidemiological data can help us to understand causes of disease in populations and also to forecast the probability (risk) of disease and its outcome in individuals. For example, we can reassure staff in institutions where

Box 2.1 The triad of epidemiological questions – time, place, and person

- How does the pattern of this disease vary over time in this population? (Time)
- How does the place in which the population lives affect the disease pattern? (Place)
- How do the personal characteristics of the people in the population affect the disease pattern? (Person)

Box 2.2 Exercise: Application of the triad to disease X

Apply the questions in Box 2.1 to disease X.

◆ Now, does this information help you to understand, or at least develop ideas on, the causes of the disease?

◆ How might you use this information to begin more detailed scientific investigation?

◆ How does the information help to plan for the control or prevention of disease?

disease X is present that their chance of developing disease is low. In studies to pinpoint the cause of the disease we will be looking for particular types of environmental exposure.

Epidemiological conclusions are directly applicable to the groups studied, but only indirectly to individuals, and then only to those who are reasonably typical of the population studied. For example, for populations, the causal link between smoking and lung cancer is solid and can be accurately quantified. For an individual it may not apply, for there may be environmental or genetic reasons why that person is not susceptible to

Table 2.1 The epidemiological triad of questions applied to disease X (Box 1.6) and its contribution to causal understanding

The epidemiological triad of questions	The questions applied to sickness X
How does the pattern of disease vary over time? (Time)	The sickness is a new, emergent problem It sometimes occurs as outbreaks It is seasonal It follows times of economic hardship
How does the place in which the population lives affect the disease pattern? (Place)	It is worst in people living in low-lying areas It affects people in institutions more, but only the inmates, not staff
How do the personal characteristics of the people in the population affect the disease pattern? (Person)	Living in poverty and sharecropping increase risk Being related to a person with the disease increases the risk It affects all ages, and both men and women

Moving from triad to causes

With the great variation in disease over time, between places, and by personal characteristics the evidence points to an environmental rather than a genetic cause. The various associations, e.g. emergence in the spring, the link to poverty, the effect on those living in institutions, etc. permit hypotheses to be developed and tested. Also they point to populations for study, e.g. those living in institutions and farmers practising sharecropping. At this stage no specific control or preventive actions are compelling but the disease seems to be preventable. In Chapter 1 (Table 1.3 and associated text) we favoured toxic, infectious and nutritional hypotheses. These can be tested using a mix of the epidemiological designs outline in Chapter 1 and discussed in Chapter 9. See Section 2.4 for the story of the cause of sickness.

Box 2.3 Thought exercise on prognosis (prediction of progression of illness)

- How would you assess the prognosis for a patient with a terminal illness who asks, how long have I got to live?
- How would you advise a parent of a 5-year-old son with asthma who asks, will my child have asthma for the rest of his life?

the carcinogenic effect of tobacco. The risk of disease outcomes for individuals can seldom be estimated. This contrasts with some other fields of life. For example, school examination grades can be predicted fairly accurately for an individual from previous examination achievements. Individuals can also assess the risk of being struck by a car while crossing the road, based on their own experiences. The difference is that most diseases are rare so few individuals get them; many diseases only occur once; and for disease you either have it or you do not. By constrast school grades are estimated many times and crossing the road is a daily event. Predicting the individual's risk of developing the common cold over, say, a five-year period is more feasible than predicting whether an individual will develop, say, stroke or lung cancer.

The knowledge gained by the epidemiological study still benefits individuals. Surprisingly, information gained from groups may sometimes be more helpful to individuals than information from the individuals themselves. Physicians from the time of Hippocrates have devoted much effort to prognosis, the prediction of outcome once a disease has occurred, which is essential to both the practice and the science of medicine. A great deal of attention has been paid to symptoms, signs, and tests which would indicate the prognosis of an individual, but prognosis at the individual level remains an erroneous art. Before reading on reflect on the questions in Box 2.3.

Even in the dying person, the outcome is difficult to predict accurately. In a study in Chicago hospices of the terminally ill, experienced physicians overestimated survival by a factor of 5.3. The likelihood of an individual child with asthma continuing to have it in adulthood cannot be predicted from the signs and symptoms or characteristics of the individual. Prognosis can, however, be expressed as a probability derived from population studies. This probability only informs the individual what happens on average, although the physician may use the individual's data to try to refine the prediction. Imperfect and unsatisfactory as this extrapolation from the population to the individual is, the approach has been widely adopted within medicine as the best available pending the development of accurate measures of prognosis based on the characteristics of individuals (this is a massive challenge for future clinical research which will, hopefully, be greatly assisted by advances in genetics). The potential and progress of personalized medicine is a hot topic in both scientific journals and the mass media. To date, the experience does not instil optimism. Epidemiology will remain the dominant means of prediction of risk and prognosis for the foreseeable future, at least in conditions that are chronic, and not recurrent.

Where a disease occurs repeatedly in the same person, individual-based prediction becomes possible, and is likely to be superior to epidemiological predictions. For example, the experience of a child who has an asthma attack once or twice a week, mostly at nights, can be used to predict the occurrence, timing, and outcome of the next attack. By contrast the occurrence and outcome of meningococcal meningitis, which is rare, is only predictable from population studies.

Information about the demographic and socio-economic characteristics of a population tells us about the health of individuals within that population. For example, knowing that a population is rich predicts a pattern of death for most individuals that is dominated by heart disease, stroke and cancer and not by infections and nutritional deficiency disorders. These generalizations are possible as population characteristics influence individuals risk of disease, as discussed next.

2.2 Harnessing variety in individual and group-level disease and risk factor patterns

Epidemiology is interested in the factors that cause population patterns of disease as in disease X in Box 1.6. These factors are usually complex interactions between individuals, their physical environment, and their society. To understand the pattern, therefore, needs understanding of the circumstances in which the population lives.

Investigation of disease patterns should be, therefore, on populations defined in terms of location, size, age and sex structure, and a wide range of data on the life and environmental circumstances of the people. The idea is to define and utilize the inherent variety of populations, and measure characteristics that are potential explanations for disease variation. In studying variation in chronic bronchitis, for example, we need to know whether the populations studied are exposed to air pollution, tobacco, poverty or poor housing. This is the central message in the famous quotation from Hippocrates (Chapter 1, p. 1), and in most definitions of epidemiology. Do the exercise in Box 2.4 before reading on.

Box 2.4 Heterogeneity (dissimilarity) and homogeneity (similarity) of exposure to potential causes of disease in epidemiology

- How would epidemiology study the link between tobacco and lung cancer in a society where every adult smoked 20 cigarettes per day?

- How would one investigate epidemiologically the effect of the gas nitrogen on human health? What about oxygen?

- Neutrinos are cosmic particles which penetrate deep into the Earth. How would we investigate, epidemiologically, their impact on health?

In a society where everyone smoked cigarettes, say 20 per day, epidemiology would be virtually powerless to assess the effect, for while lung cancer would be common, the exposure to the major cause would be uniform. The key strategy of comparing and contrasting the disease pattern in people with and without the postulated cause (exposure) is not possible. The solution would be to persuade some of the population to decrease or stop smoking, in other words, to do an experiment. Experiments usually need to be justified by data supporting the hypothesis; in the circumstances described this would be difficult.

While experimentation might be possible for tobacco, it could not be accomplished easily with respect to oxygen, nitrogen and neutrinos, for experimentally stopping, or even substantially reducing, exposure to these substances would not be feasible except for short periods of time. The effects of such gases and particles on long-term human health are not open to rigorous epidemiological study. Nonetheless, useful information might come from studies on animals or cell cultures.

Paradoxically, the variety so vital to epidemiology poses challenges in interpreting and applying research. While tobacco and alcohol, for example, are damaging to health in populations as a whole, there are people and groups for whom these substances are harmless and perhaps even beneficial in some respects. For example, tobacco use is linked to fewer problems with ulcerative colitis, and suppresses the appetite and prevents weight gain. Alcohol in small amounts reduces the risk of atherosclerotic heart disease. Whether, for a particular individual, tobacco or alcohol consumption is advisable or not is beyond epidemiology, which only permits valid judgements at the population level. The health damage caused by tobacco in populations far outweighs the health benefits. The position in regard to alcohol consumption is less clear, but the harm and damage at a population level, in most societies, is certainly more in balance than that for tobacco.

The next section will discuss why the disease and risk factor patterns in populations are more than the sum of measures in the individuals in the population.

2.3 Disease patterns as an outcome of individuals living in changing social groups

Diseases are expressed biologically in individuals. It is tempting, therefore, to assume that the causes of diseases and the solutions to their control and prevention are also biological and lie at the individual level. Many diseases, however, are caused only by the interaction of individuals, and most are profoundly influenced by such interactions. In other words the causes of disease are often social.

Individuals shape society, and in turn society exerts a powerful influence on individuals, including in attitudes, behaviour, and diseases.

Do the exercise in Box 2.5 before reading on.

Chapter 1 introduced the idea that disease patterns were influenced by the interaction of social, environmental and individual level factors. The examples were of infections. This central concept applies to many diseases. Suicide is a clear-cut example. While suicide and parasuicide are linked to psychotic disorders, particularly depression, they are

Box 2.5 Impact of social organization on disease patterns in populations

Imagine a world where humans lived an isolated lifestyle, avoiding others whenever possible, using technologies to communicate, and using physical barriers to reduce contact. Children would be raised by one parent, perhaps. Imagine that the physical and economic environment remained similar to that we experience now; that is, people lived in housing of similar quality and used similar cars etc.

◆ What would be the effect on disease patterns?

◆ Which diseases would be more common and which less so?

◆ What would be the the the influences on lifestyles?

hugely influenced by convention. Durkheim, a French sociologist working in the nineteenth century, held that common values underlie social order, and that the loss of such values leads to social and individual instability and suicide. Durkheim's studies (1951) showed huge variations in suicide which he believed to be an attribute of the society, or social reality, which in turn determined the suicide-related behaviour of individuals. This principle, that society influences mortality, has now been demonstrated in wider circumstances, and most recently in the context of inequalities in health.

Mortality rates generally, and for some specific causes of death, are associated with increasing inequality of wealth in society. For a given level of wealth, societies that distribute the wealth more equally have higher life expectancy (and other health outcomes are better) than those that distribute wealth less equally. Economically unequal societies also have poorer mental and physical health than expected. Such societies show an excess of both overtly social problems such as murder and accidents, and other apparently biological problems such as cardiovascular diseases. The explanations for these observations are complex and controversial. The main hypothesis under examination is that unequal societies are less likely to invest in activities that improve health, and/or that they undermine social cohesion and increase stress. There is some evidence that the adverse effects of income inequality are greatest in the poorer and middle income groups and least in the wealthiest groups. In short, being poor is associated with poor health, and being poor in an economically unequal society adds a further burden on health. Many industrialized countries, including the UK and US, have become both wealthier and more unequal in the last 30 years or so, so these observations have particular relevance to modern public health.

Society even has an impact on genetic diseases. Down's syndrome, a genetic disorder called trisomy 21, shows how social expectations and behaviours alter disease patterns. Societies that encourage birth at older ages will have a higher rate of Down's syndrome than those that encourage childbirth in the young because the genetic abnormality becomes more common as the mother ages. Prenatal screening is available for this disorder, and the choice of abortion of the affected fetus is possible. So, the number of people with Down's syndrome depends on age of the mother at conception, availability and uptake of screening, and the acceptability of abortion—all socially determined. The pattern of disease depends, therefore, on the way society is organized.

Individuals and their societies live in a physical environment which is the prime determinant of health and illness in populations (an argument developed in Chapter 4 on causal thinking).

In the imaginary future world in Box 2.5, which is feasible, diseases that are transmitted from person to person would occur rarely. So, an isolated individual or small group would not develop diseases such as tuberculosis, leprosy, influenza, the common cold, measles, mumps, AIDS, and sexually transmitted diseases. Some of the microorganisms causing these diseases are exclusively human pathogens (e.g. the leprosy bacillus, mumps virus, measles virus) so they would not survive, and would become extinct. If humans also isolated themselves from animals, the zoonoses (diseases transmitted from animals to humans), including Lyme disease and brucellosis, would not occur. The human–animal cycle necessary for the propagation of parasitic diseases would be broken. The effect would not just be on the highly contagious diseases. Ulcers associated with infection by the bacterium *Helicobacter pylori* would be less common. Cancers linked to microorganisms would not occur or their incidence would be profoundly reduced; for example, cervical cancer, which is primarily caused by human papillomavirus transmitted sexually, and gastric cancer, often a consequence of *Helicobacter pylori* infection.

The pattern of mental health problems would be profoundly different. The stresses of living in complex societies would be replaced by problems of isolation and loneliness.

The influence on cancer and heart disease would also be huge, mostly from changes in behaviours which are influenced by social and peer pressures; for example, smoking, alcohol drinking and the amount and content of diet. The pattern of behaviour would change hugely, causing massive alterations in the pattern of disease.

The thought exercise in Box 2.5 is not theoretical. For most of their history humans have lived as small groups of 20–100 hunter-gatherers and not in large settled communities. There are still humans who are effectively isolated. Influenza and measles are killing disorders in populations previously unexposed to them and, therefore, lacking in immunity. Smallpox, a scourge for any society, was near genocidal in isolated populations exposed to it. Over the last few hundred years isolated human groups have been rapidly exposed to populations of strangers with devastating consequences for their health. The Tasmanian aborigines were made extinct by their interaction with European settlers and North American Indians were decimated by the new patterns of disease arising from both their interaction with Europeans, and later the new social expectations and roles imposed upon them. As a form of germ warfare, European settlers gave American Indians 'presents' of blankets that had been contaminated with material from smallpox patients. In more modern times, in 1857 the British colonized the Andaman Islands (east of India, west of Thailand) where the tribe Great Andamanese comprised 5000 people. In 1988, 28 were left. Measles and influenza took their toll. The Jarawa tribe remains isolated on the Andaman Islands but is making contact with the outside world. In the first edition of this book I wrote that the result is predictable. Since then, there have been measles outbreaks and continuing encroachment of territory despite an Indian Supreme Court injunction, hitherto ignored, that the main road into the Jarawa territory be closed.

The swift move to urbanization following the industrial revolution in the eighteenth century, still continuing in the industrialized nations and accelerating in the developing ones, has exposed billions of people to new environments, disease agents and different forms of human interaction. Migration and population mixing has a profound effect on the disease patterns of society. As a generalization, over some generations, the migrant population takes on the pattern of disease of the host country. The process of change is usually slow, but it can be fast and surprising. Emigrants from India to wealthy industrialized countries develop chronic diseases such as heart disease and diabetes at a level far higher than predictable from the rate of disease in India and from the pattern of their causal factors. The explanations for this are under study. Migration also changes disease on a local scale. For example, the strongest explanation for the observed high rates of childhood leukaemia around nuclear power stations is based on the pattern of childhood infections. There was substantial population mixing because of the inward migration of workers into the relatively isolated communities hosting power stations. If the hypothesis is correct, local migration changing the pattern of childhood infection, and not radiation from power stations, is the fundamental cause of the excess of leukaemia in these areas (see Kinlen *et al.* 1995).

The twenty-first century may see a reversal, at least in wealthy industrialized countries, of population mixing. First, easier transport and new communications technology are offering people the chance of enjoying the benefits of the city while mostly living in isolation, either in the countryside or within fenced and guarded compounds in the city. Computer links at home, work that can be done solo, environmental concerns and an increase in costs of office space in cities are likely to accelerate these trends. Secondly, with increasing inequality in income the wealthiest people have both the resources and incentives to isolate themselves geographically from their societies.

The population, then, has patterns of health and disease which are caused by the interactions of individuals living in a complex, organized society. Some diseases would not arise at all in isolated individuals and small groups. For nearly all diseases the pattern would be greatly different if the social organization differed. Disease patterns are generated in, and by, populations so need to be described, explained and predicted in populations. While all individuals must sicken and die, the nature of the population they live in has a profound effect on which sicknesses they develop, when they develop them, and at what age they are likely to die within the range determined by biological processes. The close link of epidemiology to public health, which is defined as the science and art of prolonging life, preventing disease and promoting health through the organized efforts of society, is clear in this context. This sets the stage for considering the late Geoffrey Rose's idea of the sick population.

2.4 Sick populations and sick individuals

Rose proposed a radical and still controversial vision in his book, *Rose's Strategy of Preventive Medicine* (Rose 1994). His central proposition was that people with overt diseases and health problems—people with hypertension, alcohol problems or obesity –were simply at one end

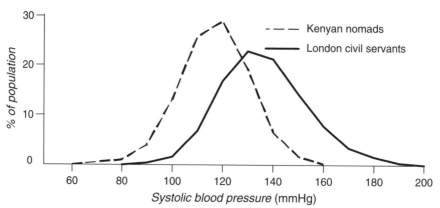

Fig. 2.2 Distribution of systolic blood pressures in middle-aged men in two populations (Source: Rose *Int J Epidemiol* 1985; 14, 32–8, see Permissions).

of the spectrum, or distribution. They are not deviant, but an integral part of the whole. To prevent such problems required changes in the population, with a shifting of the whole distribution of risk factors. For example, on Rose's argument, prevention of alcoholism requires that the entire distribution of alcohol consumption shifts, so the average and total consumption declines. To quote Rose, 'the supposedly "normal" majority needs to accept responsibility for its deviant minority—however loth it may be to do so'.

Rose developed the idea of sick and healthy populations, distinct from sick or healthy individuals, by reflecting on questions arising from international studies of high blood pressure and cardiovascular disease, and the exercise that follows is based on that.

Box 2.6 Reflection on the distribution of blood pressure values in Kenyan nomads and London civil servants

Examine Fig. 2.2 and reflect on these questions:

◆ In what ways do the shapes of the distributions differ (if at all) in the two populations?

◆ Roughly, what percentage of Kenyans and London civil servants have hypertension, i.e. systolic blood pressure of 140 mmHg or above?

◆ Is there any suggestion from Fig. 2.2 that the cause of high blood pressure in an individual Kenyan nomad and a London civil servant is likely to differ?

◆ What are the causes of the different distribution of blood pressure, in general terms, in the two populations?

◆ Are the causes of high blood pressure in the population, reflected in the distribution, different from those in the individual?

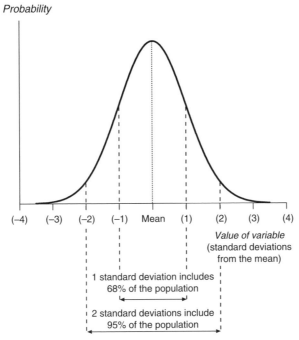

Fig. 2.3 The normal distribution.

Currently a systolic blood pressure of 140 mmHg or more is considered a matter of concern and one of 160 mmHg would cause some alarm. In the exercise consider a value of 140 mm as *indicative* of hypertension. Before reading on, reflect carefully, but broadly, on Fig. 2.2 using the questions in Box 2.6. Figure 2.2 is a graph showing the systolic blood pressure on the *x*-axis and the percentage of the population with that level of pressure in each of two populations.

Figure 2.2 shows that the shape of the two distributions of blood pressure is similar, and of the shape that is described as a normal (or Gaussian) distribution as shown in Fig. 2.3 (normal distributions are symmetric, the mean, median and mode values are the same, and 68 per cent of the population lies within one standard deviation of the mean value, and 95 per cent within two standard deviations—see glossary). The distribution of blood pressure in London civil servants is far to the right of that of Kenyan nomads. One simple indication of the impact of this on the amount of disease is the percentage of the population with hypertension. Based on the cut-off of 140 mmHg, a large percentage of civil servants have hypertension (about 40 per cent) and a small number of nomads do (about 10 per cent). Based on a cut-off of 160 mmHg substantial numbers of civil servants have hypertension (about 15 per cent) while such values are rare in nomads. Rose and Day (1990) showed that the population mean (average) predicts the number of people with the health problem. For systolic blood pressure their data predicted a 10 per cent increase in the percentage of the population with hypertension for every 10 mmHg increase in mean systolic blood pressure.

The cause of high blood pressure in individuals is usually not pinpointed and is named essential hypertension. In about 10 per cent of cases a specific cause (such as a kidney problem) is found. While Fig. 2.2 does not inform us about the causes of hypertension in individuals, the similarity in the shape of the distribution, and the range of difference between the two extremes, suggest similarities in the forces that shape the distribution. Rose surmises that the specific causes of hypertension in nomads may be the same genetic, environmental, and behavioural factors as those operating on civil servants. Certainly, renal failure will cause hypertension in a Kenyan and a Londoner alike.

The stark difference is in the location, as opposed to the shape, of the blood pressure distributions. Explaining this is a typical epidemiological challenge. It is likely that the nomads are closer to the normal pattern for humans and the Londoners' distribution has shifted rightwards. The question of what causes this difference between populations is a different one from what causes hypertension in an individual. We can speculate that the causes of the rightward shift are dietary factors (including high fat, high salt, high calories), obesity, insufficient exercise, stress and relationships between these and genetic factors. Such factors are acting on the population. The question of causes, therefore, needs to be studied in relation to the population and not just individuals. The causes of sickness in the population—for example, London civil servants who comprise a group with an abnormal blood pressure distribution—are conceptually different from the causes of sickness in the individual, and need to be studied differently too. Rose emphasizes that information on the population distribution of the risk factors (as in Fig. 2.2), and the shape of the risk factor–disease outcome relationship (see dose–response, Chapter 5) is vital to the population approach to preventive medicine.

Similar analysis could be done for many other health problems such as alcoholism, obesity and diabetes. Before reading on reflect on alcohol and alcoholic liver disease. While the cause of alcoholic liver cirrhosis is alcohol (by circularity of argument in the definition) its incidence varies hugely between populations and indeed within subgroups of the population. What is the cause of this population variation? Plainly, there are differences in populations in the consumption of alcohol. Why are there such differences?

The individual may be an alcoholic as a response to anxiety, depression, unemployment, or simply a fondness for alcoholic beverages that led to addiction. Populations, however, have high and low consumption for different reasons including stigma, religion, tradition, customs of hospitality, availability, income and taxes.

Understanding causes of phenomena in the population is the primary responsibility of population scientists, and in regard to health and disease, of epidemiologists.

Rose referred to the causes of population variations as the causes of the causes. The major cause of lung cancer is tobacco. What causes people to take up smoking even when they are knowledgeable about its harm? Why does the amount of smoking vary so much between populations? The causes of the causes, reflected in these questions, tend to be social and environmental, not biological.

The idea that the causes of diseases in individuals differ from causes in populations, leads to a radically different strategy for disease control based on both the causes, and the causes of the causes. The goal becomes changing the distribution of risk factors in populations as

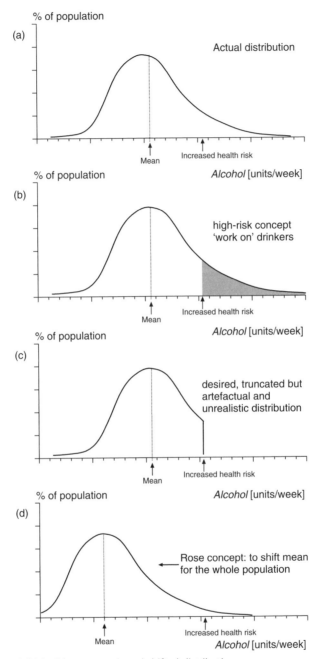

Fig. 2.4 The actual, high-risk, truncated, and shifted distributions.

Box 2.7 Sickness X: individual and population perspective

◆ Was sickness X (Box 1.6) a disease of sick individuals or of sick populations?

◆ What might have been the causes of the causes in sickness X?

opposed to individuals. Figure 2.4 illustrates the strategic difference between the so-called high-risk and population-based approaches. A distribution of alcohol consumption is shown in part (a), with the level at which health risk increases (say risk of alcoholic liver damage). Part (b) of the figure shades the high risk group. The high-risk approach concentrates on this group. If the strategy is successful, the end result would be as shown in (c), a highly artificial result that has never been seen. The population approach concedes that a distribution like (c) is not feasible. To achieve a similar result in terms of reducing risk, we shift the entire distribution leftwards. Such shifts require social action whereby the average levels of consumption are based on reducing the harm, not merely in individuals, but the population as a whole. This matter is discussed again in Section 2.8. Do the exercise in Box 2.7 on whether sickness X is a disease of individuals or of populations, before reading the material in Table 2.2. (You may wish to re-read the material in Box 1.6, p. 12.)

Isolated cases of sickness X did occur, usually in the mentally ill or in people with addictions such as alcohol. More usually it occurred in outbreak or epidemic form in whole communities. Knowledge of the specific 'causal' agent did not achieve control of the disease at the population level though it did cure the individual treated.

Sickness X is pellagra, a disease caused by deficiency of a vitamin now called niacin. The investigation of the causes of pellagra by Joseph Goldberger starting in 1914 is a compelling, classic tale. At that time an infectious cause was favoured, but Goldberger's traditional review of the scientific literature in 1914 led him, rapidly, to a nutritional cause, even though in 1914 a USA government commission had concluded otherwise.

Table 2.2 Some observations on disease X as a sickness of populations

Sickness X
Never occurred in humans free to choose their own way of life
Occurred after populations were thrown into poverty
Did not decline even after its specific cause was well understood in biological terms
Continued to occur, in hundreds of thousands of people every year, in some extremely rich countries that would not accept that the cause had been discovered even though other countries virtually eliminated the problem by acting upon available knowledge
Declined when a war led to a change in the mode of life in the USA
Declined when economic disaster led to a marked change in the mode of living and working in rural areas
Was virtually defeated by government action

Goldberger (and a colleague, Edgar Sydenstricker) pursued the investigation over more than 20 years with a mix of epidemiological designs (including a cohort study and trial), and in addition laboratory-based animal research. The biology of the disease is now clear. But, to say the cause of pellagra is niacin deficiency, or even a nutritional deficiency, is a simplification, particularly as it does not provide a course of action for controlling the disease in the population. The characteristics of the disease in a population context, some of which are identified in Table 2.2, give clues to the wider causes of the cause (niacin deficiency): poverty, loss of freedom of populations and individuals to choose their diet, and eating too narrow a range of foods. The causes of the disease are, therefore, nutritional deficiency of niacin, lack of milk and meat in the diet, lack of variation of foods in the diet, poverty, farming practices inappropriate to the needs of the population, and loss of the freedom to farm according to one's own judgement.

The effective actions to bring the disease under control have included: treatment of individuals with niacin, free distribution of yeast which is rich in niacin to supplement niacin intake, increasing the range of foods offered to captive populations, phasing out the type of farming called sharecropping, flour enrichment, reduced unemployment, military service and food rationing. In the USA flour enrichment started in 1941 and this action virtually wiped out pellagra. Pellagra outbreaks continue to occur, but are now rare. A pellagra outbreak with 908 cases between July 1999 and February 2000 occurred in Kuito, Angola, mostly in war refugees.

2.5 Individual and population-level epidemiological variables

Information collected carefully and precisely at the individual level may not portray the true state of the population. Equally, information on a population or the environment may not have meaning at an individual level. Before reading on reflect on the questions in Box 2.8.

Individual attributes such as age, age at death, blood pressure and serum cholesterol can usually be aggregated and meaningfully used to describe the population. To provide a meaningful picture the data must be from either the whole population or a characteristic (representative) sample. If this is not the case the description of the population's health status may be grossly inaccurate, even though the individual measures are accurate.

Imagine a study of the mean value of cholesterol in a population aged 18–64 where methods ensured accurate measurement. If the investigators call for volunteers to

Box 2.8 Individual and population measures

Under what circumstances might individual measures be meaningfully applied to populations and vice versa? Reflect on such measures as age (individual), sex (individual), blood pressure (individual), household size (not individual), population density (area), and gross national product (national).

participate, the population data may be erroneous because the people studied are untypical. For this reason epidemiology is generally based on studies of the entire population of interest and, when this is too large, on representative samples (e.g. by random sampling, stratified sampling, etc.). The investigator exerts control of who is studied. As representativeness is a key requirement in epidemiology, particularly for measuring the burden of disease and risk factors, small studies on representative samples may be of greater value than large ones on unrepresentative samples. Typically the response rate in population studies would be 60–70 per cent of those invited, sometimes repeatedly, to participate. Participation is usually least in young poor men living in the inner city. Even with excellent measurements and best practice in sample selection, therefore, the end result may be inaccurate as a population measure.

The population needs to be described by both the frequency distribution of their health status and summaries such as the mean and standard deviation (see Fig. 2.3, and Chapter 9 for further guidance on analysis of data). The population distribution of most biological measures follows a normal or Gaussian distribution as shown in Fig. 2.3. The mean, median and mode value is then the same. One standard deviation includes about 68 per cent of the population, and two standard deviations include 95 per cent of the population. This underlies many statistical tests. In epidemiological studies the population distribution must be examined to assess whether it follows the normal distribution. If it does, the mean and standard deviation provide an accurate picture of the distribution, i.e. like Fig. 2.3. If not, the distribution should be shown because summary statistics do not envision it accurately. The measures made on representative samples of individuals usually provide meaningful information on the whole population.

Sometimes individual measures have no value when aggregated. Table 2.3(a) lists fingerprint patterns and personality as examples of measures that are meaningful and useful at an individual level but not in aggregate. Societies do not have a personality or a fingerprint pattern and applying individual data to groups is purposeless quantification.

Measures of the population or the environment also may be meaningless when applied to the individual. Epidemiological findings based on such variables may be applicable only at the population level. Some population and environment level variables of this kind are listed in Table 2.3(b). It is a paradox that some data collected from individuals (e.g. the number of people who live in the household), when used in aggregate (e.g. as population density of an area), cease to be meaningful at the individual level.

Table 2.3(a) Some individual measures which, conceptually, have no meaningful epidemiological interpretation when aggregated into populations

Fingerprint patterns
Personality
Eye colour
Loneliness

Table 2.3(b) Some population and environmental variables which, conceptually, have no direct and meaningful individual interpretation

Population variables	Environmental variables
Population density	Air quality
Income and wealth inequality index	Road traffic density
% of population unemployed	Ambient temperature
Indexes of socio-economic deprivation	Hardness of the water
Gross national product	Land use

While social variables are usually measured in individuals, environmental variables are usually not so measured. Contemporary challenges in epidemiology include the accurate measurement of environmental exposures in individuals, and the measurement of social characteristics in aggregate. Social characteristics including cohesion in society, team-work and the state of economic transition, are likely to have profound effects on health and yet be incompletely captured and described through the usual individualized approaches to measurement. Methods in epidemiology are underpinned by the concept of population (see also Chapter 9). The next section examines the interdependence of demography and epidemiology.

2.6 Epidemiology and demography: interdependent population sciences

Demography is the study of population structure, including the impact of birth, death, fertility, marriage, migration and other social factors.

There is an obvious overlap in epidemiology and demography. Epidemiology is hugely dependent on demography and is difficult when demographic data are not available or wrong. To understand the importance of demography in epidemiology try the exercise in Box 2.9 before reading on.

Box 2.9 The importance of demography to epidemiology

- Imagine a country or region where there was no demographic data, so the number of people and the age and sex composition of the population were unknown.
- Imagine also that an epidemic (say of pneumonia or food poisoning) is suspected.
- You are asked to develop a plan to prevent and control the epidemic in the area.
- You are also asked to advise on the future needs for medical personnel in the area.
- How would you do this and what obstacles can you foresee?

It is hard to imagine a place without demographic data, for in modern times we are bombarded with population statistics. A census of population is fundamental to modern life. The US census has taken place every ten years since 1790 and the UK one since 1801. Indeed, our first epidemiological public health action in a society without a population count would probably be to undertake a survey of population size (census) or setting up a population register. Accurate population counts are hardest to obtain in fast-changing societies and in places where people do not live in built homes on land they own or rent.

Even in the industrialized world there may be a lack of reliable population size data in the inner city, in economically deprived areas, in holiday towns where there is a flux of population, holiday theme parks (although these may operate turnstile counts), war zones, refugee camps, or at major public gatherings such as pop festivals. Some industrialized countries, e.g. Holland, do not have a census but rely on compulsory registration of population to get demographic data. In most developing countries census data are usually available but may not be reliable, particularly for small localities.

Lebanon is an advanced middle-income country in the Middle East. It is unusual in not having had a census since the 1930s. The reason is political. Population size and structure is, nonetheless, estimated in various ways. With the recent civil war, the continuing border battles and the large number of refugees and soldiers, an accurate population count is not possible. Furthermore, registration of deaths takes place at the locality of family origin as registered in the last census and not at the place of residence or death. A medical diagnosis is not a requirement for a death certificate. Without such basic information, describing disease patterns on a national scale and monitoring trends is difficult. The circumstances of a refugee camp, though extreme, illustrate the principles well.

Imagine that the epidemic referred to in Box 2.9 occurs in a refugee camp, where the population size is variable and where there has been a large intake in recent days (the camp population is represented in Fig. 2.5 with each circle being a person and cases

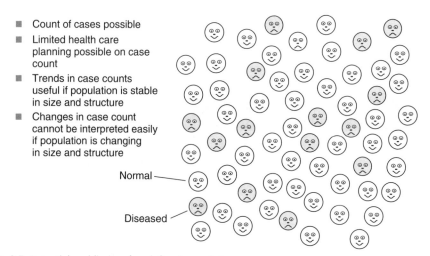

Fig. 2.5 Potential and limits of undefined populations.

of sickness/disease are shaded). An outbreak of pneumonia is suspected. What can the epidemiologist do? This scenario illustrates the key principles that apply in large populations but that are often glossed over.

The epidemiologist can count the cases, and relate this information to the date of disease onset, date of diagnosis, and the age and sex of the patients. This information is useful to assess need for care. For example, if there are 20 cases who become sick today perhaps we can assume there will be a similar number tomorrow. So, facilities can be organized and supplies ordered. What if the number of cases per day declines or rises? The daily trend can be described and used to make a prediction and the facilities and supply order adjusted. Using information on the age, sex or other characteristics of cases, appropriate refinements can be made to the plan of needs. So, if 90 per cent of the cases are children, the need for antibiotics can be adjusted, because they need small doses and possibly different drugs. This is a useful and practical application of epidemiology. Nonetheless, the information is sorely limited.

Without a knowledge of population size and composition, we cannot estimate the number of cases that are to be expected in normal circumstances, so we cannot say whether there are more than expected, and hence whether an epidemic is underway. Changes in daily numbers may simply be reflecting changes in population size. We cannot assess whether the disease is affecting some groups, such as men more than women, or whether it is commoner in some parts of the camp than others. The number of cases over time gives some, but not definitive, insight into whether the disease is controlled or not, for a rise may occur if the population is increasing, even in the face of successful control. Only if the population size is stable can changes in the number of cases reflect change in disease incidence. Epidemiological investigations into the reasons why outbreaks (here pneumonia) occur usually focus on comparing cases with controls. This work is impeded by lack of information about the population of potential cases and potential controls, as will be discussed in Chapter 9 on study design. In these circumstances a rational, epidemiologically based disease control strategy is hard to design, implement and monitor. Try the exercise in Box 2.10 before reading on.

The first step is to set boundaries (Fig. 2.6). Where does the camp begin and end? The second step is to define a time for the census. The count is likely to differ by time of year, day of week and probably time of day. The third step is to define who is to be included. It is likely that some people are visitors, others are helpers, some are staff, and some refugees will move in and out of the camp. The fourth step is to decide what information is to be collected and how. Once these decisions are made, the number, age

Box 2.10 Developing a population profile

Imagine that accurate information on the age and sex composition of the inhabitants is to be collected. How will this be done?

- Set a boundary
- Decision about those on the boundary
- Define a time
- Count the population
- Describe the population
- Count migrations, births and deaths
- Link population counts to health data to calculate birth and death rates, and disease-specific rates
- Surveillance by time, place and person
- Monitoring
- Design of studies to understand the burden and causes of disease

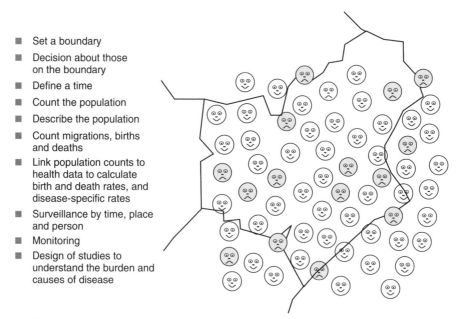

Fig. 2.6 Defining a population by setting a boundary.

and sex of the inhabitants can be ascertained. Now that we have done a census the case numbers can be expressed as a proportion of the population from which they arose. The number of cases per unit of population can be calculated either overall or separately by the characteristics of the people in the camp (e.g. by age, sex, type of resident etc.). Chapters 7 and 8 consider the epidemiological approach to collecting and analysing such data.

If there is a change in the number of cases over time, there are two main explanations: either the number or type of people has changed or the rate of disease has changed. Since the population is unlikely to remain stable for long in a refugee camp, the number of cases will change due to population size fluctuations. The obvious answer is to recount the population regularly, perhaps weekly, but this will be impractical in a camp and in most real-life circumstances. In practice, the occasional census needs to be supplemented by keeping track of population changes, which requires recording deaths, births and migration. These 'vital' statistics permit the census data to be updated routinely.

The collection of vital statistics is, in practice, incomplete and error prone, so population counts become out of date, particularly in small geographical areas, and the census needs to be repeated. In the setting of a camp this need may arise monthly. Most nations repeat the census every 5–10 years or so. Cities where population change is rapid generally need counts between census years. Reflect on the questions in the exercise in Box 2.11 before reading on.

Box 2.11 A public health and epidemiological framework for solving the problem of the epidemic in the camp

Imagine yourself as the health officer of this camp responsible for controlling the epidemic.

◆ Which questions do you need to answer to bring to bear a rational control strategy and to declare the problem controlled?

◆ Which epidemiological data do you need, in general terms, to answer the questions?

◆ How does the census help you?

The questions the health officer needs to ask and the answers are summarized in Table 2.4. These questions are generalizable to a multiplicity of epidemiological problems. The data will come from a variety of sources and study designs, although in the specific context of a refugee camp the epidemiology is likely to be fairly basic. With the population count by age and sex, basic but important epidemiological questions of whether the disease frequency has altered, and is altering in the face of control measures, can be answered (see part (a) of Table 2.4). For understanding of cause (part (b) of Table 2.4) the level of information needed is greater. For designing, implementing and evaluating effective strategies for the prevention and control of disease, knowledge of the culture and politics of the refugee camp and the society it is in will need to be integrated with the epidemiology.

The work of demographers and statisticians who calculate disease rates clearly overlaps with that of epidemiologists and yet it differs in one important goal: epidemiology needs to understand, explain and use, and not just describe, the patterns of disease. That means understanding enough about the population to generate and test causal hypotheses. The epidemiological population, as with a demographic one, is usually defined using geographical boundaries (Fig. 2.6). The epidemiological population may also be defined by the characteristics of the population such as age and sex, or consist of, say, people with diabetes, children attending a particular school, or the homeless. The epidemiological population also needs to be bounded by time limits. In addition to population size estimates, epidemiology needs an understanding of the social and environmental circumstances of the people under study.

The idea of generalization (applicability elsewhere) is crucial to many scholarly disciplines and sciences. Ideally, epidemiological conclusions should be applicable not just to the people actually studied but also to others similar to them elsewhere. In practice, as human populations are highly variable in biological, environmental and social ways, generalization is fraught with difficulty. Figure 2.1 has deliberately shown human figures, for it is too easy to forget people when using symbols (of which numbers are the

Table 2.4 Answering public health and epidemiological questions using data and study methods

The public health and epidemiological questions	Data needs	Study design usually used (Chapter 9)
(a) Frequency and pattern		
How common is this problem?	Case numbers alone are often sufficient for rare diseases and when the population is stable, otherwise population counts are essential	Disease registers Cross-sectional studies Cohort studies
Is the problem increasing, decreasing, or about the same?	Accurate numbers of cases and population counts are essential	Repeat above studies/ analyses over time
Where does the problem occur most?	Case numbers and population counts by area are essential	Analyse data by place
Who is affected most?	Case numbers and population counts by population characteristics such as age, sex, economic status, and ethnic group are essential	Analyse data by person
(b) Understanding the cause		
What are the causes of the problem?	Detailed information on the population and its social and environmental context is essential The data need to be collected to test hypotheses on causation	Case–control study Cohort study Trials
(c) Control		
What strategy is needed to prevent or control the problem?	Understanding of what has worked elsewhere, the causal chain of the disease and of the resources available, together with understanding of the population in its social context	Literature review, preferably systematic
Are control measures working?	Case numbers and population data are usually essential for monitoring effectiveness of control measures; together with understanding of other changes occurring in the population and environment	Evaluation using pragmatic designs, e.g. before and after analyses of disease Repeat cross-sectional studies Trials

prime example), but for simplicity most figures in this book use ovals to represent human beings. A clear and detailed description of the population, in its environmental and social context, is essential to assess the potential for generalization. Unfortunately, it is common for investigators to ignore this cardinal rule, to fail to provide the contextual data needed for generalization, to generalize too readily and to err. When generalization is not appropriate, epidemiological data can still be used for local assessment and improvement of the health state of the people actually studied.

2.7 **The dynamic nature of human population**

In natural communities the size and composition of populations is constantly changing owing to deaths, births and migrations. However, even when the population size remains fixed, the population is still changing. Tackle the exercise in Box 2.12 before reading on.

Box 2.12 Implications of changes in populations for studying epidemiology

Before reading on reflect on this dynamism in human populations, and its implications for studying the pattern of disease in the population. In what way is the population changing even when the number of people is relatively constant?

Obviously, the individuals are getting older so the average age increases, changing the pattern of disease. In the industrialized world we have witnessed increasing lifespan from better socio-economic conditions, nutrition, environment, and health care. The average lifespan has increased by several decades in the last two hundred years or so (and continues to rise). Simultaneously, such societies typically have smaller families, in some countries too small to replace those dying. This has led to societies where the population is, on average, ageing. This is labelled the demographic transition. The accompanying shift in the pattern of diseases is called the epidemiological transition.

Imagine, however, a place where the number of people is fixed, and whenever an individual dies, or leaves, they are replaced. Imagine that the age, sex and ethnic composition of the group stays much the same. A place of this kind might be a jail or a nursing home. Even then, the population's health patterns are not fixed because human behaviours are evolving and their environments changing. The jail environment in the UK has changed by, for example, the introduction of television, alteration in diet, and the development of a drug-taking culture. The wider social trends in behaviour, including smoking, influence these enclosed populations. In short, for epidemiological purposes there is no fixed human population, only dynamic ones, always in transition. Epidemiology is studying the pattern of disease in changing populations.

While human populations are dynamic, the concept of a fixed population is helpful in thinking about the measurement of disease occurrence. Cohort studies (discussed in Chapter 9) are an attempt to create a defined or 'closed' population, while studies on vital statistics are on natural living or 'open' populations. In closed populations people who are dying and migrating are not replaced. In open populations there are gains as well as losses, as people are born and migrate into the population. The change in size of the closed population can be predicted from the death and emigration rates. The prediction of the size of the open population is more difficult and requires, in addition to the above, estimates of immigration and fertility patterns. If the number of people entering a population is balanced by the number exiting, the population is in a steady, but not unchanging, state.

Changes in the environment and behaviour lead to time-period influences on disease patterns. For example, 30–40-year-old women were less likely to be smokers in the decade 1920–1930 than 30–40-year-old women in 1950–1960. In an examination of the relationship between age group and lung cancer, say in 2008, the investigator would need to consider both the direct effect of ageing, and the time period effect (called the cohort effect—see section 9.8) of changing exposures to the causes of lung cancer over time.

The combination of the demographic transition and the effects of wider influences on health (wealth, environment, behaviour, etc.), leads to a profound change in the pattern of disease, with the dominance of chronic diseases. This epidemiological transition is emerging rapidly in middle-income countries such as Mauritius, Chile and urban India. For epidemiology these transitions are a boon, because they have led to greater variation in disease patterns and exposures to causes, and provide the fuel for the epidemiological engine.

In relatively wealthy and stable countries, improvements in most indices of health have been dramatic. This must not lead to complacency. In the face of economic, political, and social disturbance, health gains can be rapidly reversed. The decline in recent decades in life expectancy in men in particular in Russia and other East European countries, and men and women in much of Sub-Saharan Africa, is a perfect example of the epidemiological transition in reverse.

2.8 Applications of the epidemiological population concept

The epidemiological concept of population has a huge influence on every aspect of epidemiology in practice and health care, but it is often implicit. Health policy is nearly always based on the concept of population. Policy is usually directed either at the whole population or at subgroups identified by some important characteristic, such as geographical location (a nation, a city, or economically deprived area), the age group or gender, or some other characteristic such as ethnic or racial group.

Traditionally, health care systems have been designed for those who voice their need by consulting a doctor or other healer. Increasingly, health care systems are incorporating goals of improving the health of the whole population by using the concept of population. They are planning services based on the pattern of health problems in the population, taking into account variations in the health of subgroups within the population, and not just of users of the service. They are delivering modified services to sub-groups of the population who differ in their needs, for example the homeless, those in rural areas, or those who speak a foreign language. By using knowledge of population trends in health status they are anticipating the need for future services.

Health promotion is based on the population idea. Indeed, the social sciences and psychology, which underpin health promotion theory, emphasize how peer influences dominate the actions of individuals.

The population concepts of epidemiology, particularly as interpreted by Rose, may lead to a radical shift in practice. The concepts shift attention away from individual-orientated programmes to the population. The concept requires a radical idea: the targeting of interventions at people in the middle of the distribution (the average person) and not the extremes of the distribution (the deviants as described by Rose).

In the nineteenth century epidemiology established its credentials in medicine and is now considered as an essential part of clinical research and practice. Clinical practice based on the epidemiological concept of population is potentially transformed. The clinician is presented with new challenges, a means of increasing the impact of medical science, personal responsibility to the wider society, and acute ethical dilemmas. Clearly, the purpose of the health professions is greater than just the alleviation of the pain and illnesses of individuals. Their purpose includes the acquisition of knowledge (research) and organization of care for the benefit of people who access the service, the people who need the service but do not access it, and the generations to come.

For the individual clinician the people to be served are primarily those who consult, whether in the 'walk-in' manner of the American health care system or by registration with the general practitioner and referral as in the British NHS. Clinicians have or develop a list of people for whom they are responsible. For clinicians, collectively, the list comprises all the people in the society within which they live and work. This population philosophy provides the foundation for clinical epidemiology and evidence-based health care.

The example of diabetes care illustrates the need for and power of this approach. Diabetes is a chronic disabling disease with a prolonged progression (natural history, which is discussed in Chapter 6) which may be diagnosed after the damaging effects have occurred. Many people with diabetes are diagnosed late. This poses a huge problem for clinicians managing diabetes. The traditional form of clinical care would involve awaiting the development of symptoms and problems severe enough to lead the person with diabetes to present for clinical care, for example infections, fatigue, blindness, renal failure, or even coma. The population approach is to take advantage of epidemiological knowledge to promote early diagnosis of disease and the prevention of complications. Diabetes physicians are among the early adopters of the population perspective and are increasingly assessing their effectiveness in terms of how well diabetes is detected, diagnosed, prevented, and controlled in the population and not just in individual patients.

This requires them to identify all people with diabetes and to have means of indirectly influencing them through other health care providers. Practising population-based medicine requires diabeticians to study health and disease in the community setting, to understand the epidemiology of the disease and to have access to information on the impact of their work in the population setting. The key tool for achieving all this is a population register of patients with diabetes. In future, such registers may also include people with impaired glucose tolerance and impaired fasting glucose, which are for many people a precursor of diabetes.

Biomedical scientists can use and apply the population concepts of epidemiology. First, they can use hypotheses generated by epidemiological observations in populations for their own studies whether on cells, organs, animals, or individual human beings. Secondly, they can test out hypotheses based on their research by seeing whether disease patterns in the populations are in line with their predictions. Thirdly, they can ground their own work in a defined sample of population and not rely on cells, organs, and other specimens from volunteers, or from selected patients.

2.9 **Conclusion**

The concept of population drives epidemiology and its applications. Population thinking emphasizes that disease patterns are the outcome of the interaction between groups of individuals and their environment. It emphasizes that effective understanding of the causes and control of disease needs to be based on these interactions and not on an analysis of individuals in isolation. The population approach promises to enhance the impact and effectiveness of clinical endeavour, by providing a broad scientific rationale to practice. The concept underlies the discipline of health and health-care needs assessment. No policy document or health care plan is complete without a population view, and health promotion and health education work also thrive within the population perspective. Clinical practice is embracing the idea. Medical science has always had the ambition of being generalizable to the whole population and is increasingly moving from the study of the individual and the organs, to studying these in the context of representative samples of the population.

The underlying theories that support this chapter are that disease patterns in individuals and societies are profoundly influenced by the mode of interaction of individuals with each other, animals, and the wider environment; and that the pattern of disease in society is more than the sum of disease in individuals. The central principle that can be drawn from this chapter is that the causes of disease lie in populations and their societies as much as in individuals and their biology.

Summary

Epidemiology is a population science in several senses. First, it studies disease patterns, which are hugely influenced by the interaction of individuals living in communities. Secondly, it depends heavily upon demographic population data to achieve its goals. Thirdly, its findings are drawn from, and applied to, groups (or populations) of people. Conclusions and recommendations from epidemiological data may be applied to individuals with caution (in a probabilistic way), and with open acknowledgement of individual variation.

Epidemiology without demographic data is limited in its scope, for then disease patterns can only be studied in populations which are stable in size and composition. Even then interpretation of comparisons between population groups is possible only when there are stark differences. Epidemiological studies do not work well, and are hard to interpret, without an understanding of the composition of the population under study. Serious errors in interpretation of data may arise from the use of erroneous demographic statistics.

One prime purpose of epidemiology is applying findings in health promotion, health care, and health policy to improve the health of populations. The focus on population in epidemiology distinguishes it from clinical research and the other medical sciences, which primarily study the individual, the organ, and the cell.

Sample examination questions

Give yourself 10 minutes for every 25% of marks

Question 1 Why is the population size and structure, as measured at census, so important in epidemiology? (25%)

Answer A census of population, providing data on age, sex and the social and economic structure of the population, is fundamental to modern epidemiology. Without such base information calculating disease rates, describing and interpreting disease patterns on a national scale, and monitoring trends, is extremely difficult.

Without knowledge of population size and structure, we cannot estimate the number of cases that are to be expected in normal circumstances, so we cannot say with certainty whether there are more than expected, and hence whether an epidemic is underway. We cannot assess whether the disease is affecting some groups, e.g., men more than women, or whether it is commoner in some places than others. In these circumstances a rational, epidemiologically based disease control strategy is hard to design, implement and monitor.

Question 2 Geoffrey Rose wrote that the causes of disease in populations may not be the same as the causes of disease in individuals. What did he mean? (25%)

Answer Rose meant that the causes of diseases in populations are often above and beyond the individual and relate to the way society is organized and the state of our environment. For example, the causes of asthma in populations relate to the way our housing is built, the state of the economy, the amount of allergens people are exposed to, the chemicals used, family size and structures, the hygiene of the environment etc. This is another and broader perspective on considering the wider determinants of disease in individuals. In Rose's vision it is not enough to consider disease causation at an individual level as, often, the solution does not lie there.

Question 3 Epidemiology is said to be a population science. Explain the meaning of this description in relation to *either* smoking or lung cancer. (25%)

Answer Epidemiology as population science studies populations or subpopulations, e.g. smoking in the UK uses population data to construct rates or risk factors of disease, compares populations over time, between places, and by population characteristics, and seeks improvement to health on a population basis, e.g. Rose's concept of shifting populations' distribution of risk factors points to differences between causes of disease in individuals versus causes of disease in the population.

Chapter 3

Variation in disease by time, place, and person
A framework for analysis of genetic and environmental effects

Objectives

On completion of this chapter you should understand:

- that variations generate observations of associations, which in turn spark causal hypotheses;
- that virtually all diseases vary in their frequency over time, across geographical areas and between population subgroups;
- that disease variations can be artefacts of errors or changes in data collection systems;
- that variations must be analysed systematically to check that they are real;
- the potential role of genes in causing variations in disease;
- that real variations are caused by environmental and social change over the short term, with a genetic contribution in the long term;
- that real variations, which are natural experiments, provide a potentially powerful means of understanding the causal pathways of disease;
- that study of clusters and outbreaks, i.e. abrupt changes in disease frequency, may yield both causal knowledge, and information to control the public health problem;
- that real variations help to develop and target health policy and health care.

3.1 Introduction

Diseases vary in their population frequency over time and between populations. This simple but profoundly important observation, virtually without exception, is one of the axioms of epidemiology. Medical and public health practice are often credited for bringing about a decline in disease when it is due to natural causes (but they rarely take the blame for rising disease rates). Diseases which have undergone massive natural change in incidence within the last 100 years include peptic ulcer, stroke, gastric cancer, AIDS, and infections including tuberculosis.

This chapter emphasizes a systematic framework of analysis of disease variations, particularly to ensure that observations of variation are real, and not products of data errors and artefacts. The framework applies to all measures of disease frequency. For reasons discussed in Chapter 7 (Sections 7.2 and 7.3, Table 7.2), for causal investigations, the soundest measure is the incidence rate, based on new cases. The likelihood of artefact causing disease variations is greater with prevalence measures of existing disease than with incidence rates.

3.2 Reasons for analysing disease variations: environment and genetics

Consider the questions in Box 3.1 before reading further.

There are five principal reasons for investigating a change in disease frequency:

1 To help control an abrupt rise in disease incidence, especially of a suspected cluster or outbreak of an infectious or environmental disease.

2 For understanding the factors which change disease frequency, and hence gaining insight into the causes of disease.

3 To use the time trend in disease, and its causes, to develop health policy and health care plans.

4 To predict the future course of the disease.

5 To reduce, if not eradicate, the disease.

The investigation of a decline in disease frequency is, for understanding causes, as worthy of investigation as an increase. In practice, a rise in disease incidence is a problem, while a decline is not, and so is given lesser priority.

The key strategy in epidemiology is to seek and quantify disease variations, and then develop and test hypotheses to understand their causes. The key question is why does the disease vary over time, between places, and between populations? In the first analysis, as discussed in Chapter 5, causes are distinguished as genetic and environmental, the latter broadly meaning everything that is not genetic.

Before reading on, do the exercise in Box 3.2.

Variation in disease occurs over time and place in populations because the characteristics of the people or of their environment alter unequally. As such changes are not geographically uniform, this generates different patterns of disease in different places. In addition, within apparently homogeneous populations the disease experience of subgroups usually varies too because of differences in their characteristics, including genetic inheritance, behaviour, and local environment. Even if the social and physical environment were constant, however, some changes in population patterns of disease over time would still occur, albeit much more slowly, for genetic changes are inevitable and will influence disease.

All humans belong to one species, with mating and reproduction of healthy offspring occurring between all human populations in natural circumstances, so genetic variation

---

Box 3.1 Benefits of studying variations in disease

◆ What potential benefits are there from investigation of changes in disease frequency?

◆ Is a decline in disease as worthy of investigation as a rise?

Box 3.2 Reasons for variation

- Why, in general terms, do diseases vary over time, between places, and between subgroups of the populations?
- What is the relative importance of genetic and environmental influences in bringing about population differences in disease?

between populations is small in scale. Genetic change arises from a number of processes including genetic drift and genetic mutation, which cause random variation in gene frequency from generation to generation. In small populations genetic drift can lead to important genetically driven disease differences.

In large populations, however, genetic make-up is relatively stable. Changes in disease frequency in large populations occurring over short periods of time, meaning years or a few decades, are almost wholly environmental. There must, of course, be the genetic potential to develop a disease for it to occur. For example, hypertension is extremely common in urban-living Africans, especially those living in wealthy, industrialized countries, but not in rural Africans living in traditional lifestyles. Diabetes is common in urbanized Australian Aborigines but not in those living traditional lifestyles. The increase in disease prevalence in urban settings is due to changes in environmental circumstances in populations with a genetic potential to develop these diseases. Most diseases result from an interaction of environmental and genetic factors.

Though changes over longer time periods, meaning several hundreds or thousands of years or more, may be due to genetic factors, even they are much more likely to be due to environmental ones. The varying genetic potential for disease in different populations is acquired (and lost) over evolutionary timescales i.e. thousands, hundreds of thousands and, for biological traits underpinning disease, millions of years. (The main exception to this principle is infectious diseases where the genetic change is in the microorganisms—genetic changes in microbes can occur quickly.)

To take an analogy from theatre, in shaping the pattern of disease in large populations, the environment is the leading player and genetics the stage. This is not to deny the importance of genetic and hence biological factors in disease occurrence. The main cause of lung cancer is the farming and distribution, and then consumption by inhalation, of tobacco. If humans were not biologically susceptible to the carcinogens in tobacco, then tobacco would not cause lung cancer in populations. In individuals, as opposed to populations, genetic make-up is profoundly important, for genetic variation between individuals is great. This is a public health paradox: for populations the environment is the dominant influence on the pattern of disease, for individuals genetic inheritance may be equally or more important. Disease is, to repeat, caused by the interaction of the genome and the environment. Nonetheless, the control of disease does not usually involve influencing this interaction, but in choosing between genetic or environmental manipulation, the latter usually being easier than the former. With advances in genetic techniques, genetic epidemiology is advancing, growing, and even dominating the broader discipline. The next section (new in this edition) provides the fundamental biological and epidemiological principles to follow the literature.

As already discussed in Section 2.7, in the last few hundred years change in the environment has rapidly and profoundly changed disease patterns, particularly in populations which have industrialized and become wealthy. A decline in birth rates and death rates has led to the demographic transition and together with other changes to the epidemiological transition. In a few decades, infectious disease can decline dramatically and chronic diseases such as coronary heart disease, stroke, diabetes and cancers of the lung, breast, and colon, can become dominant. This transition is reversible, for when poverty strikes either as a result of economic or political turmoil or in war, infectious diseases return.

International differences in disease patterns mainly, though not wholly, reflect that the populations are at different stages in the demographic and epidemiological transitions. Some of the differences, however, are due to local environmental factors (e.g. climate) and some to genetic factors. International variations, and ethnic differences within populations, will be much reduced, though not eliminated, as the demographic and epidemiological transitions progress. The same underlying principles apply to differences in disease patterns in other types of subgroups within a geographically defined population. Disease differences between social classes or ethnic groups, for example, largely reflect differences in the environment and not in genetic composition. These differences, too, can be conceptualized as a result of subpopulations being at different stages of the demographic and epidemiological transition.

3.3 Introducing human genetic variation and genetic epidemiology

3.3.1 The human genome

The genome, comprising all of the genes and associated material in DNA, is the blueprint for human biology. In humans there are about 30,000 genes, the basic units holding the code for the blueprint. Most of the genes are in the 23 pairs of chromosomes in the cell's nucleus. In addition, there are a small number of genes in the mitochondria which are cellular components that are in the cell's cytoplasm, i.e. the part outside the nucleus. These mitochondria are remnants of primitive bacteria that live in symbiosis within the cell, performing the crucial task of energy production. They are important to human health but, for simplicity, the remainder of this discussion considers the genes in chromosomes in the nucleus.

Twenty-two pairs of the forty-six human chromosomes are called autosomal chromosomes, and one pair the sex chromosomes. One of each pair is inherited from each parent. As implied by the name, the sex chromosomes differ in men and women. Though this is a simplification, men have one sex chromosome called X and one called Y, while women have two X chromosomes. This difference, alone, determines the biological differences between men and women and it illustrates the power of genetics in shaping biology. Damage to and faults in the chromosomes usually have extremely serious consequences, with survival being imperilled. It is no surprise, therefore, that all normal and fully healthy human populations are identical in terms of chromosomal number and basic structure. Chromosomal differences are common in different species, and that is one of the major reasons why cross-species (healthy) reproduction does not occur in nature.

Each chromosome consists of two chains of so-called bases, like a train track, with a varying number of genes. Chromosomes, and hence genes, consist of deoxyribonucleic acid, or DNA for short. DNA is a double strand of several chemicals but the code is in the nucleic acids, of which there are four: adenine, guanine, cytosine, and thymine. These are known as nucleotides, and bases, and base pairs. Each of these four chemicals lines up, on this train track, with its natural pair, adenine with thymine, and guanine with cytosine. This pairing is the key to replication of DNA and the creation of RNA (ribonucleic acid) which takes the code to where it is needed in the cell. The nucleic acids provide the code for amino acids, the chemicals that make proteins. A sequence of three nucleic acids provide a code for an amino acid. A string of such triplets (known as codons) will, therefore, give the sequence for a string of amino acids. Twenty different amino acids make all the thousands of different human proteins, when assembled in a particular order in the cellular machinery. These proteins (in the form of enzymes, structural proteins, receptors, signalling proteins etc.), in turn, function to create all the other compounds required for life.

The rail track of the bases of the double strand of DNA is twisted like a spiral staircase, giving rise to the figurative description of the double helix. The double helix is packed up tightly, and is uncoiled (partially) when a protein is to be made, and uncoiled fully for reproduction (see below).

To make proteins, the DNA structure is used to create RNA or ribonucleic acid, which (unlike DNA) is single stranded. The RNA is transportable, leaving the nucleus to give instructions to the cell's protein-making systems. In RNA the nucleic acid thymine is replaced by one called uracil. Just as DNA can give rise to RNA, so RNA can be converted back to DNA.

Genes, therefore, contain the code for proteins. Genes also contain a great deal of other code, the function of which is not fully understood. Contrary to long-standing expectation, each gene can make several proteins (via different transcripts), depending on needs and circumstances. Genes also vary in their precise composition, while remaining functional, although function varies too.

Reproduction requires that the DNA in the sperm cell enters the ovum (egg cell). As each cell consist of two chromosomes (including the fertilized egg cell), both the sperm cell and the ovum need to shed one set of chromosomes, leaving 23 rather than 46, prior to such a union. The cells with 23 chromosomes are known as gametes.

In the process of forming gametes, a crucially important process takes place that underlies the concept of Mendelian randomization, that is contributing so much to contemporary genetic epidemiology. Essentially, prior to discarding one set of chromosomes, the pairs of chromosomes exchange blocks (or sequences) of genetic code comprising many genes. The gamete consists of a single chromosome, not a pair, but it is now a mix of the former pair. In this way the single chromosome consists of a mix of grand-maternal and grand-paternal genes. The process of mixing is essentially, but not completely, random (because the exchange between chromosomes is in blocks of genetic code, and not single genes).

Imagine that in the original pair of chromosomes the grand-maternal chromosome coded for a gene variant that leads to high serum cholesterol level, while the grand-paternal version leads to low serum cholesterol. The fertilizing ovum (or, alternatively, sperm) has a 50:50 chance of containing either grand-maternal or grand-paternal variants.

Only the sex cells i.e. sperm and ova, undergo this process—called meiosis—while all other cells divide by the simpler process of mitosis where all the original 46 chromosomes are in the resulting cell. The union of male and female gametes, therefore, creates a fertilized ovum with 23 pairs of chromosomes, one from the sperm (father) and one from the ovum (mother). The children, therefore, inherit more or less equally from the mother and father. If the fertilizing sperm contains the Y rather than the X chromosome the offspring will be male. Since the X chromosome has many, and the Y chromosome few, genes, the male has only one copy of most of the genes on the sex chromosomes.

From this basic, very simplified account readers should be able to understand the ways that the variations in the genome can lead to human variations in disease at the individual and population level.

3.3.2 Genomic variation as the basis of human disease and population variation

As already stated, chromosomal abnormalities, such as missing chromosomes, extra chromosomes or misplaced parts of chromosomes, are extremely serious. Mostly, the fertilized ovum will not progress to a viable pregnancy. Some abnormalities of this kind, nonetheless, lead to relatively small effects, e.g. an extra X chromosome in a woman or an extra Y in a man. Down's syndrome, or trisomy 21, where three chromosomes are seen at the twenty-first chromosome position rather than two, is one of the commonest chromosomal problems. Epidemiological studies on chromosome level variations are not common and, equally, chromosomal variations are not a major contributor to genetic epidemiology. (They are, of course, of great interest to clinical genetics.)

Variation in gene structure is very great and easily demonstrated, in both individuals and between and within populations. This variation may cause subtle or stark differences in protein production and structure and hence biology, which influences either susceptibility to disease or directly causes diseases. Using the central epidemiological strategy of linking variations in causes (here gene structure) to diseases or precursors of diseases, epidemiologists hope to understand disease causation.

The structure of genes varies because of mutations. Mutations are changes in the sequence of nucleic acids in the DNA thus changing the nature of protein production. They are caused by background errors in the process of DNA replication and repair, and mutagens that cause mutations, agents such as radiation, some drugs and chemicals, and viruses. About 175 mutations occur in each person. Mutations are central to carcinogenesis, the process underlying cancers. Mutations in cancer disrupt the normal processes regulating cell division and regulation. The importance to human health of normal gene function cannot be overstated and gene function will be centrally relevant to virtually all disease processes at the individual level. From an epidemiological perspective, however, such variations are of value only when they are systematically and consistently varying in identifiable population groups. This happens when populations are systematically differently exposed to mutagens. So, for example, uranium miners, cigarette smokers, and airline pilots and stewards are more exposed to mutagens than the general population and are more likely to have mutations that cause diseases. In these examples, the epidemiological interest is primarily in the causative exposure of radiation and cigarette smoke. The removal of the causative exposure will remove the population variation in disease. The mutations here are not a fixed and ongoing feature of the population under study although they are permanent for the individual.

For mutations to become a lasting feature of populations they have to be transmitted across generations, and this can only happen if they occur in the sperm cell or the ovum. Mutations in these cells may not be compatible with fertilization or the progression of pregnancy (so-called lethal mutations). If they are compatible with life, they may lead to: (a) no change in function; (b) impaired functioning in relation to the environmental context (perhaps the most likely outcome—and hence the reason why most mutations are not propagated) or; (c) improved functioning. In (a) the mutation will be transmitted to future generations and hence become a normal part of the population. In (b) the recipient's capacity to function, and hence reproduce, will be diminished so the mutation will not thrive and there will be pressures for it to be selected out. In (c) there may be greater reproductive success and the mutation becomes commoner across the generations. Mutations are the basis of biological evolution. The theory of evolution predicts (correctly) that inherited changes that increase survival in particular environments underlie all permanent, inheritable biological variation (anatomy, physiology, biochemistry etc.), within and between species. Unless the theory is overturned, it seems that all life on earth has a common ancestor, seemingly a simple bacterium. Mutations over billions of years have given rise to the variety of life.

The commonest difference among genes is in the location of a single nucleic acid. This is known as a single nucleotide polymorphism or SNP (pronounced 'snip'). The production of SNPs by mutations in cells (most importantly sperm and ova) is to a large extent a random process. Over evolutionary timescales, millions of such mutations have occurred and have been retained in the genome, and are observable now (no doubt many other millions occurred but were lethal or damaging so not retained). Most such mutations are seen in few people. Strictly speaking the term polymorphism (SNPs are the most common form) is for mutations with a frequency of more than 1 per cent in the population—an arbitrary distinction that is often ignored. Some are very common, being present in 15 per cent of the population or even more.

The epidemiological and clinical significance of the SNP is well illustrated by sickle cell disease. Sickle cell disease is a serious disease where the underlying abnormality is that the haemoglobin, the molecule that carries oxygen in the blood, crystallizes and distorts the red blood cell, with anaemia and other complications. The disease is caused by a variety of SNPs and mutations. For the variant known as haemoglobin S, the SNP in the gene leads to the production of a protein with a different amino acid (valine instead of glutamic acid). This was discovered in 1955. Most SNPs on the gene coding for the proteins that make haemoglobin are harmless. People with this particular SNP on both copies of the genes inherited from their parents have sickle cell disease. Those with the SNP on only one of their two chromosomes have cell trait (called allelic variation). The inheritance follows the so-called Mendelian pattern, after Gregor Mendel. This SNP causes a single gene disorder that is recessive, meaning that the gene variant is expressed only if both copies of the gene are affected. Sickle cell trait, therefore, does not usually cause serious problems.

Sickle cell trait and disease varies greatly across populations. How do we explain this disease variation? The SNPs concerned that cause such diseases (hemoglobinopathies) are very common in the Eastern Mediterranean and sub-Saharan Africa (affecting up to 30 per cent of the population) but rare in Northern Europe. Why? There must be some evolutionary, reproductive advantage that balances, indeed even outweighs, the disadvantage. The advantage is that people with blood cells with the SNP are more resistant to the malaria parasite, and therefore less likely to acquire malaria and die from it. This is an example of a so-called balanced polymorphism. The problem is that when the environment changes, or people move to a new environment (say, without malaria), the advantage is no longer balanced by the disadvantages. The same principles apply for all common polymorphisms, but we may not understand their benefits, even while the clinical problems are clear.

Obviously, mutations at a particular part of the genome occur in a few people. It takes time and evolutionary pressures to select in favour of people with them. Polymorphisms that are common are, therefore, ancient. The circumstances that favoured their selection may be long gone and, if not, are likely to be obscure. Disentangling the causes is a high-level epidemiological challenge that requires multidisciplinary work including genetics, evolutionary biology, history and paleontology.

While there are currently more than 10 million known SNPs, giving ample variety for epidemiology, the genome is remarkably similar between humans and human population groups—perhaps 199 out of every 200 of the nucleic acids that comprise the DNA are identical in their location (0.5 per cent difference). This testifies to the precision of the mechanisms copying DNA and to the importance of the protein structure to sustaining life.

The SNP is not the only way genes can vary but it exemplifies the principles most clearly. The DNA code for the protein may vary in length (the gene for the lipoprotein called Lp(a) is a good example) as well as in nucleic acid sequence. This will create a different protein, in the case of Lp(a) a longer one. The code for the protein may be interrupted by non-coding sequences in different ways. The composition of the non-nucleic acid chemicals in the DNA may be different. These differences lead to subtle effects on protein function. The way that non-nucleic acid components change and affect gene function is called epigenetics. It looks like this is crucial to the way the environment triggers changes in gene function. The changes triggered may be short term or last a lifetime, and even be transmitted across generations (but these changes are reversible). These epigenetic factors may determine which of the several proteins that the gene can code for it actually does produce at any one time, and this may change over time. A chemical reaction called DNA methylation is the best example of epigenetic effects. So, a disease can alter the functioning and structure of the genome, and of course vice versa. Therefore, the concept of reverse causality, whereby the disease outcome alters the risk factor, is applicable to genes (see also Chapter 5).

Every cell has (or has had) the entire nuclear DNA. The blueprint for the entire body is within each cell. Cells specialize by shutting down some functions, often permanently. This process is controlled by the non-nucleic components of DNA. When such controls break down, serious health problems can occur.

The genetics of diseases caused by chromosomal abnormality and of single gene disorders following Mendel's laws of inheritance are well understood. The current excitement in epidemiology is whether genetics can help us understand and control the complex, chronic diseases, and this is discussed below.

3.3.3. Susceptibility to diseases, chronic diseases and genetics

Most health problems, including diseases, run in families. A family history does not, however, equate to a genetic basis for disease. As with any other association in epidemiology, one with family history raises questions and suggests hypotheses. A family history may arise from a common genetic heritage, a common experience in the womb (which may have common features across different generations), similarities in lifestyle, and similarities in environment. However, it probably reflects a combination of these and perhaps other factors.

The complex chronic diseases such as heart disease, stroke, breast cancer, colorectal cancer, diabetes, psychosis, dementia, and osteoporosis definitely run in families. They also vary hugely in time, place and by person. It is exciting to believe that the explanations for the causes and variations lie, and will be discovered, in the variation in the human genome. A moment's thought, however, tells us that such a belief is simplistic at best and, at worst, wholly wrong. These diseases change their incidence rapidly. Many of them were non-existent or rare in the past so evolutionary pressures to select for disease genes would have been minimal or non-existent. While we can see (sometimes) the potential benefits of a physiological trait and even the resulting disease such as the sickle cell variant of haemoglobin, what evolutionary advantage would accrue from a heart attack, stroke, a cancer or dementia, or the conditions that precede them? Most of these diseases occur after the reproductive age so selection through reproduction is not possible. So, the idea of disease genes is misleading in the context of the common chronic diseases (unlike for infectious diseases that have been present over evolutionary timescales).

The critical issue is whether some gene variants code for protein variants that alter biochemistry, physiology or immunology and thereby cause susceptibility to the pathological processes that lead to chronic diseases.

Without susceptibility to the pathological processes leading to disease, diseases cannot occur in humans. This is best understood for infectious and like-diseases. The common viral foot and mouth infection that is endemic in many countries and affects animals such as sheep and cattle, does not occur in humans, or is extremely rare. Scrapie, a brain disease, is caused by a prion and it affects sheep but not humans. The closely related disease of cows, bovine spongiform encephalopathy (mad cow disease in popular terms) does affect humans, although rarely and only those with some genotypes. Measles and leprosy are among diseases that are uniquely human. These susceptibilities are genetic. Here the susceptibility can be thought of as the fit of a lock and key. Without the key, the microorganism cannot unlock the door to the human host. If there is no such susceptibility the disease cannot occur. Susceptibility can be acquired if there is a genetic change through mutation in either the infecting agent or the human host. HIV and influenza are among the human diseases arising from viruses that infect animals, initiated by such changes. A mutation permits the virus to change so that it can now invade the human host and maintain the infection in the population through spread from one person to another. Rothman has made the surprising statement that diseases are 100 per cent genetic and 100 per cent environmental. The reasoning is easy to understand for infections. Every host must have genetic susceptibility. Equally, the environment must expose every host to the infective agent. By either changing genetic susceptibility or altering the environment (so there is no exposure to the infective agent) 100 per cent of the disease could be removed.

The issues in relation to chronic diseases follow similar principles but are much more subtle, at least partly because our knowledge base is rudimentary at present.

The causes of the chronic diseases are poorly understood but are multifactorial, i.e. many factors are known to increase the risk of disease. For example, smoking cigarettes, lack of exercise, obesity, diabetes, high blood cholesterol and high blood pressure each double or triple the risk of a heart attack. These factors work primarily (but not solely) through processes that lead to atherosclerosis, which itself starts through damage to the inner lining of arteries (endothelium). If humans did not have the biological capacity to develop atherosclerosis this would not happen. Cigarettes are a new human invention. Why then do humans react to them biologically, and therefore genetically? Presumably, the genome has evolved to react to substances in nature similar to tobacco smoke, e.g. smoke in fires, particles in the air etc. This interaction between the risk factor and biological reaction is mediated by genes, in this case by those in endothelial cells and cells of the immune system that react to the signals sent by the endothelial cells. This reaction is an inflammatory response which is fundamental to the body's control and repair mechanisms.

Diseases, and precursor conditions that lead to diseases, arise through their effects on normal biological processes. Processes such as inflammation, cell division, cell death and cell repair are each governed by many genes. The effects of a single risk factor such as smoking may be mediated by dozens or hundreds of genes. Mutagens in the smoke also damage and alter tissue DNA. There are about 10 major (and a multiplicity of minor) environmental risk factors for atherosclerosis. These almost certainly act through hundreds and perhaps thousands of genes. For this reason, these complex traits are potentially easily alterable by mutations, for it is more likely that one of these many genes will have a mutation than a solitary gene as for a single gene disorder. These genes not only interact with environmental factors but also with each other i.e. gene-to-gene inter-actions. This means that as a result of one gene (A) being activated, so is another (gene B), possibly in a way that differs from the way that gene B would work if gene A was not activated. A gene may work differently in the presence of one, two or more environmental exposures. This account, though complex, is a simplification of the reality and it explains why disentangling the genetic basis of chronic diseases is such a complex task which, despite huge research efforts leading to thousands of papers, has hardly begun to shed light on the questions of cause and effect.

Epidemiologists have focused on gene variants that increase the risk of chronic diseases. This way we find people at high risk (for clinical and public health interventions) and insights into how genes influence the pathological processes leading to diseases.

Some gene variants increase chronic disease risk very substantially e.g. the gene variant known as BRCAI (one of hundreds of such variants). Women with this gene variant are much more likely to develop breast cancer than other women. Other examples include gene variants that increase cholesterol (familial hypercholesterolaemia) and those that increase the risk of colon cancer. Such single gene effects are, however, rare and account for few cases and less than 5 per cent of the total in the examples above. Just as the control of heart disease is best done through consideration of a package of risk factors (9 account for about 80–90 per cent or more of cases), so it may be with genes. It may be possible to define a package of gene variants that, in combination, raise risk substantially even though each one only raises risk by a small amount. Human characteristics such as height, skin colour, eye colour and blood pressure are also controlled by several, not a single, genes.

Small genetic effects may give important insights on biological pathways maintaining health and causing disease. To be important in public health terms, however, risk factors need to have a big effect (e.g. doubling risk) and to be common in the population (see Chapter 8, on attributable and population attributable risk). It is clear from the tens of thousands of genetic studies already reported that the common gene variants (unlike single gene defects that are rare) have small effects, e.g. raising the risk of disease by 10–20 per cent, or less. As Yang and colleagues have calculated, it would take about 20 gene variants which are present in about 25 per cent or more of the population, and which raise the disease risk by 20–50 per cent, to account for 50 per cent of the burden of disease. This is the typical burden accounted for by each one of the major environmental risk factors for chronic diseases. This illustrates the formidable task ahead for genetic epi-demiology. The tools for the task are being developed, sharpened and widely distributed, as considered next.

3.3.4 Tools of genetic epidemiology

As we will see in Chapter 9, the study designs of genetic epidemiology are essentially those used by all epidemiologists and the central strategy is the same. The difference is that the risk factors under study are genomic: 30,000 human genes make more than 100,000 proteins, which in turn make innumerable molecules. As discussed above, for a chronic disease, epidemiologists may need to study hundreds of genes found from this larger pool. That is only the first of many steps. How are they to do this?

The 'double helix' structure of DNA was discovered by Crick and Watson in 1953. In 1987 an international collaboration set the goal of mapping the entire human genome (about 3.3 billion base pairs) and in 2002, to worldwide fanfare, the goal was all but achieved. The project focused on mapping the parts of genes that code for proteins rather than the larger amount of DNA that is non-coding (so-called 'junk' DNA). Mapping exercises also focused on single nucleotide polymorphisms that are then used as genetic markers to identify genes, or groups of genes, and their functions.

The technology that has made the task possible is called the polymerase chain reaction, which permits both copying of DNA and producing it in large quantities so it can be used repeatedly and in several places.

Just as in nature genes can be snipped out and recombined (as in meiosis in germ cells as discussed above), so it is in the laboratory. Techniques are available to snip out single genes, or lengths of DNA, and replace them elsewhere (including in different types of cell from different species). These techniques are powerful in cell line and animal experiments. They also permit the study of associations between genes, their location and their variation in relation to human biological traits (phenotypes) or diseases.

Each person has a unique genotype with the exception of identical twins. Identical twins, especially if reared apart from birth, provide the primary means of disentangling the role of environmental and genetic factors. Such identical twins have an identical genome and a very similar *in utero* experience, but otherwise their environmental exposures differ. This variation between people permits us to use DNA to identify people uniquely, except for identical twins (DNA fingerprints). So, no DNA sample can be truly anonymised, with serious implications for the confidentiality of research (see Chapter 9).

In the next section we consider the potential role of genetics in explaining population level variation in the pattern of disease, using the example of race.

3.3.5 Population level differences in disease and genetics: the example of race

For about 200 years the biological concept of race, i.e. human subspecies distinguished by physical features, has been one of the important issues in a wide range of scientific disciplines (anthropology, biology, sociology, psychology, and epidemiology). The idea underpinned much of politics and social relations and, in turn, these social applications reinforced the science.

While a number of religions, philosophies and societies accepted that humans were one species (Homo sapiens sapiens), this was not obvious or easily demonstrably scientifically. The debate on whether humans were one (monogeny) or more than one (polygeny) species was fierce in the eighteenth and into the nineteenth century, when it concluded in favour of monogeny. The physical differences between humans across the world were painstakingly studied by scientists and used to create several racial classifications.

These classifications persist in the categorizations of humans as, for example, White or Caucasian, Black or Black African, Chinese, Aboriginal etc. Such categories remain a dominant feature in epidemiology, although they are being replaced by ethnic group categories.

The physical differences between such human groups, e.g. skin colour, eye colour, hair colour, type of hair (straight or crinkly) facial shape, body composition, lung size etc., are fundamentally genetic, although environmental factors will influence the end result.

Epidemiology is one of the sciences that have taken a keen interest in differences between population groups beyond physique. Epidemiologists have noted differences in the pattern of disease and in the biological and social risk factors that underpin disease, for example, in the UK people of African Caribbean origin have high rates of prostate cancer and stroke and relatively low rates of coronary heart disease. People of Indian origin have low rates of colorectal cancer and high rates of diabetes. There are hundreds, if not thousands, of such observations on a range of diseases. (Equally, there are numerous such observations on intelligence, education, psychological traits, lifestyles, skills, behaviour, and physiology.)

The question that has intrigued scientists, particularly in the nineteenth century—the heyday of race science—is whether these wider attributes might also be biological, i.e. innate. On this reasoning, the forces that shaped the genetic changes that led to difference in physique would also have shaped the susceptibility to these wider attributes. The particular environmental circumstances of sub-Saharan Africa selected for genetic variations that lead to a dark skin and curly, crinkly hair. We can speculate on the genetic advantages of these traits. We have already seen that in the same place the sickle cell trait in blood cells was advantageous so that we can now use the observation of dark skin/crinkly hair—of sub-Saharan Africa—as a marker (albeit imperfect) of increased likelihood of sickle cell trait and disease. The fair, freckled skin of Scotland can be a marker for increased risk of skin cancers, cystic fibrosis and multiple sclerosis. These kind of associations have potential scientific value (posing questions and providing model populations for study) and public health/clinical value (easing diagnosis, screening and targeting health care).

The mystery behind skin cancer/fair skin and even sickle cell disease/malaria is not deep. However, the causes of multiple sclerosis, diabetes, pancreatic cancer, and motor neuron disease are mysterious. If we can use racial and ethnic variations in disease to point to these causes that would be potentially of great value. The added benefit of studying racial and ethnic variations is that there is greater variation in disease outcome, and genetic and environmental variability, than provided by most other types of comparisons. Similar arguments have been advanced in relation to outcomes other than disease, e.g. educational attainment, criminal tendency, IQ etc.

The theoretical benefits of this line of reasoning have, unfortunately, been greatly outweighed by the harm. By the 1950s a series of UNESCO statements concluded, effectively, that the race concept had little or no utility in science. In Section 10.10.3 there is an introduction to these harms.

From an epidemiological perspective, we can summarize the problems as follows:

1 The research was done within a racist context often for racist purposes, whether this was covert or overt.

2 The variation between racial groups in the human genome is too small to generate variation at the population level in the major chronic diseases, for reasons discussed earlier.

3 The causes of chronic diseases are largely environmental so seeking causes primarily in the genome was doomed to failure (the current emphasis on gene–environment interactions is more promising).

4 Scientists did not have the tools for the task.

The Human Genome Project, and the new concepts and tools that have made it possible, are reinvigorating the study of race in biology and bioscience, including epidemiology. Among the observations already changing our thinking radically is that there is more between group variation in the non-gene parts of chromosomes than in the genes, i.e. there is more racial variation in the genome than anticipated.

Epidemiologists working in this fraught field of endeavour need to be conscious of its history and take particular care. For reasons discussed in my book *Ethnicity, race and health in multicultural societies*, the concept of ethnicity is likely to be more useful in epidemiology than race. Whatever the epidemiological variable, or risk factor, we need a logical approach to interpretation of data.

3.4 **Variations and associations: real or artefact?**

When changes in disease frequency are natural, or real, and not a result of the way diseases are diagnosed or counted, the underlying reasons are often difficult to pinpoint. Real changes are an experiment of nature, posing a challenge to science.

For understanding disease variation, the first step is to exclude artefact as the explanation. The second is to develop a hypothesis stated as an association. The third is to design a test of the hypothesis. The fourth is to assess the results using frameworks for causal thinking. Much of this chapter and Chapter 4 show how artefactual variations and associations are identified and excluded. Assessing the causal basis of such hypotheses is considered in Chapter 5.

Demonstrating variation in disease is a key step towards establishing an epidemiological association. The association is a link (or relationship) between a disease and another factor (called risk factor, see Chapter 7 for discussion), whether this factor is another disease, or a characteristic of the person or population under study. For example, in several countries, coronary heart disease (CHD) mortality rates rose steadily in the twentieth century until the 1960s/1970s when they declined. First, we measure disease rates and demonstrate the association of disease rates and time periods. We attempt to explain the association using our understanding of social, environmental, and lifestyle changes over time. Then, we develop and test specific hypotheses. One might be that the disease pattern reflects the changing levels of factors that cause CHD, for example exercise patterns, consumption of dietary fats and fruits and vegetables, and levels of blood pressure and its control in the community. Studies are then done to assess how much, if any, of the change in CHD can be explained by the changing pattern in these factors. The association fuels a process of analysis and research which either reaffirms causal understanding or raises new questions by rejecting the hypotheses. In this example, the decline in CHD was too rapid to be a result, solely, of change in the factors mentioned. Better medical treatment has contributed and there are other unexplained factors.

The association can be based on theory alone, i.e. a postulate based on first principles with no empirical backing. It may be based on observations of one or a few persons. For example, a doctor may observe a few cases of renal failure in patients taking a particular drug, as happened for phenacetin and other anti-inflammatory drugs used for arthritis. The association implies that a disease and associated factors may be causally connected. The epidemiological challenge is to demonstrate what the factors are, to quantify the association, to assess whether the association is causal, and, if so, to explain how. Ultimately, the challenge is to understand the mechanisms by which the risk factor affects disease. Understanding of mechanisms invariably requires collaboration with other laboratory, clinical, and social sciences.

The first and crucial question in the analysis is this: is an association an artefact or real? If artefact, then there is no more to explain. Before reading on, do the exercise in Box 3.3.

Most often disease variations are artefacts, arising from the following:

- Chance. The numbers of cases are varying randomly.

- Errors of observation. Biased techniques are the most common reason for making erroneous observations, and this is discussed in detail in Chapter 4.

- Changes in the size and structure of the population from which the cases arose. This was discussed in the previous chapter (see section 2.6).

- The likelihood of people seeking health care and hence being diagnosed and eventually counted in statistics. This varies with the public's level of knowledge and expectations, and the accessibility and acceptability of health care.

- The likelihood of the correct diagnosis being reached, which is dependent on availability and use of medical care, the level of skill of the doctor, and the quality of the diagnostic facilities available (Chapters 6 and 7).

- Changes in the clinical approach to diagnosis, which are dependent on changing medical trends, for example whether wheezing is to be called wheezy bronchitis or asthma.

Box 3.3 Why variations and resulting association may be artefactual

Consider the possible reasons why a variation in disease pattern might be an artefact rather than real. (You may find 7–10 reasons.) Can you group them into three or four categories of explanation?

- Changes in data collection methods; for example, when computerization of medical records takes place with structured methods of entering a diagnosis and automatic data extraction, the numbers of recorded cases is likely to rise.
- Changes in the way diseases are diagnostically coded, which is influenced by both the versions of disease codes used and the interpretation of the disease data by the coder (Chapter 7).
- Changes in the way data are analysed and presented; for example, merely altering the 'standard' population used in adjusting disease rates for differences in age and sex (Chapter 8) can spuriously alter disease incidence.

These artefactual explanations, listed in Table 3.1, can be further summarized as: chance; measurement error and bias; diagnostic variation; data processing and presentation. The role of chance is assessed using statistical probability methods (see Chapter 7) and measurement and data processing errors by quality assurance methods (see Chapter 4). Errors in population counts may be difficult to find or correct, so the key is a high level of awareness. Diagnostic activity can usually be assessed indirectly by observing changes in staffing and diagnostic facilities, or directly by counting the number of tests done. Where specialists are employed, the number of tests done for the disease that interests them will rise, and the disease frequency will appear to rise. For example, the north-east of England has an extremely high prevalence and incidence of primary biliary cirrhosis, and the prevalence rose dramatically in the late twentieth century. One potential explanation was that the number of gastroenterologists interested in this disease increased. This was demonstrated to be the case.

Diagnostic activity, measured by the number of tests, can be related to the number of cases diagnosed, to test a hypothesis that a high number of cases reflects excessive diagnostic activity. If so, we would predict a large number of tests for each case diagnosed (high test to case ratio). If, however, there was a high incidence of disease, and no

Table 3.1 Summary of potential artefactual causes of disease variations and associations

Chance
Error
Change in:
Size and structure of underlying population
Healthcare seeking behaviour
Diagnostic accuracy
Diagnostic fashion
Data collection
Coding
Analysis
Presentation

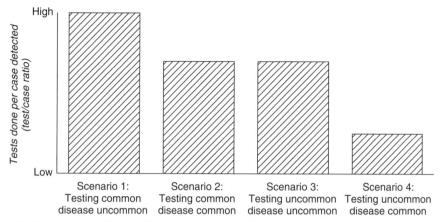

Fig. 3.1 Assessing the effect of diagnostic activity on disease frequency. (Adapted from Bhopal, *J Pub Hlth Med*, 1991, **13**, 281–9, see Permissions.)

excessive testing, then the test to case ratio would be low. Figure 3.1 illustrates this in a study of Legionnaires' disease.

Geographical variations are particularly likely to be artefact, because clinical practice varies greatly between places. One real, yet potentially misleading cause of geographical variation, is short-term fluctuation in disease incidence. Figure 3.2 illustrates the point. Over the three-year period the disease incidence in places A and B was identical. A study done in any one year, however, would have concluded that the incidence of disease varied. Short-term changes in disease incidence create geographical variation, when in the long term there is none.

If there are no artefacts, and this is usually impossible to prove, the variations in disease are real. Before reading on try the exercise in Box 3.4.

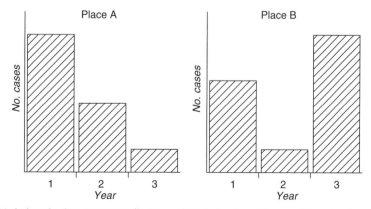

Fig. 3.2 Variations in time masquerading as variations in place. (Source: Bhopal, *J Pub Hlth Med*, 1991, **13**, 281–9, see Permissions.)

Box 3.4 Explanations for real changes in disease frequency

◆ What explanations can you think of for a real change in disease frequency?

◆ Can you group these into three or four categories of explanation?

There are numerous explanations for disease variations; for example, human beings may change their behaviour, their social interaction, or their reproductive patterns. The causes of disease might change; for example, a microorganism might mutate so that it becomes less or more virulent (as happens with influenza) or crosses the species barrier (as has probably happened with HIV infection and new variant Creutzfeldt-Jakob disease).

The composition of the cause of a disease might change; for example, the reduced tar content of modern cigarettes reduces the risk of lung cancer compared with the high tar cigarettes of the past.

The susceptibility of people to disease may change for reasons including genetic, nutritional, social, and medical factors. For example, measles immunization in childhood led to this disease occurring rarely, but increasingly in adolescence and adulthood rather than in children.

Changes in the social, chemical, or physical environment may make the disease easier or harder to contract. For example, a combination of smaller family size, the move from extended to nuclear families, and more space at home and work, have reduced the incidence of tuberculosis, even when the disease remains endemic and common in some subgroups of the population (e.g. the homeless and some migrant populations). Real changes, as summarized in Table 3.2, are caused by changes in the host (person acquiring the disease), the specific agents of disease, or the wider environment (together known as the causal triad of host, agent, and environment).

The real-artefact framework used in a study of Legionnaires' disease is summarized in Fig. 3.3. It can be applied to the systematic analysis of any population variations in disease. Section 3.5 provides the opportunity for you to apply the framework.

3.5 Applying the real/artefact framework

Imagine you are the epidemiologist responsible for surveillance of infectious diseases in a city of about 1 million people. You are examining the statistics on the numbers of cases of

Table 3.2 Summary of real explanations of disease variation and examples: the causal triad

Causal triad	examples
Host	Genetics, behaviour
Agent	Virulence
	Introduction of a new agent
Environment	Housing
	Weather

Legionnaires' disease, which is an environmentally acquired bacterial pneumonia with no person-to-person spread. This pneumonia is rare, with a reported incidence rate of about 3 cases per million population in the USA and England and of about 8 cases per million in your country.

The main sources of the causative microorganisms, the 'Legionellacae' or, for short, the legionellas, are complex water systems, particularly cooling towers and hot water systems, which are usually found in large buildings or as part of industrial machinery. The incidence rate varies geographically (between localities, cities, and nations) and over time (seasons and years).

Your surveillance system is based on voluntary reporting by clinical and laboratory colleagues who send you a copy of the laboratory test request form. Your data are entered onto a computer which provides a list of cases on a week-by-week basis but your statistical analysis is usually on monthly, quarterly, and annual statistics. The number of cases is based on numbers of reports of laboratory tests compatible with a diagnosis of Legionnaires' disease per month. Your database records the date of onset of illness when this is on the laboratory request form. You keep the original request forms in paper files.

Examine the surveillance data in Table 3.3 and use the framework and background information above to systematically analyse the pattern. Answer the questions in Box 3.5 before reading on.

Table 3.3 shows the number of cases of disease in 1984 per month, and shows a month-by-month fluctuation in the number of cases with an abrupt rise in June. At 72 cases per million population the incidence rate in this city is exceedingly high in relation to

Table 3.3 The number of cases of Legionnaires' disease by month in the City of X in 1984

Month	Cases
January	0
February	2
March	3
April	0
May	1
June	26
July	4
August	4
September	6
October	7
November	7
December	12
Total	**72**

Box 3.5 Are the variations in the number of cases of Legionnaires' disease artefactual?

◆ First, describe briefly the nature and content of Table 3.3.

◆ Now, work your way systematically through the factors listed in Table 3.1, and discussed above, for guidance. What information would help you to decide whether the variations are real or apparent?

◆ Now, make a judgement on whether the findings represent an outbreak of Legionnaires' disease.

national rates (8 per million), and cannot be ignored. There is no automatic means of judging whether an outbreak has occurred and whether some action is required. Judgement has to be exercised. In this case, chance (random fluctuation) seems to be a remote possibility. Yet, an outbreak of 26 cases in one month is a major public health problem, with serious social, political and economic repercussions, so that we must not blunder by declaring an outbreak when there isn't one. We first need to exclude explanations based on error.

Was there, for example, a problem in the techniques used to handle laboratory specimens, thereby leading to false positive results? The issue needs to be discussed with the laboratory staff and, if appropriate, the specimens need to be double checked. Once this is excluded, consider other errors. Two common errors are misdiagnosis and miscoding. On computerized databases the disease is usually given a code number. Could information on other similar diseases, say pneumococcal pneumonia or influenza, have been miscoded as Legionnaires' disease? A cross-check of the codes against the original report forms, which will have the full diagnosis, will rule out this possibility. These simple checks will prevent the embarrassment of a lengthy and inappropriate investigation arising from a pseudo-outbreak.

Has there been a batch of reports in June, possibly arising from some doctor accumulating reports over some months or even years and submitting them to you all together? Alternatively, someone doing a research project may be re-testing positive specimens from previous years. For projects large numbers of blood tests may be submitted as a batch. If the people tested are currently sick then this is an unlikely explanation. The date of onset of disease on the lab request form will help to clarify this. If the date of onset varies greatly, say it spans years, then we are not looking at an outbreak. Where the date of disease onset is not given you should ask the physician in charge. Surveillance systems should analyse cases by date of onset but unfortunately this information is often not available, leaving the epidemiologist to use the much less satisfactory date of receipt of the specimen.

Has the number of people at risk altered? A change in the size of the population from which the cases are drawn can change the number of cases, though the rate remains the same. This is important for popular tourist areas where the population can increase many-fold. If the reputation of the doctors, health care system, or laboratory becomes enhanced, patients can be referred from a wider catchment area, effectively increasing the population size. This is an unlikely explanation for the data in Table 3.3, the change having occurred so fast. However, one possibility worth considering for environmentally acquired disease is travel abroad. An increase in international travel can increase the number of cases. Information on the number of travellers is not readily available. The rise in cases in June could reflect a travel-associated outbreak. The cases could be returning from a package tour. Question the cases about their whereabouts. In fact, the data in Table 3.3 are on locally infected cases only.

Has the likelihood of diagnosis increased, either because of greater vigilance by doctors or of people using the health care system? A common problem which causes pseudo-outbreaks is the newly appointed doctor who is unusually thorough in reporting certain diseases, either because of a diligent commitment to the concept of disease surveillance or because of a research interest in these diseases. (It is worth noting that there may be a fee for notification to a health authority of certain diseases.) This diligence causes problems because the surveillance of disease is normally incomplete, due to a mixture of non-diagnosis and non-reporting. Effective surveillance relies more on stability in the levels of reporting, than on the absolute levels of reporting. Local knowledge about the doctors and their reporting habits helps you to assess this possibility. Research projects increase the likelihood of the correct diagnosis being reached both because of greater awareness of the diagnosis among the doctors involved and more resources and techniques being available to make the diagnosis. As research may be of a personal nature, and may not be recorded in research databases, it may be difficult to detect that this is the cause of an apparent outbreak. The investigator will be alerted to this possibility if there is a predominance of reports from one or a small group of doctors.

Have there been changes in diagnostic fashion or disease definition? Diagnosis is not a fixed or rigid entity but relies on medical knowledge, beliefs about how to manage patients, facilities to practice medicine, and case definitions. The cause of, and diagnostic methods for, Legionnaires' disease were discovered in 1977. Following such a discovery, the incidence of the new disease will inevitably appear to rise and that of the other similar diseases (here, other forms of pneumonia and viral infections such as influenza) will appear to fall. Abrupt changes such as here, with a rise and fall, are unlikely to arise merely from changes in diagnostic fashion or disease definitions.

Have there been changes in the completeness of the data collection methods? Change in the process of surveillance will lead to a changed frequency of disease. For example, if following notification of a case of Legionnaires' disease a microbiologist contacts the reporting doctors to request more information and to discuss the case, the extra education and interest is likely to spur those doctors into notifying and diagnosing Legionnaires' disease in future. More obviously, during the investigation of a declared outbreak doctors are alerted by health officials of the need to report disease and to do the necessary tests for it. The greater likelihood of testing, diagnosing, and reporting is likely to last for a while. In the case of the data in Table 3.3, these explanations seem improbable for the 26 cases in June but are likely to be contributing to the cases after that.

Has there been a deliberate change in the way disease data are coded, analysed or presented? Disease coding systems change. At the time, as there was no specific code in the International Classification of Diseases for Legionnaires' disease, the codes were probably created locally. In other cases, a new edition of the code book may change the coding rules or codes. For instance, the principal global source of codes, the International Classification of Disease (ICD), is revised every ten years or so (see World Health Organisation 1992). Major fluctuations in the apparent frequency of some diseases occur in the transition period as new editions are adopted. Guidance is available on how to maximize comparability across different revisions of the ICD.

The decision on whether a change in disease frequency is real or apparent can usually be taken rapidly. The important thing is to consider the questions systematically and to judge the likelihood of each possibility. In this example, once error is excluded, the date of onset of illness in the cases has been checked, and the symptoms and signs found to be of a pneumonic illness, the likelihood is that the rise in case numbers in June is real and there is an outbreak.

The challenge now is to develop a testable explanation, a hypothesis, for the rise in the disease. One crucial question is whether the cases were local or travel-acquired infections and this is easily resolved by questioning patients. The rise was, in fact, in locally acquired cases. This simple observation helps to rule out some artefacts (e.g. a laboratory or coding error would be seen in local and travel cases) and to refine the hypothesis. The same reasoning would be applied to other disorders; for example, is a rise in heart disease confined to coronary heart disease or also affecting, say, rheumatic heart disease? Specific changes are less likely than non-specific ones to arise from artefact.

The rise in locally acquired Legionnaires' disease can be analysed as follows using the host, agent, environment framework (Table 3.2), and the questions in Box 3.6.

Susceptibility to disease is genetic and acquired. Genetic factors, immunization, past exposure to organisms, nutrition, general health status and other relevant risk factors determine the susceptibility of the population. As the susceptibility of the population usually changes over long periods, and in the case of genetic factors over generations, this is not the explanation for the findings in Table 3.3. If the same data were for decades or centuries, not months, such factors might need to be considered.

Box 3.6 Changes in host, agent, and environment as explanations for the outbreak of Legionnaires' disease

Do changing susceptibility of the local population, changing virulence of the causal microorganism, or changes in the environment explain the occurrence of the outbreak? What might the nature of these changes be?

The virulence of microorganisms is very difficult to determine, and baseline data rarely exist. This is an area of microbiology that is rapidly developing with the recent capability of mapping the microbial genome, and hence in future this will change. The virulence of microorganisms is constantly changing. Virulent legionellas may have colonized water systems in May or June 1984, possibly replacing other strains, and led to the abrupt rise in disease incidence. In this instance, and indeed in most circumstances, an interaction would be required between the agent and environment. In practice, change in microbial virulence is unlikely to be demonstrated and such an explanation will be based on exclusion of other possibilities. A mutation in a microorganism that led to increased virulence could rapidly change disease incidence.

A rise in the number of cases could reflect an increase in the level of exposure to the microorganisms, either because the environment has become more hazardous or the contact between the environment and the population has become closer. In our example, the following changes could have occurred:

◆ The weather changed leading to the switching on of water systems in air conditioning units that harboured virulent legionellas.

◆ The winds and humidity changed such that virulent organisms could be delivered to a susceptible population at the infective concentration.

◆ Protective mechanisms (such as the drift elimination mechanisms or chemical decontamination procedures in a cooling tower, or temperature control in a hot water system) broke down.

Explanations of this type must be generated and tested. To re-emphasize, the key to a successful epidemiological investigation is the systematic analysis and explicit statement of the possible explanations.

In reality a rise in cases will be a result of an interaction of factors. Indeed, both real and artefactual factors will be relevant. For example, the rise in Legionnaires' disease shown in Table 3.3 probably arose because of environmental changes which permitted a virulent organism to colonize a complex water system and which permitted the organisms to be dispersed so that many people were exposed, of whom a small proportion (maybe 1 per cent) were susceptible. Once the excess of cases was publicized and case search procedures started, cases were notified which normally would have remained undiagnosed (e.g. patients originally diagnosed as pneumonia or influenza being re-tested for antibody to legionellas, even after they have recovered). This enhanced surveillance will lead to a lasting excess of cases.

In practice, teasing out the different explanations is a complex task. In studies of the geographical epidemiology of Legionnaires' disease in Scotland, 1978–1986, I prepared a case list of all 372 potential cases diagnosed over the period. The explanations for geographical variation are listed in column one of Table 3.4. The solutions generated to provide evidence to choose between the explanations are in the second column. The chart showing the plan of the studies is in Fig. 3.3. The plan clarifies which hypotheses need exploring, the studies that are to be done, and indeed which explanations remain untested. Such an overview is necessary in all investigations of disease variations, both as

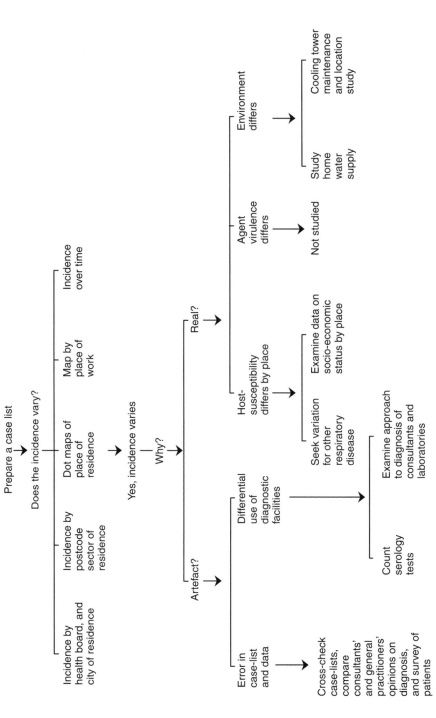

Fig. 3.3 Plan of studies of Legionnaires' disease: framework for geographical variation. (Source: Bhopal, *J Pub Hlth Med*, 1991, **13**, 281–9, see Permissions.)

Table 3.4 Summary of explanations for geographical variation in disease with solutions adopted in a study of Legionnaires' disease in Scotland

Explanations	Solutions adopted
Time variation	
Geographical variation results from varying incidence in time	A reasonably long time period was studied (1978–1986)
Artefact	
Differences in case definition	Standard case-definition applied
Missing cases/incomplete surveillance	Cross-checked case lists; used data from several sources
Errors in address data/postcodes (zip codes)	Addresses checked against medical records; all post codes confirmed using postcode directory; living patients and relatives asked to check basic details
Differential hospital admission rates	Examined hospital admission rates for other diagnoses (effect would be non-specific); compared travel and non-travel-related Legionnaires' disease cases
Differential use of diagnostic tests	Ratios of serology tests to pneumonia and serology tests to Legionnaires' disease used as an indicator; consultants' and laboratories' approach to diagnosis surveyed
True variation	
Host susceptibility differs	Assessed whether geographical variation existed for other diseases which share risk factors; assessed whether populations differed in terms of socio-economic status
Agent virulence differs	Not studied
Environmental factors differ	Developed hypotheses on most likely source; collected new data on location and maintenance of cooling towers and did association studies

Adapted from Bhopal, *J Pub Hlth Med* 1991; **13**, 281–9 (see Permissions).

a guide to the actions needed and as a means of data interpretation. The reasoning illustrated here applies to all conditions and all epidemiological investigations of variation.

3.6 **Disease clustering and clusters in epidemiology**

According to the *Oxford English Dictionary* a cluster is a collection of things of the same kind, a bunch, a number of persons close together, a group or crowd. In epidemiology, according to *Last's Dictionary*, a disease cluster is an aggregation of relatively rare events or diseases in time or place, or both. The terms clusters and clustering are not used for common diseases because clustering is inevitabe due to chance alone, or for infectious diseases that spread from person-to-person for which clustering is the norm. A disease cluster is a mini-epidemic of a rare event.

The disease cluster is a special instance of disease variation. Typical examples might be four cases of leukaemia in one street, or three cases of primary biliary cirrhosis in a single nursing home, or five cases of Legionnaires' disease in a factory. Once observed such a cluster cannot easily be ignored, and presents a difficult epidemiological puzzle. From a scientific perspective, if the factors that led to the cluster can be identified then the cause of the disease might become clearer. The cluster is a potential causal goldmine. From a public health perspective the fear is that unless the cause of the cluster is discovered and preventive action taken there may be further cases. The cluster may herald a large outbreak or even widespread epidemic. Clusters are an especially difficult problem in epidemiology, for the causes are rarely discovered so the difficulties of judging the appropriate public health action remain.

Typically, clusters are identified by a member of the public or a local health professional observing an excess of cases in a locality or over a short time period. For example, Norman Gregg observed that in 1941, cases of congenital cataract, an exceptionally rare problem, far exceeded the normal. He saw 13 cases of his own, and 7 of his colleagues. He hypothesized that this cluster was associated with a preceding outbreak of German measles (rubella). He was correct and rubella syndrome was discovered. It is possible to identify a cluster on the basis of the personal characteristics of cases. For example, if cases were in 6-year-old children we might suspect that the problem arose in a classroom setting. Similarly, if cases were in bus drivers we might suspect the cause to be at the bus depot.

Clusters may also be identified through examining routinely collected surveillance data, and this becomes easier if cases are mapped, or plotted over time. The opportunities to seek clustering of disease are expanding with automated searching on large data sets. Geographical information systems (GIS) make it easy to examine the space and time location of cases. The key data for seeking clusters are spatial coordinates usually obtained from postcodes, time (usually date of onset of disease) and personal characteristics of the case such as age, sex, occupation.

Identification of a cluster of cases is not the solution to a problem, but rather the beginning of one. Leukaemia clusters have been observed for about 100 years, but explaining them has been extremely difficult. Clustering, usually, points to environmental causes. Clustering of childhood leukaemia around nuclear power stations occurs commonly. Intuitively, the explanation would be expected to be exposure to low levels of radiation. The radiation hypothesis for such clustering has not held. The currently favoured hypothesis is that leukaemia is one rare outcome of a common childhood infection. Leukaemia clusters are possibly a consequence of a change in the pattern of such an infection resulting from the migration and population mixing that occurs when a nuclear power plant is built and put into operation.

As clustering is merely a specialized variant of disease variation the analysis of clustering follows the principles in Section 3.4. Clusters may arise from data error, or chance. One potential problem is investigators selecting cases that create a cluster, by focusing on cases that are in a cluster and ignoring others. This can be done by choosing time or geographic boundaries selectively. This is the so called 'bull's eye' or 'Texas Sharpshooter' effect (see Rothman). Clusters are, however, also easily missed in clinical practice and even by routine surveillance systems, because of either incomplete data (e.g. the date of onset of disease is missing), or the insensitivity of data presentation and analysis methods.

The concept of a cluster in epidemiology goes beyond that of merely a group of cases, as shown in Fig. 3.4, using the analogy of grapes. Do the exercise in Box 3.7 before reading on.

Box 3.7 Do the five grapes make a cluster?

Reflect on whether the five grapes in Fig. 3.4 make a cluster. What characteristics make you think that they may be a cluster? What information would lead you to change your mind?

The five grapes may or may not be part of a cluster, but they seem to be. They look the same and are close together spatially. The fact that they look equally fresh suggests that they share a common origin in time. If two of the grapes had been red and three green, one was a plastic replica and one dried and shrivelled, we would not perceive them as a cluster. So, we would probably conclude that the grapes in Fig. 3.4 are part of a cluster. The next step is to prove this. Imagine, instead of grapes, five cases of acute leukaemia are reported from a single street in a small town. The first action is to verify this observation. If all five cases are recent cases of acute leukaemia we would be inclined to judge this as a cluster. If one turns out to be a misdiagnosis (say anaemia), one occurred 15 years ago, one was chronic myeloid leukaemia and only two were acute leukaemia in childhood, we would not perceive them as a cluster. A mixed bag of diagnoses makes an unconvincing cluster, as does a mixed bag of grapes. The epidemiological challenge is to discover how the cluster came together. Do the exercise in Box 3.8 before reading on.

Evidence that the grapes had one stalk would be compelling. For diseases the common factor, that holds or bring the cluster together, provides this compelling evidence. Diseases, in contrast to grapes, have a background rate of occurrence. Five cases of leukaemia close together in time and place could occur by chance. Statistical tests help to assess the role of chance. The close occurrence of leukaemia cases could be an artefact. Just as the grapes may have come from several bunches and have been placed together, so the cases of leukaemia may come from several localities. For example, a children's hospice

Box 3.8 Assessing whether the cluster of grapes and cases of leukaemia is an artefact or whether there is a common cause

Reflecting on both the cluster of grapes and five cases of childhood leukaemia, what evidence would you seek to help you to exclude artefact and to ascertain a common cause? What would provide irrefutable evidence that the grapes are part of one cluster?

Is this a cluster?

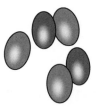

Perhaps. The challenge is
statistical and causal

Fig. 3.4 Clusters I: are these grapes in a cluster?

will bring cases together. An even more mundane explanation would be a coding error in residential postcode so that cases are wrongly being given the same but erroneous postcode. Figure 3.5 shows the grape's common stalk and leaves no doubt that the cluster is real. Similarly, if our investigation of leukaemia cases had shown that these were bound by common factors such as type of leukaemia, age group, residence, time of disease onset, and exposures to causal factors we would think the cluster is real. The next step is to explain mechanisms. This is easy for grapes; we simply study the mechanisms by which grapes grow on vines (Fig. 3.6) as clusters. For diseases, the processes are far more difficult to study. Nonetheless, the guiding concepts are similar. The investigator's job is incomplete unless these steps are achieved—but it is rare to explain why and how the cluster arose. To achieve such understanding needs epidemiology to work with sciences that study mechanisms. We now return to Legionnaires' disease.

Legionnaires' disease cases may occur in outbreaks, or in sporadic form. The cause of outbreaks has often been tracked to cooling towers or complex hot water systems, as the sources of infective aerosol. What of sporadic cases? By definition, these are solitary cases, unconnected in space and time to others. The source of infection for such cases is harder to study but epidemiology has a role to play. I studied non-outbreak, non-travel Legionnaires' disease in and around the city of Glasgow 1978–1986. The results are in Table 3.5. Before reading on do the exercise in Box 3.9.

As these were apparently sporadic cases no clustering was expected, but there was some. Nine cases occurred in July–September 1979, six in November 1983, and 36 between October 1984 and February 1985. The next step is to see whether there is

Box 3.9 Defining and assessing clusters of Legionnaires' disease

◆ On first principles, what would you expect the distribution of cases to be like in time? What possible clusters do you see in Table 3.5?

◆ What additional information would you like to assess these?

Is this a cluster?

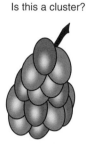

Yes, but, significance unclear
i.e. how or why the grapes
are together

The challenge is biological and causal

Fig. 3.5 Clusters II: what is the significance of this cluster? How did it come about?

clustering in space too. Table 3.6 shows these cases by postcode, the number of hospitals and the number of hospital consultant physicians in charge of each cluster, and Fig. 3.7 shows similar data on a map.

These data indicate that some supposedly sporadic cases were actually part of space–time clusters. Questions which arise include these: why were these clusters missed, and what is their cause? The findings showed that clusters can be easily missed in clinical

Is this a cluster?

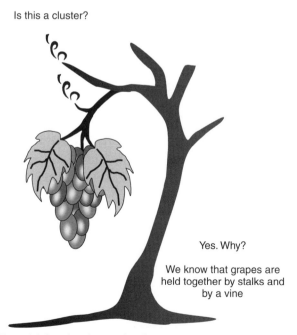

Yes. Why?

We know that grapes are
held together by stalks and
by a vine

Fig. 3.6 Clusters III: explaining the cluster: the vine.

Table 3.5 Number of non-travel, non-outbreak cases of Legionnaires' disease in Greater Glasgow Health Board by year and month

Year	Jan	Feb	Mar	Apr	May	Jun	Jul	Aug	Sep	Oct	Nov	Dec	Total
1978				1	1		1			1	3		7
1979					3		2	4	3		3		15*
1980	1			1		1			1	1			5
1981	1					1			1	1	1		5
1982							1	1	1				3
1983	2	2					1	1	3		6	1	16
1984		1	2			2	1	3	2	7	6	12	36
1985	4	7	1	2	1	1	1		1	3	4	4	29
1986										1	1		2
Total	8	10	3	4	5	5	7	9	12	14	24	17	118

* For one case neither the month of onset nor the date of serological testing was known.

Source: Bhopal *et al. British Medical Journal* (1992), **304**, pp. 1022–27, with permission from the BMJ Publishing Group.

Table 3.6 Clusters of apparently sporadic cases of Legionnaires' disease by area of residence, date of onset of disease and numbers of hospitals and consultants (hospital specialists) involved

Health Board and postcode sector of apparent cluster*	No. of cases	Date of onset	No. of hospitals	No. of individual consultants in charge of each group
Greater Glasgow				
G5.0	3	Oct, Nov 1978	2	3
G21.1, G21.3	2	Nov 1983	2	2
G11.5, G12.8	2	Nov 1983	2	2
G4.0	2	Aug, Nov 1983	1	1
G33.5	2	Sep, Dec 1983	1	2
G4.0	5	Mar, Jun, Aug, (2 cases), Oct 1984	2	5
G31.4, G31.3, G31.1	6	Oct, Nov 1984; Jan, Feb, Apr, Nov 1985	2	4
G33.3	3	Jul, Oct, Nov 1984	2	3
G13.4, G13.3	2	Sep, Dec 1984	2	2
G72.8	3	Nov, Dec 1984	2	3
G5.8, G5.9	2	Feb 1985	2	2
G21.2, G22.6, G21.4	5	Jan, Feb, Oct 1985	3	6

* Postcodes in a row are contiguous areas.

Adapted from Bhopal *et al. British Medical Journal* (1992), **304**, pp. 1022–27, with permission from the BMJ Publishing Group.

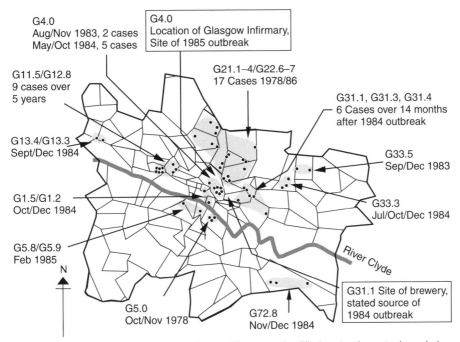

G4.0
Aug/Nov 1983, 2 cases
May/Oct 1984, 5 cases

G4.0
Location of Glasgow Infirmary,
Site of 1985 outbreak

G11.5/G12.8
9 cases over
5 years

G21.1–4/G22.6–7
17 Cases 1978/86

G31.1, G31.3, G31.4
6 Cases over 14 months
after 1984 outbreak

G13.4/G13.3
Sept/Dec 1984

G33.5
Sep/Dec 1983

G1.5/G1.2
Oct/Dec 1984

G33.3
Jul/Oct/Dec 1984

G5.8/G5.9
Feb 1985

N

River Clyde

G31.1 Site of brewery,
stated source of
1984 outbreak

G5.0
Oct/Nov 1978

G72.8
Nov/Dec 1984

Internal lines are simplified postcode sector boundaries

Fig. 3.7 Community-acquired, non-travel, and apparently sporadic cases of Legionnaires' disease in Glasgow suspected to constitute a space–time cluster. (Source: Bhopal *et al. British Medical Journal*, 1992, **304**, pp. 1022–27, with permission from the BMJ Publishing Group.)

practice, possibly because of the dispersion of small numbers of patients to several hospitals and physicians and because of incomplete data. For example, the six cases in postcode sectors G31.4, G31.3 and G31.1 in October 1984–November 1995 were spread over time, admitted to two hospitals and cared for by four hospital consultants. The routine surveillance system's data on postcode and date of onset were, in fact, incomplete. In these circumstances, identification of clustering is problematic. Effective surveillance requires proactively seeking, completing and analysing data to find patterns of disease. The final step of ascertaining cause requires us to develop and test hypotheses as to why some apparently sporadic Legionnaires' disease clusters. Aside from artefacts the principal three hypotheses generated were these:

1 People living in different parts of Glasgow are differentially susceptible to Legionnaires' disease. This seemed highly unlikely.

2 The clusters reflect the intermittent virulence of Legionella. This hypothesis seems unlikely and is extremely difficult to test.

3 That sporadic cases are either part of larger outbreaks, or are mini-outbreaks, arising from the same general sources of aerosol as for most outbreaks. This was tested by seeking an association between the location of Glasgow cooling towers and residence

of cases, as shown in Fig. 3.8. Table 3.7 summarizes these data and shows that living near a cooling tower was associated with a greater relative risk of sporadic Legionnaires' disease. This pattern was not present for travel-associated disease or lung cancer (data not shown; available in referenced paper). This work, therefore, provided a general explanation for the phenomenon of clustering, but it did not provide a specific explanation for each of the many clusters, that is, which cooling tower was involved for each cluster. That is often the best that can be accomplished epidemiologically.

3.7 Applications of observations of disease variation

Variations in disease patterns are of practical value in helping the clinician in both diagnosis and management of disease. For example, the diagnosis of myocardial infarction (heart attack) is much more likely to be correct in a man of 70 years complaining of chest pain than in a woman of 30. This is based on age and sex variations in heart attack. Clinicians can also make use of seasonal variations and of variations by ethnicity, geographical origins, occupation, and pattern of travel. So, for example, diabetic Muslim patients are most likely to have problems with control of their disease when fasting during daylight hours in the month of Ramadan than at other times of the year. Most infections have a distinct seasonal pattern; for example, influenza is more common in winter and gastroenteritis in summer. Outbreaks and clusters alert clinicians to consider a diagnosis even of rare diseases. Long-term trends are important to clinical practice; for

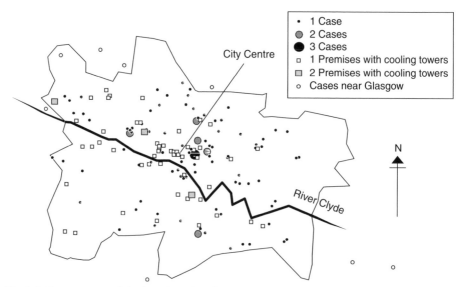

Fig. 3.8 Clusters: map of the location of cooling towers in the city of Glasgow and in relation to the residence of non-travel, community-acquired, non-outbreak cases of Legionnaires' disease. (Source: Bhopal *et al. British Medical Journal*, 1991, **320**, pp. 378–83, with permission from the BMJ Publishing Group.)

Table 3.7 Relation between distance of patients' homes from cooling tower and risk of Legionnaires' disease

Study group	Distance of home from nearest cooling tower (km)*	No. of cases observed (No. expected)	Relative risk of disease compared with group living >1.0 km from nearest cooling tower
Legionnaires' disease: no history of travel abroad (n = 107)	≤0.25	12 (4.4)	3.89
	>0.25 to ≤0.5	28 (13.2)	3.00
	>0.5 to ≤0.75	15 (17.9)	1.19
	>0.75 to ≤1.0	14 (17.9)	1.11
	>1.0	38 (53.7)	1.00

* The denominator population living within each distance category varied from year to year owing to the varying numbers of cooling towers in each year. The average denominator populations were as follows: 404 431 people lived more than 1 km from a cooling tower, 116 339 lived between 0.75 and 1 km away, 114 886 lived between 0.5 and 0.75 km away, 84 466 lived between 0.25 and 0.5 km away, and 27 884 lived less than 0.25 km away.

Adapted from Bhopal *et al. British Medical Journal* (1991), **320**, pp. 378–83, with permission from the BMJ Publishing Group.

example, the changing nature and decline of tuberculosis over the last few hundred years has led to a change in the differential diagnosis (the preliminary list of possible diagnoses) of symptoms such as coughs and fever. It is likely that within 10–20 years, assuming that the recent rise and decline in coronary heart disease continues, the differential diagnosis of chest pain will also alter. Certainly, doctors in India and other industrializing countries, where CHD is on the rise, will be much more alert to this diagnosis than hitherto. By contrast, doctors in the UK or USA may be looking for other commoner causes of chest pain.

For health policy decisions, disease variations over decades (known as secular trends) are of special importance in setting priorities and for evaluating whether health objectives have been achieved. Variation in disease by place and by socio-economic status is a guide to the level of inequity in health status. The health care planner uses disease variations to match resources to need. One simple example is the prediction that in winter, emergency admissions to hospital will rise, especially in an epidemic of influenza, and hence there will be fewer beds available for elective, non-emergency admissions.

The health promoter can tailor both the timing and the content of interventions. For example, an educational campaign on the perils of drinking and driving could be timed using information on alcohol consumption patterns by day of week, week of year, and information on the peak incidence of road traffic accidents. Spatial variations in health behaviour and disease patterns can help in assigning staff and resources to particular places; for example, community health staff may spend more time in geographical areas with low breastfeeding rates.

Analysis of disease variation is, therefore, the prime source of hypotheses on causation and also at the heart of applied epidemiology.

3.8 **Epidemiological theory underpinning or arising from this chapter**

Disease variation arises because of (a) changes in either the host, the agent of disease, or the environment; or (b) changes in interaction between the host, agent, and environment. As these changes occur at a different pace in different places and subpopulations, disease variations are inevitable. In studying these variations in epidemiology we are seeking to uncover the natural forces that caused them. (The first step, however, is to ensure that variations are not merely artefacts.)

3.9 **Conclusion**

The interpretation of change in disease frequency is difficult. Erroneous conclusions arise easily. Therefore, to avoid the twin and opposite pitfalls of (a) false alerts or (b) missed clusters, outbreaks, epidemics, and health inequalities, a systematic approach to the collection and interpretation of data is necessary. The approach outlined here provides a structure for the investigator's thoughts. It places heavy emphasis on artefactual causes of changes in disease incidence. These artefacts and related biases are discussed in more detail in the next chapter.

Summary

Diseases wax and wane in their population frequency. The underlying reasons are often difficult to detect and may remain a mystery. There are three principal reasons for investigating variations in disease frequency. First, to help bring under control an apparent abrupt rise in disease incidence (a suspected outbreak or cluster, the commonest public health emergency). Secondly, by understanding the factors which changed the disease frequency, to gain insight into the causes of disease. Thirdly, to use the knowledge of the disease trend and its causes to make predictions and plans, both in terms of health policy and health care, and the frequency of disease. Disease variations are often, however, artefactual, and arise from data errors. A systematic approach to the analysis of variation in disease begins by differentiating artefactual change from real change. Real change results from changes in host susceptibility, in the agent's capacity to cause disease, and in the influence of the environment. The epidemiological challenge here is to pinpoint the causal factors. The principles behind the investigation of clusters, outbreaks, epidemics, and inequalities in both of communicable and non-communicable diseases, are similar.

Sample examination questions

Give yourself 10 minutes for every 25% of marks.

Question 1 Define what is meant by a disease cluster and describe the factors that you would take into account when determining whether an alleged cluster (e.g. of childhood cancer in pupils of a primary school) is likely to be real. (25%)

Answer A disease cluster can be defined as a higher than expected number of cases of a relatively rare health event or disease aggregated by time or place or both, e.g. an unusually high number of cases of lymphoma occurring in residents of a small village over a period of five years.

The following factors should be taken into account when determining whether an alleged disease cluster is likely to be real:

- Are the cases all of a reasonably similar clinical problem?
- Are the cases all real i.e. correctly diagnosed, meet a sensible case definition, and correctly coded and recorded?
- Do formal statistical tests confirm that the incidence of disease in the locality/time period of interest is likely to be genuinely higher than background expected levels, i.e. that such a finding is unlikely.
- Is the aetiology of the condition understood and is there a plausible explanation of how a cluster could have arisen, e.g. known or possible exposure of the local population to accepted risk factors.

Question 2 Why do virtually all diseases vary in incidence over time, between places and between populations? (25%)

Answer The causes of disease are constantly changing e.g. time: genetic changes, weather, quality of housing etc.; place: quality of water, food, man-made environment etc.; population: health-related lifestyles and behaviours, e.g. smoking and alcohol drinking.

Chapter 4

Error, bias, confounding and risk modification/interaction in epidemiology

Objectives

On completion of the chapter you should understand:

♦ that error in measurement is crucially important in applied sciences such as epidemiology, studying free-living, human populations;

♦ that bias, considered as an error which affects comparison groups unequally, is particularly important in epidemiology;

♦ the major causes of error and bias in epidemiology can be analysed based on the chronology of a research project;

♦ that biases in posing the research question, stating hypotheses, and choosing the study population are relatively neglected but important topics in epidemiology;

♦ that errors and bias in data interpretation and publication are particularly important in epidemiology because of its health policy and health-care applications

♦ that confounding is the mis-measurement of the relationship between a risk factor and disease which potentially arises in comparisons of groups which differ;

♦ that different epidemiological study designs share many of the problems of error and bias.

4.1 Introduction

> Man approaches the unattainable truth through a succession of errors.
>
> Aldous Huxley
> 1894–1963

An error is by definition an act, assertion, or belief that is not right. In mathematics an error is the difference between a computed or measured value and a true or theoretically correct value. For example, a metre is a length fixed by agreement, but in different ways at different times: as a fraction of the length of the quadrant of the Earth's meridian through Paris, as the distance between two marks on a metal bar, and now as the path travelled by light in a vacuum in a particular time. In other words the true length of a metre is arbitrarily decided by agreeing a definition. The difference between a 'correct' metre stick and an erroneous one can, therefore, be accurately measured.

In the arena of health and disease the truth is unknown and cannot be defined or computed unequivocally. There is no 'right' body shape, height or weight. There is no 'truthful' measure of asthma, heart disease or irritable bowel syndrome. In health and disease research, including epidemiology, errors are not avoidable. If not recognized, errors generate false knowledge, which only time and deeper study will show to be wrong. Error is an inevitable and important part of human endeavour, as captured in the Huxley quotation above. These ideas have particular importance in epidemiology for reasons discussed below. Before reading on reflect on the exercise in Box 4.1.

A bias is a more subtle matter than error and is a preference or an inclination, or deviation from the truth, especially one that inhibits impartial judgement (or leads to unfairness). In science, including epidemiology, error and bias are frequently used as synonyms. Bias is the usual term applied to a range of errors in science (usually excepting random statistical error). This word frees science from producing erroneous results, only biased ones! In this book bias in epidemiology is conceptualized to be error which applies unequally to comparison groups.

Error is common in science, contrary to popular view. Whether science is estimating the age of the Earth, calculating the speed of light, achieving cold fusion in the laboratory, or assessing when humans first started using weapons, errors and corrections are the norm. Epidemiology is no exception. Indeed, the provocative Popperian view is that science progresses by the rejection of hypotheses (by falsification) rather than the establishment of so-called truths (by verification) (Popper 1989). Epidemiologists must not lose heart over errors, at least those that are not deliberate or a result of shoddy work.

Biological research is difficult because of the complexity and heterogeneity of life, and because of natural variations; for example those arising from circadian rhythms. In addition, measurement techniques in epidemiology are usually limited by technology, cost, or ethical considerations. In human studies, especially those using large community-based populations, these difficulties are compounded by the rules on what measurement is ethical and what humans are willing to consent to. To take an example, the best way to make a diagnosis of Alzheimer's dementia is brain biopsy, and this may be done after death. This 'gold standard' test would not be possible in an epidemiological study to measure the prevalence of dementia in the population. We accept the error in other methods of diagnosing Alzheimer's disease, mainly based on clinical assessment and brain imaging, and forego the brain biopsy test.

Experimental manipulation to test a hypothesis is usually done late, and observation, without deliberate intervention by the investigator, is the dominant mode of investigation in epidemiology. Moreover, epidemiology is interested in health and disease in

Box 4.1 Error and bias

Reflect on the word bias. What is the difference, if any, between error and bias? Why might error and bias be particularly important in epidemiology?

human populations living normally in their natural environment, not in laboratory or institutional settings (or even clinical trials settings).

Most discussions of error and bias in epidemiology are simplified under the headings of (a) selection (of population), (b) information (collection, analysis, and interpretation of data), and (c) confounding, although this phenomenon is is sometimes considered as separate from bias. The important question of whether error and bias are inherent in the process of choosing and developing research questions and hypotheses is too seldom raised. For example, are the questions of sex or racial differences in intelligence, disease, physiology, or health biased questions? A long history of misleading and damaging research would have been avoided if questions about racial and sex differences had either not been posed at all, or not posed in the way they were. The Tuskegee Syphilis Study of the US Public Health Service (see Jones 1993), for example, followed up 600 African American men for some 40 years, to assess the natural history of disease. The underlying question was: does syphilis have different and, particularly, less serious outcomes in African Americans than Americans of European origin? The investigators deliberately denied the study subjects treatment even when it became available and was curative (penicillin). The study was based on a premise which has guided so much research on race and health: that races are biologically different in regard to a broad range of matters. This premise has repeatedly been shown to be in error. In retrospect the study question and design was unethical. The process of defining, selecting and funding research questions, which lies in the domain of the ethics of science, deserves much more attention in consideration of errors and bias in epidemiology.

Much of epidemiology is concerned with population subgroups and comparison between them. Even when an epidemiological study is of a single group, its interpretation usually rests on an understanding of, and inference about, how the group compares with the population from which it was selected. The scientific value of the work, in the sense of generating understanding about disease patterns in populations, arises from its generalizability. Furthermore, to make sense of studies where the data have only been collected from a fraction of the population of interest, sometimes due to non-response by study subjects, the interpretation rests on the assumption that the results apply, by and large, to the whole group as originally chosen. Only in recent decades have medical sciences, including epidemiology, moved away from mainly studying White, adult men, and assuming that the understanding so generated can be applied to women, other ethnic groups and other age groups. This assumption has now been shown to be over-optimistic. The choice of study population is, therefore, a crucial matter in avoiding error and bias.

One conception of bias in epidemiology, and which is close to the everyday usage of the term to mean discrimination against individuals and groups because of prejudice, is error which either:

◆ affects population or study subgroups unequally (the way it is usually used in this book); or

◆ results from the inappropriate generalization of study data to another population which differs from the population actually studied.

In this usage, bias is often an error which affects one group more than another. Bias leads to so-called differential errors, i.e. errors that differ between groups. This kind of error is usually far more serious than so-called non-differential error, which is error that is similar between groups. Figure 4.1 uses the scales of justice to symbolize and illustrate the concept of bias as unequal error in compared populations, which may lead to both wrong and unfair conclusions.

Bias is more important than random errors, which affect all comparison groups equally, so are non-differential. However, even errors which affect groups equally (non-differential errors) can mislead. Misclassification errors are discussed later to illustrate this point (section 4.2.7). Error control requires good scientific technique. Bias control needs equal attention to error control in all the population subgroups, but as error and bias cannot be fully controlled the most important need is for systematic, cautious, and critical interpretation of data (Chapter 10, Sections 10.10–10.13).

4.2 A classification of error and bias

Epidemiologists have been creative in identifying and naming biases with the creation of lengthy lists of unconnected biases. It is not appropriate for the reader to learn all possible biases: it is better to develop an understanding of their nature and effects. Errors and biases can be analysed logically by using the concepts in section 4.1

- Error is normal in science
- Researchers have their human foibles
- In epidemiology bias is unequal error in comparison populations
- Bias creates false patterns and misjudgements—either differences where none exist (a) or failure to detect differences (b)

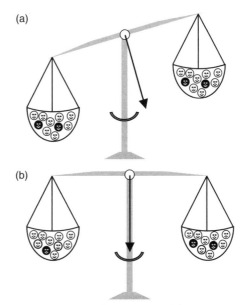

Fig. 4.1 Bias: a picture illustrating unequal errors in compared populations. (a) Error is unequal in one of these identical groups, leading to falsely detecting differences; (b) error is unequal in one of these groups leading to a failure to detect differences. (Each circle is a person—shaded circles represent cases of a disease.)

and a framework. It is a good idea for each reader to think through this matter, by trying the exercise in Box 4.2, using the chronology of a research project.

The common grouping of selection bias, information bias, and confounding is incomplete. In Table 4.1, this grouping is shown in the broader context as discussed below. There are many other biases, e.g. lead time and length bias (these two are discussed in Chapter 6 in relation to screening).

4.2.1 Bias in the research question, theme or hypothesis

Science is done by humans who often have strong views, generated both through and independently of their research. Science is as much about generating imaginative ideas and collecting data to test them as about looking to data to inspire ideas. Scientists become attached to ideas which they hope to support (and reluctantly reject) through their research. As human beings they share in the social values and beliefs of their era, including those which may, in retrospect, be considered unworthy such as class, racial, religious, and sexual prejudice.

It is worth reflecting on whether a scientific question or even a research theme can be inherently biased. In epidemiology, a biased question would adversely affect one group more than another. The question 'Are men more intelligent (or healthy) than women?' could be considered a biased question, for there is a presupposition in the way the question is written which points out that there is a case to be answered. Otherwise the question could have been whether women are more intelligent than men. The apparently neutral hypothesis here would be that there are no gender differences in intelligence. If the underlying values of the researchers are that men are more intelligent than women

---

Box 4.2 Towards a classification of errors and biases

Think through the main steps of a research project and consider how error and bias might arise at each step. Develop a set of three or four broad categories for all the errors and biases you list.

In doing this task you can consider in what ways two groups of the population might be affected unequally in terms of:

- choice and phrasing of the study question;
- choice of the study populations;
- non-participation of some individuals in a study;
- measurement of disease and factors which could cause disease;
- loss to follow-up of participants;
- measurement of outcome;
- analysis, interpretation, presentation, and publication of data.

Table 4.1 A classification of error and bias (including confounding*) based on the chronology of a research project

Potential cause of bias	Example	Specific terminology	Broad general category of bias
1 Research theme, question or hypothesis is biased	Where alternative approaches are feasible, posing a question or hypothesis in a way which shows one population in a poor light, and creating a sense of superiority and inferiority	None	The terms assumption or conceptual bias are close matches. My preferred term is research question bias
2 Choice of populations is biased	Sampling based on convenience, or cultural preferences of researcher	Population bias (volunteer bias, sex, race, or age bias)	Selection bias
3 Participation in a study	Hospital populations studied where two or more associated problems increase the chance of hospitalization	Berkson's bias	Selection bias
	Unequal time and effort spent in the invitation leading to unequal participation, unequal interest or motivation	Response bias	
4 Comparing populations which differ	Study population is older or poorer than the comparison population, leading to a false interpretation of the reason for differences in disease rates	Confounding	Confounding*
5 Mismeasurement of disease, and factors which could cause disease	Diagnostic effort, skill, and facilities unequal	Measurement error	Information
	Measurement imprecise or unequal	Measurement error	Information
	In reporting, there is unequal memory of the problem in minds of doctors	Recall bias	Information
	Effort, skill, and facilities to collect data unequal in comparison groups	Work-up bias	Information
	Interviewer extracts information differently in different groups	Interviewer bias	Information

Table 4.1 (continued) A classification of error and bias (including confounding*) based on the chronology of a research project

Potential cause of bias	Example	Specific terminology	Broad general category of bias
	Risk factors unequally memorable for respondent	Recall bias	Information
	Deception by study subject, investigator, or diagnostician	No specific name but it is scientific misconduct if the investigator or professional is involved	Misconduct or fraud
Measurement at follow-up and outcome	Unequal effort made to maintain contact by investigator or subject	No specific name	Selection
	Unequal proportion of subjects drop out	No specific name	Selection
	Intervention in health care not equal	No specific name	Intervention bias
	Participation in study alters behaviour unequally in different groups	No specific name	Participation bias may be appropriate
Analysis and interpretation of data	Preferred outcome in mind of investigator	No specific name	Interpretation or presentation
Selected findings reported	Reporting interesting findings, usually findings of difference between groups (i.e. positive results). Reporting publishable findings	Various	Publication
Interpretation, judgement and action by readers and listeners	Reader and listener interpret data in a way that suits them	No specific name	Interpretation

* In some accounts confounding is viewed as a phenomenon separate from bias.

(a view that has been widely held through much of history and is now deeply undermined, although it persists in much of the world) then the bias will remain. These values may affect the data analysis and interpretation. Researchers' beliefs and hopes do influence the conduct of research.

To quote Ruth Hubbard:

> The mythology of science asserts that with many different scientists all asking their own questions and evaluating the answers independently, whatever personal bias creeps into their individual

answers is cancelled out when the large picture is put together. This might conceivably be so if scientists were women and men from all sorts of different cultural and social backgrounds who came to science with very different ideologies and interests. But since, in fact, they have been predominantly university-trained white males from privileged social backgrounds, the bias has been narrow and the product often reveals more about the investigator than about the subject being researched.

Ruth Hubbard, Mary Sue Henifin and Barbara Fried (eds) (1979) *Women look at biology looking at women*

This issue demands more attention in the ethics of epidemiology. It is problematic to describe difference without conveying a sense of superiority and inferiority. Stigmatization may be an inevitable outcome of epidemiology, for example, in demonstration of the association between HIV and homosexuality, and cigarette smoking and disease. This potential harm has to be balanced against the potential benefits. This problem is discussed further in Chapter 10 in the context of race, ethnicity and health.

4.2.2 Choice of population—selection bias

Bias can result from the choice of populations to be studied. This is known as selection bias. Investigators are prone to include or exclude individuals and populations for reasons of convenience, cost, or preference rather than for neutral, scientific reasons. Investigators will often pick populations of convenience rather than representative ones. Volunteers are popular. The problem is that volunteers tend to be different in their attitudes, behaviours, and health status compared with those who do not volunteer. Men have been selected more often than women, for example, in studies of coronary heart disease. Sometimes investigators want to avoid the ethical problems posed by the possibility of pregnancy during the study, but sometimes the problem under study is seen as less relevant to women. Ethnic minority groups are much more likely to be excluded from major studies than the ethnic majority. These observations have led to the main USA research funding agency National Institutes for Health (NIH) requiring investigators to include women and ethnic minority groups or provide a reasoned justification.

Selection bias is affected by the source of a study population. For example, the telephone directory and the register of licensed drivers are both popular sources in the USA. Those without a telephone or without a driver's licence are excluded from the study. In the UK, the registers of electors and those registered with a general practitioner in the National Health Service are popular, but these exclude those not eligible to vote (or unwilling to divulge their details) or those not registered with the NHS, respectively. Figure 4.2 illustrates these points. In addition to the ignored population (e.g. those who do not speak English or are not on the list from which the sample is drawn), there are others who are missed, for example because they do not participate.

Populations in workplaces and institutions (schools, prisons, universities, hospitals) are popular choices for study. Some such populations may be fairly representative of their age group (e.g. schoolchildren), others not at all (e.g. university students). The attention given to these populations means that research effort is deflected away

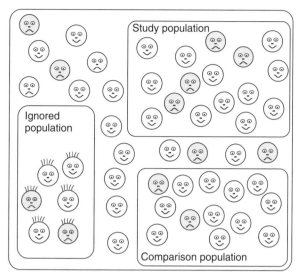

- Ignoring populations
- Questions harming one population
- Measuring unequally
- Generalizing from unrepresentative populations

Fig. 4.2 Bias in epidemiology: population concept.

from other less accessible populations. Extrapolation of results beyond those studied is the norm rather than the exception. Indeed investigators may even explicitly compare populations derived in different ways. One example is the ground-breaking survey of health and health behaviours by the Health Education Authority (1994), which studied ethnic minority groups in the UK. Typical results are given in Table 4.2. The ethnic minority groups were shown to be different compared with the UK population in several indicators. The emphasis in interpretation fell on those issues where the ethnic minority groups were worse off, thus leading to perceptions that the health of ethnic minorities was impaired, a view propagated in professional journals and newspapers. The comparisons were, however, not easy to interpret because the ethnic minority groups were drawn from small areas (enumeration districts) where at least 10 per cent of the population was born in six overseas areas of the world (e.g. India, the West Indies). Such places would

Table 4.2 Selected data, standardized for age and sex, on health and related factors from the HEA's report on black and Asian minority groups (figures are percentages)

Topic	African Caribbean	Indian	Pakistani	Bangladeshi	UK population
Describe health status as poor	17	16	20	29	8
Suffered high blood pressure	16	8	8	10	14
Current smokers	22	10	16	22	28

From Health Education Authority 1994; *Health and Lifestyles* (see Permissions).

almost invariably be in the inner city places, where the poorest people live, while the comparison 'UK' population included all areas, not just inner city ones. Irrespective of this bias, the study was at the time of value and interest, but the interpretation was potentially biased.

Berkson's bias is an example of how subtle bias can be. It specifically refers to a bias in the interpretation of hospital-based case–control studies (see Chapter 9). It arises because hospitalized cases of a disease are not usually a representative sample of cases. In fact they tend to be the more complex ones, often with other health problems. For example, a man with influenza is more likely to be admitted to hospital if he has chronic bronchitis. In comparing people admitted with and without influenza, an association between influenza and chronic bronchitis is inevitable because of this selection effect.

Selection bias matters much more in epidemiology than in biologically based medical sciences. Biological factors are usually generalizable between individuals and populations. For example, if an anatomist describes the presence of a particular muscle, or cell type, based on one human being it is likely to be present in all human beings (and possibly all mammals), for the number of models of life are few. The anatomist is likely to check that the finding applies to a few other individuals and if so will rapidly conclude that it applies universally. By contrast, epidemiological findings usually concern the interaction of social and biological factors. Because societies are made up of highly variable individuals and population groups, the outcome of the biology–environment interaction is variable and context-dependent. The result is crucially dependent on the choice of study population and the interpretation depends on proper understanding of its circumstances. For example, in nearly every population the blood pressure rises with age. It would be easy to conclude that this is a generalizable finding, possibly based on the biology of the ageing process. However, this assumption and generalization needs serious qualification, because in nomadic populations living in traditional ways in rural areas of countries such as Kenya there is little or no association between age and blood pressure. Given this caveat, it is reassuring that causal links between exposures and diseases tend to be generalizable, although the strength of the association varies.

4.2.3 Non-participation: non-response bias

Some people chosen for a study do not participate. This is non-response bias which is a type of selection bias. In studies of randomly sampled populations the non-response is typically 30–40 per cent, and sometimes much higher (even 90 per cent). It is likely that non-responders differ from responders. For example, in a written questionnaire study well-educated people may be more likely to respond than those who have difficulty in reading and writing. The effect of non-response bias can be partly understood if some information is available on those not participating, such as their age, sex, social circumstances, and why they did not respond. Investigators should seek this information as a high priority. Usually, such information is not available, enticing investigators to assume that the non-responders were not atypical. A similar problem arises in studies of health records when some records are inaccessible to the investigator. The problem is compounded when the non-response rate differs greatly in two populations that are to be compared; for example, men and women (the latter often have higher response rates), groups in different social classes (higher response in well-off people) or ethnic groups (response rates may be very low in minorities for self-completion questionnaires).

Investigators should ensure that time and effort spent in recruitment meet the need, so that comparison populations have similar response rates. The strategies for recruiting comparison populations may differ but, ideally, the type of people participating and the level of non-response should be similar. A degree of non-response bias is, however, an intrinsic limitation of the survey method and hence of epidemiology.

Formal studies of responders and non-responders have shown that the differences are usually important but seldom so great that the study is irrevocably undermined.

4.2.4 Comparing disease patterns and risk factor–disease outcome relationships in populations which differ (context for confounding)

Confounding is a difficult idea to explain and grasp (and the reader may wish to return to this section again, after reading the remainder of the book). The word confounding is derived from a Latin word meaning to mix together, a useful idea, for confounding mixes us up about causal and non-causal relationships. The word's meaning in everyday language, to confuse or puzzle, is also helpful. In epidemiology, it is the error in the estimate of the measure of association between a risk factor and disease, which may arise when there are differences in the comparison populations other than the risk factor under study. In this circumstance confounding might occur but it is not inevitable. These differences must include factors that are associated both with the disease and the risk factor under study for confounding to be present. These differences may not have been measured or they may have been measured imprecisely, so controlling for confounding may be impossible or very difficult.

Confounding is a major problem in epidemiology, and probably the most difficult one to understand, show and counteract. The potential for it to occur is there whenever the cardinal rule 'compare like-with-like' is broken. The only way to achieve this ideal, conceptually, is simultaneously to compare population X with the risk factor, and the identical population X without the risk factor. This is an example of counterfactual reasoning, where something is not observable but is a theoretical idea (see also Chapter 5, Section 5.4.2). This compare like-with-like rule is a counsel of perfection that is rarely, and perhaps never, attained, except that we get close to it in experimental research where study subjects can be randomly allocated to one group or another, a technique which employs the laws of chance to create comparable groups. If the experimental study is large the randomized populations will tend to be similar. Even with randomization there is no certainty that the groups are comparable, especially in subgroup analysis (see Chapter 9, randomized trials). The degree of confounding is the difference between the measure of risk when the study group is compared with a counterfactual population (which can never be known) and that seen in real data. The counterfactual measure of risk can, theoretically, be estimated in a perfect randomized trial (but perfection is never possible in trials, and often they cannot be done at all). Mostly, therefore, we estimate the degree of confounding by more pragmatic statistical techniques, as discussed below and in Chapter 9. The concept of confounding is best explained by examples (Table 4.3) and by illustrations as in Figs 4.3 and 4.4. Before examining these tables and figures read the next three paragraphs and then reflect on the questions in Box 4.3.

Imagine that a study follows up people who drink alcohol and observes the occurrence of lung cancer. In studying this association we can neither observe the same people without the risk factor (the counterfactual approach), nor randomize people into alcohol use/non-alcohol use groups. We use, instead, a comparison group to put the results of the study group into context.

A group of people who do not drink and are of the same age and sex provide the pragmatic (not counterfactual, and not randomized) comparison group. The study finds that lung cancer is more common in alcohol drinkers; that is, there is an association between alcohol consumption and lung cancer. Reflect on the questions in Box 4.3.

Investigators find that mortality rates in an English seaside resort are higher than in the country as a whole. Why might this be so? Is it something to do with the environmental

Table 4.3 Examples of confounding

The confounded association	One possible explanation	The confounded factor	The confounding (possibly causal) factor	To check the assumption
(a) People who drink alcohol apparently have a raised risk of lung cancer	Alcohol drinking and smoking are behaviours which go together	Alcohol, which is a marker for, on average, smoking more cigarettes	Tobacco, which is associated with both alcohol and with the disease	See if the alcohol–lung cancer relationship holds in people not exposed to tobacco: if yes, tobacco is not a confounder (stratified analysis, see Chapter 7)
(b) People living in an affluent seaside resort apparently have a higher mortality rate than the country as a whole	A holiday town attracts the elderly, so has a comparatively old population	Living in a resort is a marker for being, on average, older	Age, which is associated with both living in a resort and with death	Look at each age group specifically, or use age standardization to take into account age differences (see Chapters 7 and 8)
(c) African Americans are apparently heavier users of crack cocaine than 'White' Americans	Poor people living in the American inner city are particularly likely to become dependent on illicit drugs	Belonging to the racial category 'African American'	Poverty and the pressures of inner-city living, including the easy availability of drugs	Use statistical techniques to adjust for the influence of a number of complex socio-economic factors (see Chapter 8)

Box 4.3 Some questions to assess confounding

In each of the above examples ask these questions:

- Have the investigators compared like with like?
- Is a counterfactual comparison group or randomiaation of the risk factor possible?
- In what ways that are associated with the risk factor and disease under study might the two comparison populations differ?
- What are the potential explanations for the findings, other than the self-evident ones (i.e. alcohol causes lung cancer, living in an English seaside resort is a risk, and African Americans are prone to the crack cocaine habit)?
- What is the confounding factor?
- What is the confounded, non-causal factor?
- How can we check out that our understanding is correct?

or social conditions associated with living in the resort or is there another explanation? In what ways might the population of the resort differ from the country as a whole and in a way that affects mortality? Reflect on the questions in Box 4.3.

African Americans were demonstrated to be more likely to use crack cocaine than White Americans (see Lillie-Blanton *et al.* 1993). Is this a racial or ethnic difference in attitudes or behaviour in relation to this drug? In what ways relevant to this observation might the two populations differ from each other? Compare your answers with Table 4.4.

Figure 4.3 offers a pictorial representation of confounding. The relationship between disease, the associated risk factor under study, and the confounding factor is shown as a triangular one. The confounding factor, shown at the apex of the triangle in Fig. 4.3, is associated both with the factor being examined and the disease. The right-hand line is shown in bold to signify the solidity of this link. Note that the arrow on the left-hand line points in both directions, showing a relationship in both directions. The arrow in the right-hand line points in one direction because we believe that the confounding factor is on the pathway that causes the disease or at least the association, but not vice versa. The arrow at the bottom is a broken line to symbolize the non-causal, confounded nature of the relationship. Figure 4.4 illustrates this with the example of alcohol, smoking, and lung cancer. There is an association between the confounding (smoking) and confounded (alcohol) factor. Do the exercise in Box 4.4 before reading on.

In the association between living in the resort and mortality, age (confounding factor) would be at the apex and living in the resort at the left-hand angle. In the association between African American race and crack cocaine use, socio-economic status would be at the apex and race at the left-hand angle. These interpretations are alternative and simplified explanations of a complex reality and, in turn, need to be subjected to test.

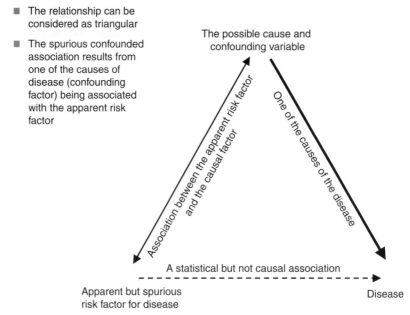

Fig. 4.3 Confounding variable: a pictorial representation.

The first key analysis in all epidemiological studies is to compare the characteristics of the populations under study, paying particular attention to factors that are thought to be on the disease's causal pathway. Simply because the groups are similar on the characteristics actually measured does not imply they are similar on all relevant characteristics. For example, two groups may be comparable on age, sex, smoking, and exercise habits but

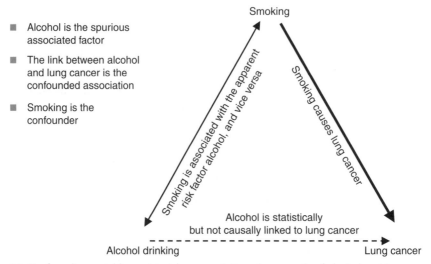

Fig. 4.4 Confounding variable, a pictorial representation: the example of alcohol and lung cancer.

Box 4.4 Pictorial presentation of associations in Table 4.3

Draw and analyse the associations (Table 4.3) between living in a seaside resort and high mortality, and between being African American and using crack cocaine, using the approach shown in Figs 4.3 and 4.4. What is the nature of the relationship between confounding and confounded factors here?

---

differ in the type of housing they live in, a variable on which data are often not collected. If the study is of accidents, infections, or respiratory disease, for example, differences in housing may matter greatly.

This same principle applies to all subgroup analysis. A comparison of two populations may show that they are virtually identical in age structure. The investigator may wish to examine the disease experience of men and women separately. The age structure of each sex must again be shown to be similar and this must not be assumed.

Serious problems with confounding are likely if it is not considered at the stage of designing the study, analysing the data, and interpreting the findings. A combination of methods is usually applied to handle confounding. In recent years the trend has been to control for confounding at the analysis stage but it is best to consider it at each stage and take one or more of the appropriate actions as shown in Table 4.4. Whatever is done the possibility of confounding can rarely be dismissed and, along with chance, it usually remains an alternative interpretation of epidemiological findings.

We will look at confounding factors in the context of age standardization in Chapter 8.

4.2.5 **Risk/effect modification, susceptibility and interaction**

This section introduces concepts that are not biases, but which are both relevant to error and bias (including confounding), and in some ways conceptually similar. However, as this theme relates to causation, readers might wish to read Chapter 5 first.

We have already considered, briefly, the idea of disease susceptibility, e.g. in the extreme case where some diseases rarely, or never, occur, because humans have no susceptibility to them. Even for human diseases, exposure to the causes is often common but the disease is rare. The fact that some people who are exposed to the known causes get disease, and others do not, implies there are other factors that determine the outcome (in Chapter 5, this kind of reasoning is extended).

Whether we consider trivial problems such as the common cold, or serious diseases such as CHD, it is clear that some individuals are more susceptible than others. Epidemiology cannot help with understanding such individual differences. The same, however, applies to populations, where epidemiology can shed some light. In the case of the common cold the reasons tend to be fairly obvious: populations living in overcrowded conditions are more susceptible to exposure to the common cold virus, and therefore

Table 4.4 Possible actions to control confounding

Possible action	Example	Benefit	Cost/disadvantage
Study design: randomize individual subjects or units of populations, e.g. schools	To determine the effectiveness of sex education in schools in reducing the incidence of teenage pregnancy, half of the schools in a city could be in the intervention group, the other half in a control group. The allocation of the group would be determined by chance (see Chapter 9, Section 7)	Selection biases bypassed Avoids schools selecting themselves into the intervention group for they would be different from those which chose the control group	Limited to research questions where randomization is possible, and acceptable to subjects and professionals Comparability may not be achieved, especially in small samples Effective only in large studies
Study design: select comparable groups/restrict entry into study	Study only subjects who are 35 years of age Study non-smokers only e.g. in studying the health effects of air pollution	Vagaries of chance and selection bias bypassed	Creates extra work in finding the chosen population Findings may not apply to populations not studied Erroneous conclusions may be reached e.g. air pollution has no effect on health when it might affect smokers but not non-smokers Practical applications of findings in health policy etc. are reduced
Study design: match individuals or whole populations	Select subjects and controls on pre-determined criteria e.g. age, sex, race, smoking Select populations on basis of population statistics e.g. unemployment levels, type of housing	Investigators' judgements and knowledge of confounding factors is used	The result is not a population sample so there are problems of representativeness Practical applications of data may be less Needs statistical analysis designed for matched populations Overmatching can lead to false conclusions
Analysis: analyse subgroups separately	Compare disease experience of each age group, sex, race etc. separately (stratified analysis)	Direct control and observation of possible confounding factors	Makes assimilation of results difficult In most studies, there are insufficient subjects to make detailed stratification possible
Analysis: adjust data statistically	Use techniques to amalgamate results of	Summary measures possible	Hard for non-statisticians to understand and do well

(continued)

Table 4.4 (continued) Possible actions to control confounding

Possible action	Example	Benefit	Cost/disadvantage
	stratified analysis e.g direct or indirect standardization (Chapter 8), Mantel Haensel technique and multiple regression modelling (consult an introductory statistics or intermediate epidemiology textbook)	Computers and statistical software make this relatively quick to do	Actual data are hidden behind summary figures, which are distorted by the process (see Chapter 8) Outputs are not easily used for health care policy and planning May lead to false sense of complacency that confounders are controlled

more likely to get ill. A combination of exposure to the virus and exposure to psychological stress and physical cold temperatures both increase the risk of getting the common cold disproportionately.

For CHD it is not at all clear why, to take one of many potential comparisons, Indian-born women in England and Wales should have more CHD than (predominantly White) women born in England and Wales. This observation seems real, and not a data artefact. In fact, on first principles we would expect the opposite (because of less smoking in Indian born women for example). Just as with the common cold, there must be one or more factors that increase Indian-born women's risk. These factors might be obvious ones like age, smoking, high blood pressure etc. It is commonplace in epidemiology to treat such factors as confounding variables, to try to find the 'independent' effect of the factor under study, here ethnicity, as indicated by country of birth. Typically, in studies of ethnic variations in CHD, the known risk factors do not appear to explain such differences, although at least part of this may be due to difficulties in measuring risk factors precisely (see, for example, the next section). There may also be other factors that are unknown that cause these differences in risk of CHD. Such unknown factors may even modify the risk of CHD through known risk factors, e.g. hypertension may be a more potent cause of CHD in one ethnic group than in another. If that were true, the question of why this is so still remains. At this point, speculation is usually required, e.g. unknown genetic variations, or life-course effects, that alter susceptibility to the effects of high blood pressure.

This is an example of how enhanced or reduced susceptibility can affect the influence of an exposure on risk of an outcome. The factor that influences susceptibility is known as a risk modifier or effect modifier and there is said to be an interaction between the study exposure and the effect modifier on outcome. Risk and effect is judged in epidemiology by how the incidence of disease is changed by exposure to the risk factor (Chapter 7), and it is quantified using either absolute or relative measures of risk (Chapter 7 and Chapter 8).

Risk or effect modification is different from confounding. It occurs when two factors (which can each be causal or protective) interact to reduce or increase risk. When two (or more) causal risk factors coexist, what is the likely effect on the outcome? For example, say that smoking cigarettes triples the risk of cancer X, and drinking alcohol also triples the risk. What is the risk of cancer X in a population where people both smoke cigarettes and drink alcohol? Let us say that the incidence of disease in people who do not drink or smoke is 100 per 10,000 people. In those that smoke, the risk is 300 per 10,000 people, 200 extra cases being contributed by smoking (relative risk 3, excess risk 2, where excess risk is relative risk minus the baseline risk, which is by definition 1), and similarly for those that drink alcohol (200 extra cases per 10,000 people, relative risk 3, excess risk 2). Assume the four groups of people—those who do not smoke or drink, those who smoke, those who drink, and those who both smoke and drink—are identical in every other respect, i.e. there is no confounding. Now imagine we have 10,000 people who all drink alcohol and smoke cigarettes. What are the possible combined effects? You may wish to prepare an appropriate table to test your thinking, before looking at Table 4.5a, which summarizes the text below.

The possible combined effects are that the coexistence of these factors can lead to the addition of the individual risks, less than the addition of the two risks (antagonism, or negative interaction), or more than the addition of the two risks (synergy, or positive interaction). Our default situation, and expectation on first principles, is that the two

Table 4.5 Effect modification for (a) cancer x (imaginary) and (b) lung cancer (real)

Exposure	Cancer x incidence/10 000		Relative risk	
(a) Imaginary data	Actual	Excess*	Actual	Excess
No smoking, no alcohol**	100	0	1	0
Smoking, no alcohol	300	200	3	2
Alcohol, no smoking	300	200	3	2
Smoking and alcohol				
No effect modification	500	400	5	4
Effect modification (example)	750	650	9	8
(b) Based on classic example (Hammond et al)	Lung cancer Death rates/100 000		Relative risk	
	Actial	excess	Actial	excess
No smoking or asbestos	11.3	0	1	0
Smoking, no asbestos	58.4	47.1	5.2	4.2
Asbestos, no smoking	122.6	111.3	10.9	9.9
Asbestos and smoking				
no effect modification (as expected) if no interaction	169.7	158.4	15.1	14.1
with effect modification (as found)	601.6	590.3	53.2	52.2

*Over baseline
**Baseline

risks will be combined, the additive concept of effect modification. There are good reasons for basing biomedical and public health research and practice on this model (readers should consult Kenneth Rothman for the arguments—see references—but be aware that this is still a slightly controversial area). In this case, if there is no effect modification or interaction, the risk in this population is 100 (baseline) plus 200 (excess from smoking) plus 200 (excess from alcohol) i.e. 500 per 10,000. If our research shows a different result—say 800 per 10,000, and it is not a result of chance, error or bias (including confounding), then we have risk modification. The two risk factors, smoking and alcohol, are combining to give a result other than the intuitive and expected one of the additive effect.

Where the additive model does not apply we can say that the presence of one factor has modified the effect of the other. A simple definition of effect modification is this: the association between a risk factor and an outcome differs in subgroups of the population. In this example, above, the association between smoking and cancer X has been altered by the presence of alcohol, and vice versa, and this alteration only occurs in some populations, where both risk factors are present.

The two risks might have large modifying effects, perhaps even so much that the effects are multiplicative or more i.e. the two factors smoking and alcohol together increase risk by ninefold ($1 \times 3 \times 3$; the 1 signifying baseline risk, in the absence of the two risk factors) and not by fivefold ($1 + 2 + 2$). If a third factor (say a gene variant) also tripled risk, people with the 3 factors would have a 27-fold risk ($1 \times 3 \times 3 \times 3$) and not a sevenfold risk as for the addition of risks ($1 + 2 + 2 + 2$).

In fact, this multiplication effect is often seen. As a result, sometimes interaction is defined as a departure from the expectation of multiplication of risks. Investigators can wrongly conclude that there is no effect modification, simply because there is no departure from multiplication of risks. Logically, if there is no interaction on the additive scale then there must be interaction on the multiplicative scale (negative interaction), and if there is positive interaction on the multiplicative scale then there must be interaction on the additive scale also.

The combined effects might be even bigger than 27. Then we would have effect modification demonstrable even using statistical methods that are based on the multiplication of risks. It is exceptional to demonstrate such large interactive effects in epidemiology.

The way that risk factors are modifying each other needs to be checked out empirically. These additive and multiplicative considerations in relation to risk are important to the proper analysis of data, the choice of statistical methods and analysis programmes, and interpretation of data. Statistical models often assume a multiplicative model of risks. They may use logarithms, where addition is equal to multiplication, e.g. for logarithms on base 10, where 0 is 1 in ordinary numbers, and 1 is 10 in ordinary numbers, the addition of the logarithms 1 plus 1 is equivalent to 100 in ordinary numbers. (The multiple logistic regression model uses logarithms.)

In epidemiology and statistics, the concept of effect modification is increasingly discussed as interaction. Interaction may be demonstrable often on the additive scale (relating to the biological and public health concept of interaction) but rarely on the multiplicative scale (relating to statistical concept of interaction).

In the classic and most commonly cited example of effect modification (interaction) between smoking (tenfold increased risk) and asbestos (fivefold increased risk), the combined effect on lung cancer is multiplicative with a combined increased risk over 50-fold (compared with 15.1 i.e. 1 plus 9.9 plus 4.2, on the additive model). This result, summarized in Table 4.5b, has been shown by Hammond *et al.* (1979). If this interaction had been tested out using modern approaches of statistical analysis, based on the multiplication of risks as the standard approach, investigators could wrongly have concluded that there was no effect modification. If the combined effect had been substantially more than 50 there would also have been interaction on a multiplicative scale. The risk of lung cancer in smokers who are exposed to asbestos is much higher than in those not so exposed. In this case both smoking and asbestos are causal factors, and neither are confounders.

One difference between confounding and effect modification is that the exposure–outcome association would be similar in all levels (strata) of a confounder but that the exposure–outcome association differs in different levels (strata) of an effect modifier. Confounding is an obstacle to proper interpretation that should be controlled but effect modification is of causal and public health interest and should not be "controlled" i.e. lost in the analysis. (A variable can act as both a confounder and an effect modifier in different circumstances e.g. age.)

As we will discuss in Chapter 8, there are two main ways of presenting risk data—by absolute/actual risk, and relative/comparative risk. In discussing interactions we should clarify which approach and analysis we intend to pursue, our prior definition of interaction and the causal model we are assuming. In the above classic example involving smoking and asbestos in lung cancer, the interaction is clear if the causal model is an additive one. If, however, the chosen causal model (arguably, wrongly) presumes a multiplication of risks, then there is no departure from that. The latter cannot be correct, as this is the prime example of interaction in epidemiology.

Interaction can also occur when the outcome is a continuous variable, e.g. blood pressure or cholesterol levels.

The promise of the new genetics is to clarify the nature of individual and group-level susceptibility to diseases, and the variable response to treatments. Gene variants can act as effect modifiers/interactive factors of the relationship between an environmental exposure and an outcome. The problem is that studies that can accurately assess interaction need to be very large, especially when effects are small (as with most gene variants). Mostly, studies that report there is no interaction are too small to reach such a conclusion, and many others have applied the wrong conceptual approach. If there is heterogeneity in the effects of a risk factor within populations, as is highly likely, there must be effect modification/interaction and vice versa.

Failure to measure accurately and control confounding factors can lead to spurious findings of risk modification (see below in the section on misclassification bias) and failure to seek or notice risk modification can lead to a false measure of population risk and the possibility of missing an important finding, at least for subgroups of the population.

4.2.6 Measurement errors: differential and non-differential

Measurement errors and biases fall into the huge category of information bias. Before reading on you may wish to reflect on the questions in Box 4.5 on measurement errors in epidemiological research.

Unlike measuring the length of a red cell, an atom, or even the orbit of the moon, which are also error-prone, assessing disease in living humans requires a judgement. It is a subjective matter, aided by imprecise measures of biological indicators and information provided by the patient or study subject. After death the accuracy of the diagnosis can be improved or verified by autopsy but the patient is no longer available for questioning, and some tests, particularly dynamic ones (e.g. an exercise ECG for heart disease), are no longer possible. A combination of clinical and autopsy data is sometimes essential to reach a diagnosis.

Similar problems apply to most measurements of exposures thought to be causing the disease, and to confounding factors. For example, measuring socio-economic circumstances, ethnic group, cigarette-smoking habits, or alcohol consumption are complex matters. Even measures such as height, weight, and blood pressure are difficult, particularly in large studies where numerous people may be making measurements in different places. Accuracy in biochemical and other laboratory tests, though easier to achieve than disease, exposure or physical measures, is still problematic. Issues such as the quality of the specimen, and changing laboratory reagents and techniques come into play. For environmental exposures such as air pollution, past circumstances will need to be estimated and not directly measured.

Measurement error is compounded by biological variation, which is not error but may be confused with it. For example, blood pressure varies from moment to moment in response to activity, in a 24-hour (circadian) cycle with lowered pressure in the night, and with the air temperature. To examine the relationship between blood pressure and disease we need a meaningful and true summary estimate of the blood pressure. There is, however, no readily available estimate. The usual compromise is taking the blood pressure in standard conditions, measuring it on several occasions, and taking an average of the readings. The value is useful in clinical practice and epidemiology for predicting disease outcomes, but it is not an accurate summary of the constantly varying blood pressure. For that we need long-term recordings of blood pressure over several days (ambulatory blood pressure)—a method sometimes used in clinical practice but seldom in epidemiology.

Box 4.5 Measurement errors in epidemiology

Why are measurement errors in epidemiology likely to be both more common and more important than in other scientific disciplines, say, physics, anatomy, biochemistry, or animal physiology?

Biological variations can cause bias. Imagine two populations with identical blood pressures. If blood pressure measurements on one population were made in the morning and the other in the evening, the average blood pressure in the two populations would seem to be different when it is not.

For some variables the natural variation is so great that making estimates is extremely difficult, for example, in diet, alcohol consumption, and the level of stress.

Measurement errors include those arising from machine imprecision and inaccurate observation by the investigator or diagnostician. Measurements of the 'causal' factors and confounding factors are often obtained from the subject alone, whereas information on the disease is obtained from the patient's account, the physician's examination, and laboratory tests. Measurement errors in the former, therefore, are more likely to occur than in the latter.

Measurement errors which occur unequally in the comparison populations are, in line with earlier discussion of bias, considered as epidemiological biases. They can irreversibly destroy a study. For example, in a study where one population is interviewed face-to-face and the comparison population completes a self-completion questionnaire, the results are unlikely to be comparable. Inequality in follow-up arising from unequal interest by subjects or from the investigators can lead to both selection and information bias, and will compound the problem of confounding.

Imagine that the sphygmomanometer in one town is faulty and is underestimating the blood pressure by 10 mmHg. In this town, many people who are hypertensive will be misclassified as not hypertensive, and very few the other way round. This is a systematic error, known as a differential misclassification bias. The degree to which a measure leads to a correct classification can be quantified using the concepts of sensitivity and specificity, and these are discussed in Chapter 6 in relation to screening tests.

These kinds of differential misclassification errors or biases may be hard to find, but the damage they do is self-evident. Measurement errors which are equal in all comparison populations, or non-differential errors or biases, are also important, as discussed in the section below.

4.2.7 Misclassification bias: non-differential measurement errors and regression to the mean

Misclassification error occurs when a person is put into the wrong category (or population subgroup), usually as a result of faulty measurement. For example, imagine a survey of hypertension in two towns. Inevitably, some people who are hypertensive will be misclassified as normal, others who are normal will be misclassified as hypertensive. The misclassification may be random, with as many misclassified in one direction as the other. The total number of people with hypertension may be about right. This error is known as a non-differential misclassification bias, in that it affects all subgroups equally (non-differentially).

The consequences of misclassification can be severe in both clinical practice and in epidemiology. Clinically, misclassified persons will be treated wrongly. Information from epidemiological surveys is often sent with the permission of the study subject to the personal physician. Epidemiological mismeasurements can, therefore, trigger off unnecessary clinical investigations and treatments (false positive), or, alternatively, convey that there is no problem (false negative).

Differential errors deeply undermine epidemiological studies. If differential misclassification errors occur the study may need to be abandoned, unless the extent of the error can be quantified and data corrected. In the example in section 4.2.6, if we find the sphygmomanometer in one town always measured blood pressure 10 mmHg too low then we could add 10 mmHg to the recorded values. A correction can often be made for measures of physical attributes and for laboratory test measures. It is more difficult to correct for misclassification in social information collected by questionnaire or interview, and it is usually impossible for diagnostic information collected from medical records.

The effect of non-differential misclassification is more subtle than for differential error, and therefore more likely to be overlooked, particularly if there is little or no effect on the final prevalence figure. In measuring the strength of associations between exposures and disease outcomes, however, non-differential misclassification error has an important, and not always predictable, effect. If the misclassification only applies to disease outcome then the strength of the association is always reduced, so the main problem is failing to find associations that, in reality, exist. Misclassification, however, affects exposure and confounding variables, and the combined effect of the mixture of misclassifications is not so predictable. This is best illustrated with a fictitious example.

Imagine a study of 20,000 women, 10,000 are cigarette smokers and the rest not. Our interest is in the occurrence of new cases of cardiovascular disease over 10 years (incidence of disease). Say that over 10 years 20 per cent of cigarette smokers develop a cardiovascular disease (CVD) compared with 10 per cent of those not smoking. The rate of disease in the smoking group is doubled (relative risk 20%/10% = 2). Table 4.6 shows the true results, given no misclassification.

Let us assume that misclassification in exposure occured 20 per cent of the time, so that 20 per cent of women actually smoking cigarettes were classified as not smoking, and that 20 per cent who were not cigarette smokers were classified as smoking cigarettes. Assume that there is no misclassification of disease outcome, and the disease incidence remains the same. Before reading on, you should modify the figures in Table 4.5 and recalculate relative risk of disease given this misclassification.

Tables 4.7(a) and 4.7(b) give the results. Table 4.7(a) shows the reality of the effects of misclassification. The investigator does not, however, usually know how much misclassification there is. For the investigator the data look like Table 4.8. The reason for this is shown by the reorganization of the data in Table 4.7(a) into 4.7(b), and then into 4.8.

The risk of CVD in the 'smoking group' with 20 per cent misclassification is 1800/10 000. In the 'not cigarette smokers group' it is 1200/10 000. So the relative risk is 1.5 (with misclassification), rather than 2 (without misclassification).

$$\frac{1800/10\,000}{1200/10\,000} = \frac{0.18}{0.12} = 1.5$$

Table 4.6 Imaginary, perfect and therefore impossible, study of cardiovascular outcome and cigarette smoking: no misclassification

True classification of cigarette smoking status	Cardiovascular disease		Total
	Yes	No	
Yes	2000 (20%)	8000	10 000
No	1000 (10%)	9000	10 000
	3000	17 000	20 000

This illustrates the general principle that when the misclassification is of exposure then the strength of the association (measured here by the relative risk) is reduced. Misclassification will, inevitably, also arise in measurement of the disease outcome. At the end of this chapter you will find an exercise on misclassification that gives you practice for both exposure and outcome misclassification.

In reality there will be misclassification simultaneously in both measurement of exposure and in disease, and this will distort the results even more. Generally, non-differential misclassification error weakens the association and so lowers the relative risk. This general principle may break down when misclassification occurs in confounding variables with unpredictable results. The demonstration of this is beyond this book, but there is a reference to a paper by Greenland (1980) giving access to the literature.

Other than awareness, what can investigators do about misclassification bias? The answer is to do studies to measure its extent and then adjust the data accordingly. To do this requires validity studies that assess to what extent measures are accurate (i.e. valid). The concepts here are discussed again in section 6.5 within the context of screening and screening tests, and in particular sensitivity and specificity of tests.

A closely related problem, and one that combines selection and measurement biases is regression to the mean, a phrase coined by Francis Galton (1822–1911), where regression means 'to revert to' to or 'return to'. This bias has come to light from the observation that

Table 4.7 (a) Smoking and cardiovascular disease: 20% misclassification of cigarette smoking-the figures as actually collected

Actual classification of smoking with 20% error	Cardiovascular disease		Total
	Yes	No	
Yes, classified right (incidence 20%)–smoker	1600	6400	8000
Yes, classified wrong (incidence 20%)–'non-smoker'	400	1600	2000
Subtotal	2000	8000	10 000
No, classified right (incidence 10%)-non-smoker	800	7200	8000
No, classified wrong (incidence 10%)-'smoker'	200	1800	2000
Subtotal	1000	9000	10 000
Total of subtotals	3000	17 000	20 000

Table 4.7 (b) Smoking and cardiovascular disease: 20% misclassification of cigarette smoking. The rows shown in bold show the data as the investigator sees

Classification of cigarette smoking status	Cardiovascular disease		Total
	Yes	No	
Yes, classified right (smoking cigarettes) so incidence rate is 20%	1600	6400	8000
Yes, classified wrong (actually not cigarette smokers) so incidence rate is 10%	200	1800	2000
Subtotal—results as seen by investigator	1800	8200	10 000
No, classified right (not cigarette smokers) so incidence rate is 10%	800	7200	8000
No, classified wrong (actually smoking cigarettes) so incidence rate is 20%	400	1600	2000
Subtotal—results as seen by investigator	1200	8800	10 000
Total	3000	17 000	20 000

measurements that initially lie at the extremes tend to move nearer the average on subsequent measurements. Wherever appropriate or possible, the population across the range of measures should be studied rather than taking a sample from one end of the spectrum. Of course, this may not be appropriate where the focus of interest is in those at the extremes rather than the average.

The phenomenon can also be observed across generations, the classic example being that the offspring of very tall, clever, obese, short, energetic, sporting, beautiful (etc.) people tend to be less so in each respect than their parents, rather than equally or even more so. Offspring of parents who are short on these qualities tend to have more of them than their parents. Such a general phenomenon must have a general cause. Before reading on, reflect on some possible explanations.

In essence, the cause is random error. Imagine that we have measured the waistline to find overweight people for a study to prevent obesity. Let us say that we set a value of 90 cm (36 inches) as the cut-off of interest. We measure the waist using a tape measure. We follow instructions on how to do this complex task. In 1000 people we find 200 who

Table 4.8 Smoking and cardiovascular disease: 20% misclassification of cigarette smoking—as the investigator sees it in summary

Apparent classification of cigarette smoking	Cardiovascular disease		Total
	Yes	No	
Yes	1800	8200	10 000
No	1200	8800	10 000
Total	3000	17 000	20 000

exceed this cut-off. We call them back for a repeat measure in 72 hours. Why might there be fewer than 200 people exceeding the cut-off? Leave aside the possibility that they lost weight in the interim, that they had been fasting prior to measurement or even that the measurements have been made with a different protocol (all good explanations, but even if they did not occur, regression to the mean would still be there).

The fundamental answer is that some of the 200 people had been mismeasured because of random error. Those who had been mismeasured with too low a waist (i.e. truly over 90 cm but mismeasured as less so) are not in our group of 200 who have returned, but those mismeasured too high are back. When they return for the second measurement some of these 200 will be measured too low because of mismeasurement error. Some of those previously measured too high will now be measured correctly, i.e. less than 90 cm. Our group of 200 people may dwindle to 180 people or even less.

If, rather than calling back the 200 sample, we had re-measured all 1000 people, some of the 800 who had a waist of ≤90 cm (36 inches) would now have one above the cut-off for the same reasons. Then, the total number of people with a waist of ≥90 cm may well still have been about 200, but they would not have been exactly the original 200 people.

In the example of offspring having less extreme characteristics than their parents, the explanation is that those characteristics arise partly from chance events that are unlikely to be repeated. The reasons why a person is clever are complex—numerous genes, nutritional factors and environmental and social stimuli will be important. Some of these will be chance effects. Their repetition across the generations is unlikely.

Regression to the mean is of particular importance in epidemiology when subsamples of the population are followed over time, either to examine the effects of interventions (when the apparent effect may be misleading) or when the association between risk factors and outcomes is to be studied (the effects are underestimated by just using the original measure, just as is usually the case for mismeasurement). The solution here, apart from awareness, is to assess the extent of the bias through repeat measurements, usually in a subsample, and then to adjust the results for the whole population.

In these examples the association is generally reduced or diluted. The phenomena known as regression dilution bias and attenuation bias relate to these errors, and arise in regression and correlation analyses (see Chapter 5), respectively.

4.2.8 Analysis and interpretation

In virtually every project the potential for data analysis is far greater than that actually done. The choice of which data to analyse, the way to analyse them, and how to present the findings are usually left to the investigator. Clearly, the choices will be informed by the prior interests (and biases) and expertise of the researcher. These choices will usually be good ones. Sometimes the choices will be poor, misleading, negligent, malicious, and even fraudulent.

There is no easy solution to this potential problem. External scrutiny by objective advisers of the research protocol, including the plan for data analysis and interpretation, is one important safeguard. This is done increasingly, especially for clinical trials.

Another step, more difficult to achieve, would be the inclusion of objective, uninvolved people in the research team at the data analysis and interpretation stage.

As a minimum, investigators should ensure that their analysis is driven by prior stated hypotheses, research questions, and analysis strategies. One controversial proposal, being implemented slowly, is that investigators should make public their data collection proforma e.g. questionnaire, data, analysis strategy, and other information required to replicate the analysis. Then anyone could check the work or analyse the data differently. Some scientific journals require that authors of manuscripts reporting original research make the data available on request. In practice, this requirement is rarely imposed, and is unlikely to be except in the case of suspected fraud.

Given these safeguards, statistical analysis of data can proceed. There are numerous pitfalls in the process, so much so that readers of this book will need to turn to specialist courses and books. A brief overview is, however, given in Chapter 9.

4.2.9 **Publication**

The pressure to make choices is intensified at the stage of publication, particularly in scientific journals. The article will usually be written in 1500–5000 words (the most prestigious journals are usually at the shorter end of the spectrum). Research submitted as a short report may be 500–700 words, and as a letter to the editor, even shorter. Choices on the data to be presented will be combined with choices on emphasis and interpretation. Convention dictates that the authors indicate their preferred interpretation, and that data are never published without discussion (the ultimate but impractical solution to the problem of bias in interpretation). Editorial guidelines usually indicate that originality, interest, and readability will be key criteria for publication. Researchers write accordingly, by highlighting the points of interest to themselves, editors, and readers. Exaggeration of the novelty or interest of the work is probably the norm rather than the exception, because without it the chances of publication in prestigious journals is diminished.

In epidemiology the usual point of interest, determined by the dominant paradigm, is the difference in the pattern of disease between compared populations, and the potential to understand disease causation. Other perspectives and interpretations are usually secondary. Similarities between populations are too seldom commented on.

Manuscripts showing interesting findings (positive results in trials, differences in disease patterns in most epidemiology) are most likely to be published in widely read journals, others are often unpublished or published in specialist journals or as reports to the funding agency, which may be confidential or difficult to get. There is, nonetheless, a good case for research to be written as a full report with fewer constraints on the word limits from which papers are later published, especially if both report and papers were available to the reader on the Internet.

The result of these problems with publication is a biased understanding of the differences and similarities in the disease patterns of populations and an exaggerated view of the importance of associations between risk factors and disease outcomes. This has huge importance for systematic reviews and meta-analyses (see Chapter 10).

4.2.10 **Judgement and action**

The summary results and interpretation of epidemiology will probably need to be examined by decision-makers, whether the population as a whole, politicians, industrialists, policy-makers or other researchers. It is likely that controversial interpretations, especially those proposing changes that threaten powerful interests, will be contested. Interpretation is a matter of judgement which depends on the prior values, beliefs, and interests of the observer. A pattern seen by one observer as clear evidence of the detrimental effect of smoking on respiratory health may be seen by another as due to error, bias, confounding, or another cause such as air pollution. According to Thomas Kuhn (1996), a key characteristic of science is that the scientist and the peer group are the sole arbiters of the meaning and validity of the theory and data. Epidemiology differs from other physical and biomedical sciences in that the data are usually of direct interest to a wide range of people and, moreover, are much more amenable to interpretation. As a result epidemiologists are not the sole arbiters of the theory and data. Epidemiologists have, therefore, the dual responsibilities of minimizing the impact of their own biases and preventing the misinterpretation of data and misleading recommendations by those with vested interests. Sound data interpretation rests on sharp critical appraisal skills (see Chapter 10).

4.3 **A practical application of the research chronology schema of bias and error**

The above 'research cycle'-based discussion of bias in epidemiology is now illustrated by a study of the possible impact of industrial air pollution in Teesside on the health of populations living close by. Box 4.6 gives the title and abstract of the study. Using the list of potential causes of bias in column 1 of Table 4.1, analyse the information in Box 4.6. Do this exercise before reading on. Unusually, this study was followed by a formal examination of the impact of the research; again interested readers may wish to read how the study report was perceived (Moffat *et al.* 2000, b). Table 4.9 provides some answers to the exercise for comparison with yours.

4.4 **Conclusion**

Error is inevitable in all sciences but is particularly important and likely in those studying humans. Scientists need to be particularly careful about errors that may be applied in health settings, and hence damage health (at worst) or waste resources (at best). Bias is a more subtle issue and both more likely to be overlooked or, even when sought, remain undetected. In this chapter I have utilized the central epidemiological strategy—comparison of populations—to discuss bias. Bias, in an epidemiological context, arises when errors affect comparison groups unequally. Since this is often the case, perhaps always the case, bias is a central issue in epidemiology. Confounding is a special and difficult aspect of bias. It remains one of the critical issues for all aspects of epidemiology. Strictly speaking, effect modification is neither an error nor a bias but, since it can lead

Box 4.6 Analysis of an environment and health study based on the research-cycle approach to bias

Title

Does living close to a constellation of industries impair health? A study of health, illness and the environment in north-east England.

Study objective

To assess whether public and professional concerns that industrial air pollution from petrochemical and steel industries in Teesside, north-east England, contributed to poor health, particularly high mortality rates.

Design

Populations which were similar on a broad range of census indicators of social and economic circumstances, but which varied in the distance of the home from major industries were compared on a broad range of health indicators including mortality, morbidity, self-reported health, health-related lifestyles, occupational histories, social circumstances, and attitudes to industry. The underlying hypothesis was that respiratory health, in particular, would show gradients with the worst health in those populations living closest to industry.

Setting

Twenty-seven housing estates, nineteen in Teesside and eight in Sunderland, two conurbations in the north-east of England, were the focus of the study. The estates were aggregated, on the basis of distance and direction from industry, into zones (designated as A, B and C in Teesside where A is closest to industry, and S in Sunderland).

Main measures

Census data (1981 and 1991), and mortality (1981–1991), cancer registration (1983–1994), birthweight and stillbirth (1981–1991) and fetal abnormality (1986–1993) statistics were compiled for all 27 areas. General practitioner consultation data (1989–1994) were studied in 2201 subjects in 12 Teesside estates. A population-based sample survey in 1993 based on self-completion questionnaires of 9115 subjects provided data on social circumstances, lifestyle, occupation, and health status. Current pollution levels were estimated by air quality measures and computer modelling of emissions from industrial, road traffic, and other sources; estimates of past exposure were made from a twentieth-century land-use survey and historical pollution data.

Main results

The estates chosen for study were extremely economically deprived and comparable on a broad range of indicators including residential histories and unemployment, especially when grouped into zones. Mortality rates were high but there were no

(continued)

Box 4.6 Analysis of an environment and health study based on the research-cycle approach to bias *(continued)*

consistent and statistically and epidemiologically significant differences in all cause, or all age mortality, or for most specific causes. Lung cancer in women was, however, highest closest to industry (Zone A SMR (Standardised Mortality Ratio) = 393, Zone B = 251, Zone C = 242, Zone S = 185; where the standard population had a value of 100 (see Chapter 8 for details on the SMR). A less striking gradient was observed for respiratory disorders. Lung cancer registration ratios were consistent with mortality data.

There were no associations between proximity to industry and birthweights, stillbirths, fetal abnormality, and general practice consultation rates. On a broad range of measures of both respiratory and non-respiratory health, including asthma, there were no important variations across the study zones. Smoking habits across the populations compared were similar.

Land-use data showed prominent heavy industry in the Teesside area, and that the contemporary proximity of the housing estates to industry was echoed in the past. Air quality data indicated major improvements in air quality in the preceding 20 years. Levels of major pollutants were generally below guide values.

Conclusions

Living close to a constellation of major petrochemical and steel industries was not associated with most health indicators, whether mortality or morbidity, including disorders such as asthma which had been a cause of concern to health professionals. Lung cancer in women was an important exception. In the absence of plausible explanations based on differences in social and lifestyle factors, exposure to past industrial pollution is the prime explanation. Further research and monitoring of lung cancer rates is warranted.

Note: This abstract is similar to that in Bhopal *et al.* 1998, *Occupational and Environmental Medicine*, 55, pp. 812–22, published with permission from the BMJ Publishing Group.

to erroneous interpretation and it has conceptual overlaps with confounding, it is considered in this chapter. As Chapter 9 on study design discusses, most epidemiological studies have similar problems in controlling error and bias and mostly these are inherent in the survey and disease registration methods which underly epidemiology. Before reading on, do the exercise in Box 4.7 then look at the answers in Table 4.10.

When epidemiological data are applied to provide health advice to individuals and to shape public health policy, error and bias are especially important. The implication of this is that the rudiments of critical appraisal (see Chapter 10) are essential for those

Box 4.7 Exercise on assessing the impact of repeating the study, removing errors and biases, and removing confounding factors and effect modifiers on associations

What happens to an association when the following actions are taken?

◆ Evaluate the role of chance by repeating the study on a larger population

◆ Remove errors and biases

◆ Repeat the study in a population where the confounding factor is absent

◆ Repeat the study where an effect modifier is removed

Table 4.9 The research cycle framework for bias in epidemiology and the Teesside Study of health and the environment

Bias	Examples of source of bias
Research question	The question focused on industrial air pollution, the interest of the investigating team and the people of Teesside, but not of the local industry and local authority who would have preferred a focus on road traffic pollution, or a focus on all forms of pollution
Choice of populations	The study questions focused on one population living closest to industry (the population of interest living in Zone A). Another population was included because of the interests of the local authority, but investigators chose certain parts of the area Zone B in which this second population lived to maximize comparability with the population living closest to industry. Other populations were chosen on their comparability to the population of interest (living in Zones C and S).
Participation in a study	Unequal interest in the issue of industrial air pollution was reflected in unequal response rates with higher response in the three Teesside areas than in the comparison area in Sunderland (Zone S).
Comparing populations which differ	While the populations were very similar on a wide range of relevant indicators it would be impossible to show they were comparable on all potentially important exposures, say living near an asbestos plant 30 years before the study.
Assessment of disease	The comparison rests on the assumption that the diagnostic effort, skill, and facilities were equal in the areas studied; a reasonable assumption in this case. The assumption is that subjects close to industry do not report health problems with more diligence; an assumption which cannot be accepted without testing In view of funding and time constraints, general practice records were not studied in the Sunderland area
Assessment of factors which could cause disease	As for assessment of disease Misinformation is a potential problem for, arguably, the populations living close to the industry have a vested interest in showing an association between pollution and ill-health while the local industries had the opposite interest.
Follow-up	Not applicable

(continued)

Table 4.9 (*continued*) The research cycle framework for bias in epidemiology and the Teesside Study of health and the environment

Bias	Examples of source of bias
Outcome	Not an issue affecting the interpretation of the study
Analysis and interpretation of data	Many potential alternative analyses of the huge data set were avoided despite extreme pressures to veer away from the central hypotheses. A focus on the study questions was maintained by referring to the study proposal. While the investigators were trying to keep an open mind, for some the expectation and preferred outcome was an association between industrial air pollution and health, for others the opposite The analysis was searching, with detailed subgroup analysis going beyond the stated hypotheses, to seek such associations
Interpretation by readers and listeners	The complex findings were interpreted by industry as showing no causal association Health and local authorities preferred to focus on the issue of poverty rather than on air pollution Most of the researchers interpreted the data as showing that air pollution from industry was important to health and that more research was warranted

using epidemiological research in health areas. Equally, knowing that there may be health care implications, and health professionals and policy makers may be using their work, epidemiologists need to make explicit the potential errors and biases—hence limitations—of the work. This action may, however, undermine the prospects of publication (see section 4.2.9). Epidemiology has identified many types of errors and biases, and hundreds have been listed. The epidemiological approach has been pragmatic rather than theoretical, such that problems have been identified and solutions developed. I am not aware of an epidemiological theory on why error and bias occur. To develop such a theoretically based understanding, one might start with statistical and social science perspectives on these topics. Statistical theory is, to a large extent, about random (chance) variations. The theory is used in epidemiology to define the probability that a finding of difference, or one more extreme than that *actually found*, occurs by chance

Table 4.10 Effects of actions to test role of chance, error and bias–confounding and effect modification–interaction in assessing associations

Action	Effect on association
Repeat the study	Association usually disappears if it was chance
Remove error and bias	Association usually disappears if it arose from error or bias
Repeat study where confounding factor is absent	Association usually disappears
Effect modifier–interacting factor removed	Association remains (but reduced in strength)

alone (i.e. in truth there is no difference). The result is usually given as a P-value, p for probability, often misleadingly said to be a 'significance level'. Bias cannot be studied in this kind of statistical way. One of the most fundamental observations of social sciences on the nature of science is that the scientific endeavour is not wholly objective but is open to the influence of society and context. This view helps to explain many scientific actions that lead to error and bias, e.g. the Tuskegee Study mentioned above and discussed in Chapter 10. In studying and classifying bias I have promoted the framework provided by the chronology and structure of a research project.

The main principles which apply to all studies and help to minimize these errors include:

- develop research questions and hypotheses which help to benefit all the population or at least those studied and will minimize harm
- study a representative population, whenever possible
- measure accurately and with equal care across comparison groups
- compare like-with-like
- check for the main findings in subgroups before assuming that inferences and generalizations apply across all groups
- check for and take into account confounding and interaction
- a single study should only exceptionally be accepted as accurate
- in interpreting associations, first consider artefact
- maintain a critical stance.

Summary

Epidemiological studies are prone to error, because they usually study human populations in natural settings and not in laboratory conditions. The large size of many epidemiological studies imposes time and cost constraints which may promote errors. Bias in epidemiology may be thought of as error which affects comparison groups unequally or leads to inappropriate inferences about one group compared with another. Error and bias may be inherent in the research question and the hypothesis, but this is a relatively neglected matter.

Three broad problems confront epidemiologists: selection of study populations, quality of information, and confounding. Confounding causes an error in the assessment of the association between a disease and risk factor. It results from comparing groups which differ in characteristics that are associated with the disease and the risk factor under study, without fully accounting for such differences.

The different epidemiological research designs have similar problems with error and bias, which are mostly inherent in the survey and disease registration methods. Principles which apply to all studies and help to minimize these errors include: construct research questions and hypotheses carefully; study representative populations; measure accurately and with equal care across groups; compare like with like; take into account confounding and interaction; and check before assuming that inferences and generalizations apply across groups. The chronology and structure of a research project offers a natural framework for the systematic analysis of error and bias.

Sample examination questions

Give yourself 10 minutes for every 25% of marks. Many of the questions at the end of Chapter 9 are highly relevant to this chapter.

Question 1 What is misclassification bias, and why is it important in measuring risk factor–disease outcome relationships? (25%)
Answer Misclassification bias occurs when we categorize a person wrongly, e.g. a smoker is classified as a non-smoker, or a person with rheumatoid arthritis is classified as having osteoarthritis.

Misclassification can occur in both risk factors and outcome variables. Where risk factor–outcome relations are under study we are usually interested in the relative risk of the outcome in those with and without the risk factor. If misclassification is greater in one of these two groups, the relative risk will be exaggerated. The study may be irreversibly destroyed.

Where classification occurs equally in those with and without the risk factors, the relative risk is usually diminished. The study may reach a wrong conclusion, but the damage is sometimes repairable by adjusting for the degree of misclassification.

Question 2 How can we control confounding in epidemiology? (25%)
Answer We can control for confounding by, above all, awareness, foresight and planning. This will alert us to compare like with like wherever possible. Strategies to do this include restriction of who is recruited to the study, and matching. In trials random allocation of people into intervention and control groups is of great help. Further control of confounding is achievable by stratified analysis, standardization methods, and multivariable analysis where confounding factors are entered as covariates.

Question 3 Why might bias occur in the wording of an epidemiological research question? What can you do to minimize such a bias? Illustrate your answer with at least one example. (25%)
Answer Bias in epidemiology arises from errors that are not equal in the compared populations. Errors can arise from prejudices (conscious or subconscious), stereotypes, or lack of awareness and they can affect the research question. For example, imagine we are interested in the question of hygiene and its relationship to gastrointestinal infections in children of unemployed families. The question could be posed as:

(a) Are the higher rates of gastrointestinal infections in children of unemployed parents related to their poorer hygiene? Or

(b) Are there any differences in the hygiene practices of children that are directly associated with the employment status of their parents?

An issue such as this is open to bias. While bias in the minds of investigators is not easily set aside, the second question, written in a neutral way, reduces the potential for bias.

Question 4 What biases may arise in a cohort study assessing a possible association between a risk factor and disease, e.g. dietary salt intake and the development of hypertension? (25%)

Answer Bias is a type of error that affects comparison groups unequally so that the risk factor or intervention effect under study tends to be systematically over or under-estimated and hence erroneous conclusions drawn.

Biases can be categorized according to the chronology of a research project:

- Question bias. Processed food industry funding studies might aim to discredit the importance of dietary salt in blood pressure control.
- Selection bias. Restricting study participants by gender, age group, ethnicity, or volunteer status.
- Participation bias. Differential non-response/participation rates or loss to follow-up.
- Information bias. Diet and blood pressure are both difficult to measure accurately.
- Intervention bias. Although cohort studies do not impose an intervention as such, differential treatment of risk factor and control groups, e.g. in frequency or intensity of follow-up, may bias results.
- Interpretation bias. Unintentional or intentional misinterpretation of results to reflect researchers' preferred outcome is a form of bias.
- Publication bias. Only putting forward preferred results for publication leads to biased availability of evidence.
- Confounding. The risk factor and control groups may be dissimilar in other factors that influence the development of hypertension. Diet is linked to a range of other health behaviours, e.g. alcohol intake, that may influence blood pressure. Confounding may be considered as a special form of bias.

Question 5 What is publication bias? Why is it important in epidemiology? (25%)

Answer The pressures and difficulties of publication, particularly in scientific journals, can generate biases. The article will usually need to be short. Choices on the data to be presented will be combined with choices on emphasis and interpretation. Editorial guidelines usually indicate that originality, interest and readability will be key criteria for publication. Researchers write accordingly, by highlighting the points of interest to themselves, editors and readers. Manuscripts showing interesting findings (positive results in trials, differences in disease patterns in most epidemiology) are most likely to be submitted for publication, and to be accepted for publication, in widely read journals, while others are often left unpublished or published in specialist journals or as reports to the funding agency. The result is a biased understanding of the differences and similarities in the disease patterns of populations and an exaggerated view of the importance of associations between risk factors and disease outcomes.

Further exercises

Misclassification

Imagine a study of 20 000 women, 10 000 on the contraceptive pill and the rest not. Our interest is in the occurrence of new cases of cardiovascular disease over 10 years (incidence of disease). Say that over 10 years 20 per cent of those on the pill develop a cardiovascular disease (CVD) compared with 10 per cent of those not on the pill. The rate of disease in the oral contraceptive group is doubled (relative risk = 2). Table 4.6 shows the true results, given no misclassification.

Let us assume that misclassification in exposure occured 10 per cent of the time, so that 10 per cent of women actually on the pill were classified as not on the pill, and that 10 per cent who were not on the pill were classified as on the pill. Assume that there is no misclassification of disease outcome, and the disease incidence remains the same. Before reading on, you should modify the figures in Table A1 and recalculate relative risk of disease given this misclassification. Table A1(a) and A1(b) give the results.

Table A1 Imaginary and perfect but impossible study of cardiovascular outcome and pill use: no misclassification

True classification of pill use status	Cardiovascular disease		Total
	Yes	No	
Yes	2000	8000	10 000
No	1000	9000	10 000
	3000	17 000	20 000

Table A1(a) Pill and cardiovascular disease with an imperfect but possible study: 10% misclassification of of pill use

True classification	Cardiovascular disease		Total
	Yes	No	
Yes, classified right (incidence 20%)	1800	7200	9000
Yes, classified wrong (incidence 20%)	200	800	1000
Subtotal	**2000**	**8000**	**10 000**
No, classified right (incidence of 10%)	900	8100	9000
No, classified wrong (incidence 10%)	100	900	1000
Subtotal	**1000**	**9000**	**10 000**
Total of subtotals	**3000**	**17 000**	**20 000**

Table A1(a) shows the reality of the effects of misclassification. The investigator does not, however, know how much misclassification there is. For the investigator the data look like Table A1(c). The reason for this is shown by the reorganization of the data in Table A1(a) and A1(b), and then into A1(c).

The risk of CVD in the cigarette-smoking group with 10 per cent misclassification is 1900/10 000. In the 'not on the pill group' it is 1100/10,000. So the relative risk is

$$\frac{1900/10\,000 =}{1100/10\,000} \quad \frac{0.19 =}{0.11} \quad 1.7$$

Misclassification will, inevitably, arise in measurement of the disease outcome also. Let us now assume that there is 10 per cent misclassification bias there. For simplicity, assume there is no misclassification of cigarette smoking (so use Table A1 as the

Table A1(b) Pill and cardiovascular disease: 10% misclassification of pill use, bold rows as seen by the investigator

Classification of pill use status	Cardiovascular disease		Total
	Yes	No	
Yes, classified right (on the pill so incidence rate is 20%)	1800	7200	9000
Yes, classified wrong (actually not on the pill so incidence rate is 10%)	100	900	1000
Subtotal	**1900**	**8100**	**10 000**
No, classified right (not on the pill so incidence rate is 10%)	900	8100	9000
No, classified wrong (actually on the pill so incidence rate is 20%)	200	800	1000
Subtotal	**1100**	**8900**	**10 000**
Total	3000	17 000	20 000

Table A1(c) Pill and cardiovascular disease: 10% misclassification of pill use and as the investigator sees it

Apparent classification of pill use	Cardiovascular disease		Total
	Yes	No	
Yes	1900	8100	10 000
No	1100	8900	10 000
Total	3000	17 000	20 000

Table A2(a) Pill and cardiovascular disease. Ten per cent misclassification in measurement of disease outcome: reorganization of Table 4.5

True classification of pill status	Cardiovascular disease						Subtotal	Total of subtotals
	Yes			No				
	Classified right	Classified wrong	Subtotal	Classified right	Classified wrong	Subtotal		
Yes	1800	200	2000	7200	800	8000	10 000	
No	900	100	1000	8100	900	9000	10 000	
	2700	300	3000	15 300	1700	17 000	20 000	

Table A2(b) Pill and cardiovascular disease: 10% misclassification in measurement of disease outcome: reorganization of table A1(a)

Oral contraceptive	Cardiovascular disease				Total
	Yes		No		
	Yes correctly classified as CVD	Misclassified as yes	CVD, but misclassified as no	No CVD, correctly classified	
Yes	1800	800*	200†	7200	10 000
No	900	900‡	100§	8100	10 000
	2700	1700	300	15 300	20 000

* 10% of 8000 (row 1, column 3, Table A1); † 10% of 2000 (row 1, column 2, Table A1);
‡ 10% of 9000 (row 2, column 3, Table A1); § 10% of 1000 (row 2, column 2, Table A1).

Table A2(c) Pill and cardiovascular disease. Ten per cent misclassification in measurement of disease outcome: reorganization of table A2(b) to show results as investigator perceives them

Oral contraceptive	Cardiovascular disease		Total
	Yes	No	
Yes	2600	7400	10 000
No	1800	8200	10 000
	4400	15600	20 000

starting point). Before reading on, try to work out the result. Tables A2, b and c give the results.

Before reading on calculate the effects of 10% misclassification of outcome—see Table A2 b.

Now the relative risk is

$$\frac{2600/10\,000 =}{1800/10\,000} \quad \frac{0.26 =}{0.18} \quad 1.44$$

Chapter 5

Cause and effect
The epidemiological approach

Objectives

On completion of the chapter you should understand:

- that the purpose of studying cause and effect in epidemiology is to generate knowledge to prevent, cure, treat and control disease;
- that cause and effect understanding is particularly difficult to achieve in epidemiology because of the long natural history of diseases and because of ethical restraints on human experimentation;
- how causal thinking in epidemiology depends on and contributes to other domains of knowledge, both scientific and non-scientific;
- the potential contributions of epidemiological study designs for making contributions to causal knowledge;
- how to use a systematic approach, which checks for error, chance and bias before reaching judgements on cause and effect;
- that epidemiological approaches to, and guidelines for, causality are not a checklist and therefore conclusions must be carefully judged and tentative;
- the value of synthesizing data from epidemiological studies and other disciplines before reaching conclusions.

5.1 Introduction: causality in science and philosophy

Cause and effect understanding is the highest achievement (the jewel in the crown) of scientific knowledge, including epidemiology. Causal knowledge permits rational plans and actions to break the links between the factors causing disease, and disease itself. It helps to predict the outcome of an intervention and helps to treat disease. To quote Hippocrates, 'To know the causes of a disease and to understand the use of the various methods by which the disease may be prevented amounts to the same thing as being able to cure the disease' (see Chadwick and Mann 1950). This is only a modest exaggeration.

Epidemiology enjoys the status of a science. As in sciences including physics and chemistry, epidemiological understanding of cause and effect does not have to be 100 per cent complete or accurate to permit useful application. Arguably, more so than in other sciences, in epidemiology even partial understanding must be applied as quickly as possible, for it may be a life and death matter. There is, therefore, an ethical responsibility to apply knowledge even when, from a scientific point of view, further research is advised. Yet, this ethical imperative may be perilous.

Early knowledge sometimes has devastating effects and sometimes beneficial effects. Sylvia Tesh (1988) gives two examples. The public health endeavours of the nineteenth century, including the building of sewers, the delivery of clean water, and the improvement of the sanitary conditions of the home and workplace, were driven by the 'miasma' theory of health and disease. This presumed that noxious air was the cause of most of the prevalent diseases, including cholera. Though wrong, the miasma theory worked.

By contrast, according to Tesh, the contagion theory was both correct and dominant in explaining the occurrence of plague. Jews were incriminated in a poorly understood causal pathway of contagion and thousands were executed in a vain attempt to control plague. Tesh gives a figure of 16 000 Jews killed in Strasbourg alone. (Roy Porter gives a figure of 2000 Jews slaughtered in Strasbourg and 12 000 in Mainz.) The contagion theory was ineffective and its crude application was outrageous.

The effective application of incomplete knowledge requires art and science. Epidemiology is one of the principle sciences that public health policy draws upon. Recent examples of major policy decisions requiring the application of incomplete data include: whether to ban consumption of beef products in the light of the epidemic of bovine spongiform encephalopathy in cattle; what action to take in the light of evidence that living near a nuclear power plant is associated with raised risk of childhood leukaemia; what proportion of daily energy intake should be consumed as fat; what is the recommended daily salt intake; whether we should strive to increase the average birth-weight of newborn babies; and whether women should or should not take the contraceptive pill to reduce post-menopausal problems and chronic diseases.

To the study of causality, epidemiology has contributed:

- a philosophy of health and disease
- models that illustrate that philosophy
- frameworks for interpreting and applying the evidence
- study designs to produce quantitative evidence for cause and effect
- information on the relationships between numerous factors and diseases.

The first of these contributions is discussed in Chapters 1 and 2, the second and third are the subject of this chapter (continuing a theme introduced in Chapters 3 and 4), the fourth is the subject of Chapter 9, and the last is a recurrent theme.

Scientific thinking encourages turning empirical observations into theories and hypotheses that permit generalizable cause and effect judgements. This applies to epidemiology, physics and microbiology alike. Epidemiological reasoning on cause and effect is embedded in observations of disease variation, the discovery of associations between putative causes of the variation and the disease and ways of testing hypotheses so associations can progress towards causation. Epidemiology draws upon the reasoning of other disciplines including philosophy and microbiology. Epidemiology shares similar problems of disentangling cause and effect relationships with other disciplines (particularly those mainly reliant on observation of naturally occurring events). Solutions to problems are likely to arise from sharing of ideas among such disciplines.

This understanding is necessary to counter the criticism that epidemiological reasoning on cause and effect is empirical and atheoretical. On a pragmatic note, epidemiological debates on cause and effect are often in the public eye and, more so than most other sciences, non-epidemiologists become involved in the interpretation of data and making judgement on their meaning. This requires that epidemiological approaches to analysis of cause and effect are easy to understand.

The first and difficult question is, what is a cause? Before reading on reflect on this apparently obvious question.

In simple terms, a cause is something which has an effect, that is, it brings about or produces something. In epidemiology a cause can be considered to be something that alters the frequency of disease, health status, or associated factors in a population. These are pragmatic definitions, but it is worth knowing more about the broader debates and controversies on cause, and where such simple ideas fit. This is important so that epidemiologists can converse about cause and effect in multidisciplinary settings, where pragmatic definitions may be questioned or even derided.

Philosophers have grappled with the nature of causality for thousands of years (Cottingham 1996). Aristotle, for example, held a broad view that there were four elements to cause, which have been re-considered in the context of a house by John Dreker, as extracted in Cottingham. The causes of a house are the material (the stone, brick, or wood), the formal (the plan), the efficient (the thing which puts it into effect, here the builder), and the final (the purpose being to create a comfortable home).

Aristotle foresaw one effect could have several causes. The cause of Legionnaires' disease is, at its simplest, exposure to the causal bacteria. From an Aristotelian point of view the four causes would be the existence of living bacteria (material), the essence of the nature of the relationship between bacteria and humans (the formal), the delivery of an infective dose by some mechanism, such as a cooling tower (the efficient), the need for bacteria to survive (they cannot do so for long in aerosol) and the human quest for efficient industrial processes and human comfort that leads to complex water systems such as cooling towers (final).

David Hume's philosophy has also been influential. Hume's view that a cause cannot be deduced logically from the fact that two events are linked, but needs to be experienced or perceived, is crucially important to epidemiology. Just because thunder follows lightning does not mean thunder is caused by lightning (indeed, it is not as we discuss later). When we flick a light switch the light may go on but this does not prove that the one act causes the other. To stretch the imagination, can you think of alternative explanations, no matter how absurd they seem?

Perhaps there is someone observing you and as soon as you flick the switch he puts the light on. This is, indeed, absurd, but it is possible. To someone who had no understanding of electrical circuits it might seem more plausible than the truth. When we understand the mechanism of electrical circuits we accept that there is cause and effect.

This perspective is echoed in the axiom 'association is not causation'. Cause and effect deductions need more than *linkage*; they need understanding. Hume's thoughts are relevant to the debate on black box epidemiology. The black box metaphor comes from the increasing availability of technology as a closed unit, not amenable to easy opening and exploration, e.g. a DVD player, modem or mobile telephone. The unit works, or if it does not it is discarded and replaced, without regard to what the problem is. This has become an apt metaphor for epidemiological research based on the study of associations (risk factor epidemiology) and the evaluation of complex interventions. The late Petr Skrabanek (1994) described it as epidemiology where the causal mechanism behind an association remained unknown but hidden (black) but the inference was that the causal mechanism was within the association (box). Skrabanek argued that the purpose of science is to open and understand the black box, which epidemiology too often failed to do.

The contribution of another philosopher, John Stuart Mill, captured in his canons, is so similar to the modern ideas of epidemiology that it is discussed in the section on guidelines for causality. Philosophical discussion on the nature of causality, questioning whether causes can be stated definitively or only as a matter of probability, is of central importance to epidemiology, but is beyond the scope of this book.

5.2 Epidemiological causal strategy and reasoning: the example of Semmelweis

The epidemiological idea is simple. To reiterate, diseases form patterns, which are ever-changing. Over short time periods the changes are largely, but not exclusively, caused by environmental changes. Over long time periods genetic variation also changes the pattern of disease. Clues to the causes of disease are inherent within these patterns. These patterns, therefore, can be studied both to generate and test ideas on causation and to test out ideas developed in other fields of enquiry. The combination of epidemiological and other types of observation is particularly potent.

The epidemiological mode of reasoning is illustrated by the discovery by Ignaz Semmelweis of the general cause of puerperal fever. Semmelweis (1818–1865) was training in obstetrics in Vienna when he observed that the mortality from childbed fever (now known as puerperal fever) was lower in women attending clinic 2, run by midwives, than in those attending clinic 1, run by doctors. He also noted that women who gave birth in the street, or prematurely, had a lower mortality than those in clinic 1. The statistics he collected are given in Table 5.1. Do these figures spark off any ideas of causation in your mind? Reflect on this question before reading on.

He also noted that while the cases in clinic 2 were sporadic, in clinic 1 a whole row of patients might be sick. Semmelweis was perplexed but saw that the pattern he observed meant an endemic cause, that is, the cause lay within the clinic itself. He tried, unsuccessfully, to solve the problem by delivering the mothers by lying them on their sides rather than on their backs.

Table 5.1 Births, deaths, and mortality rates (%) for all patients at the two clinics of the Vienna maternity hospital from 1841 to 1846

First clinic (doctors)			Second clinic (midwives)		
Births	Deaths	Rate	Births	Deaths	Rate
20042	1989	9.92	17791	691	3.38

Extracted and adapted from Semmelweis as reprinted in Buck *et al*. (p. 47).

A year or so later, in 1847, his colleague and friend Professor Kolletschka died following a fingerprick with a knife used at an autopsy. Kolletschka's own autopsy showed inflammation to be widespread, with peritonitis and meningitis. Semmelweis's mind was alert and he connected the disease in women with that of his friend. He wrote

> Day and night I was haunted by the image of Kolletschka's disease and was forced to recognise, ever more decisively that the disease from which Kolletschka died was identical to that from which so many maternity patients died.

Semmelweis (1983, p. 52)

Semmelweis was 'compelled to ask' whether cadaverous particles had been introduced into the vascular systems of maternity patients, as in the case of his friend.

Semmelweis's inspired idea was that particles had been transferred from the scalpel to the vascular system of his friend and that the same kind of particles were killing maternity patients. He foresaw that the particles could be transferred from the hands of medical students and doctors to the women during pelvic examinations. If so, something stronger than ordinary soap was needed for handwashing. He introduced chlorina liquida, and then for economy, chlorinated lime. The maternal mortality rate plummeted, reaching the level of the midwives' clinic.

Although Semmelweis was not the first to link puerperal fever to lack of hygiene, his contribution was huge, particularly because of the systematic evidence he accumulated and the way he tested his ideas (hypotheses). The epidemiological observations outlined the problem and prepared the mind to seek a solution, itself inspired by clinical and autopsy observation, and tested by experimentation and epidemiological monitoring.

Two great principles are illustrated by this work. First, deep and generalizable knowledge lies in the explanation of disease patterns, rather than in their description. The questioning mind may solve the riddle inherent in the pattern. Second, inspiration is needed, and may come from unexpected sources, as here from Kolletschka's autopsy. Such inspiration needs to be converted into a scientific hypothesis so it can be tested by scientific observation or experiment, as by Semmelweis's intervention of handwashing with chlorinated lime.

Most disease patterns remain unexplained, despite lengthy study, and others are never explored fully (so called cul-de-sac epidemiology). Those that are explained usually lead to profound insights. Epidemiology does not, however, have the tools to demonstrate disease mechanisms. Whether the cause is biochemical, as in scurvy, or social, as in the rise of suicide in populations hit by unemployment, epidemiologists are reliant on other sciences to be equal partners in pursuit of the mechanisms. Action cannot always await understanding of the mechanism. A contemporary example of this is the use of epidemiological data showing that lying an infant on its front (prone position) to sleep raises the risk of 'cot death' or sudden infant death syndrome. Yet the prone position was long advocated as a means of avoiding the potential danger of infants inhaling their own vomit. A campaign to persuade parents to lay their infants on their backs has halved the incidence of cot death. In countries where the evidence has not been implemented we have seen no such change. The mechanism is yet to be fully explained.

5.3 Models of cause in epidemiology

5.3.1 Interplay of host, agent, and environment

The idea that disease is virtually *always* a result of the interplay of the environment, the genetic and physical make-up of the individual, and the agent of disease, is one of the most important of the cause and effect ideas underpinned by epidemiology. This theory applies both to diseases said to be multifactorial (e.g. cancers or heart disease) and to diseases which are by their definition a result of a single cause, such as tuberculosis, a drug side-effect or an overdose.

Diseases attributed to single causes are invariably so by definition. For example, tuberculosis is a disease which has many manifestations. It is characterized by a multiplicity of diffuse signs and symptoms which affect nearly every part of the body. Some diseases, for example sarcoidosis, are often indistinguishable from tuberculosis clinically, while the microscopic finding in Crohn's disease looks very similar to tuberculosis. In some ways tuberculosis is a number of diseases (e.g. pulmonary tuberculosis, cutaneous tuberculosis, tuberculous meningitis), some of which are indistinguishable from other diseases. The fact that 'tuberculosis' is 'caused' by the tubercle bacillus is a matter of definition. In fact the causes of tuberculosis are many, including malnutrition and overcrowding.

This idea is captured by several well-known disease causation models, such as the line, the triangle, the wheel, and the web. These models help to organize ideas about causes and about strategies to prevent and control disease. Figure 5.1 illustrates the idea of the line of causation. First, an arbitrary division is made between genetic and all other causes, categorized by convention as the environment. The line conceptualizes causes as lying

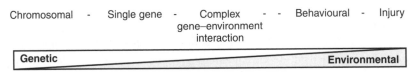

Fig. 5.1 Line of causation—a simple tool for considering genetic and environmental factors.

on a spectrum from being wholly caused by genetic factors or by environmental ones. Although the interaction of the genome and the environment is the key to understanding causation, the gene—environment division, though artificial, is widely used as a simple first step in analysing causes. At one extreme lie disorders which are almost entirely genetic, such as Down's syndrome (trisomy 21). At the other extreme lies injury arising from a road traffic accident. Most disorders lie in between. One of the early judgements required on diseases of unknown cause is the likely relative importance of genetic and environmental factors, for the preventive or control strategy will be fundamentally different. Try the exercise in Box 5.1 before reading on.

Figure 5.2 shows how epidemiology can help to make judgements on the question in Box 5.1. Diseases where the incidence varies rapidly over time or is much different in genetically similar groups are strongly influenced by environmental factors, while diseases which have a stable incidence or are clustered in blood relatives are more likely to have strong genetic influences. Figure 5.3 places some diseases on this spectrum.

In analysing causes it is advisable to move from simple to complex models. The triangle, wheel, and the web are more complex versions of the same concept as the epidemiological line. Each model has its strengths and limitations for helping to clarify causal thinking. Each model is, however, a simplification. The categories of host, agent, and environment (Fig. 5.4) are arbitrary. While the meaning of the words host and agent of disease are self-evident, or can be illustrated with simple examples (Tables 5.2 and 5.3), this is not the case for the environment, which has an immensely broad meaning (Table 5.4). The host and agent are, of course, both part of the environment. The environment, in this context, is arbitrarily defined to mean factors other than the host and the agent of disease. The environment, in particular, can be split to some benefit into several categories, such as the chemical or physical environment.

Tables 5.2, 5.3 and 5.4 list some of the many host, agent, and environmental factors which are generally important causes of individual and population level variations in human disease. Of the factors listed in Table 5.2, age is the most powerful, and for many diseases, particularly of the reproductive tract, sex equally so.

In using epidemiological comparisons to spark *new* understanding of disease causation, it is essential that the populations compared are alike in *known* causal factors, of which age and sex are the most important. Hence the almost routine use of age and sex

Box 5.1 Exercise on gene—environment interaction

Think about three or four health problems or diseases that you or your friends or relatives have had. Place them on the line of causation. (Use these diseases for the following exercises too.)

Think through the cause of disease X using this model (Box 1.6, Chapter 1). What is your judgement? Is disease X likely to be genetic or environmental? Why?

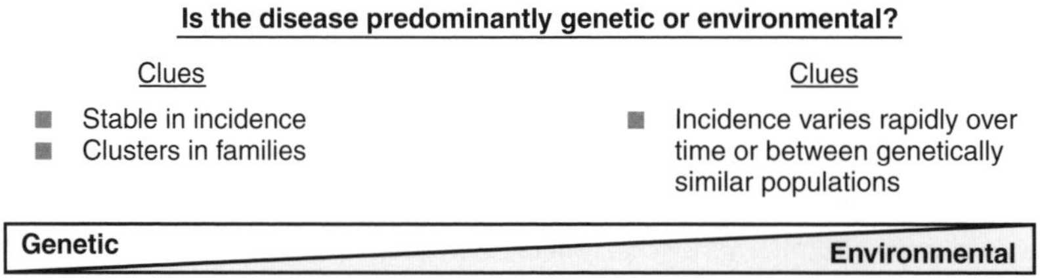

Is the disease predominantly genetic or environmental?

Clues

- Stable in incidence
- Clusters in families

Clues

- Incidence varies rapidly over time or between genetically similar populations

Genetic ———————————————————————— Environmental

Fig. 5.2 Line of causation: epidemiological clues to environment or genetic causation.

matching or adjustment techniques in causal epidemiology (Chapter 7). This said, even for variables such as age and sex, the causal effects and mechanisms are complex and cannot usually be specified as biosocial mechanisms. For example, at any age, women have a lower incidence of cardiovascular diseases such as myocardial infarction (heart attack). This sex difference is well characterized but the mechanisms cannot be specified and are likely to involve a mix of genetic, behavioural, and social factors. The human genome project is expected to lead to rapid growth in such understanding.

Before reading on do the exercise in Box 5.2.

The triangle is a useful model for analysing interactive causal relationships and to derive public health strategies, as shown in Figs 5.5 and 5.6, for example, for the control of Legionnaires' disease. In this and other infectious diseases the concept of the disease agent is central to causation, and usually a specific agent can be identified or assumed.

Box 5.2 Analysing disease using the triangle of causations

Reconsider your chosen health problems (Box 5.1) using the triangle of causation (Fig. 5.4). Also, think through the cause of disease X (Box 1.6, Chapter 1) using this model.

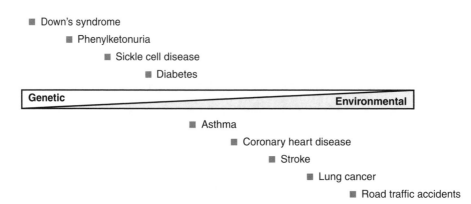

- Down's syndrome
  - Phenylketonuria
    - Sickle cell disease
      - Diabetes

Genetic ———————————————————————— Environmental

- Asthma
  - Coronary heart disease
    - Stroke
      - Lung cancer
        - Road traffic accidents

Fig. 5.3 Line of causation: examples of disease/health problems.

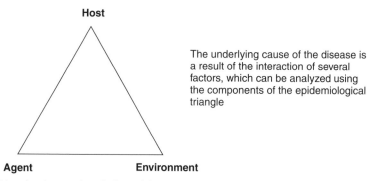

Host

The underlying cause of the disease is a result of the interaction of several factors, which can be analyzed using the components of the epidemiological triangle

Agent   **Environment**

Fig. 5.4 Triangle of causation. (Adapted from Mausner and Kramer 1985; see Permissions).

In explaining population differences in the pattern of disease, agent factors, examples of which are in Table 5.3, arguably receive less attention than they deserve. This is possibly because in infectious disease epidemiology characterizing the virulence of organisms is difficult and sometimes impossible, and in other diseases conceptualizing the cause as an agent is not easy. The issue of agent virulence is likely to be considered more carefully in future. The reason is that the genome of most pathogenic bacteria is being mapped and understanding of gene variants associated with virulence is growing fast. The bacterium *Helicobacter pylori*, for example, is associated with severe inflammation and duodenal ulceration in 89 per cent of infections with the VacAsla strains and 20 per cent of infections with the vac s2 strain. Virulence genes can be identified and can be removed to create organisms that are not pathogenic to humans.

Traditionally the concept of the disease agent has been applied to infections. It works well with many non-infectious agents; for example, cigarettes, motor cars, and alcohol can be considered as the agents of disease and injury. A reduction of the tar content of cigarettes, and hence their virulence (in the literal sense of being toxic or very harmful to health) could be responsible for some of the recent reduction of lung cancer incidence. The interaction of the host, agent, and environment is rarely understood. For example, the effect of cigarette smoking is substantially greater in poor people than in rich people. The reason is unclear. It may be that there is an interaction between the agent

Table 5.2 Causes of diseases: examples of host factors

Age
Sex
Previous disability
Behaviours (such as smoking)
Genetic inheritance
Height and weight

Table 5.3 Causes of diseases: examples of agent factors

Virulence of organism
Serotype of organism
Antibiotic resistance
Cigarette—tar content
Type of glass in motor car windscreen

(cigarettes), susceptibility due to host factors such as nutritional status, or environmental factors such as air quality in the home, in the residential neighbourhood or in the workplace. These ideas are illustrated below in the simpler context of Legionnaires' disease.

Legionnaires' disease is a pneumonia (an inflammation of the lungs) which presents with some atypical features. It results from the inhalation, by susceptible people, of virulent organisms belonging to the genus Legionellacae (legionellas for short). The organisms which cause Legionnaires' disease are environmentally acquired. The causal microorganism is found in most natural waters and is usually harmless. It is, therefore, a simplification to say that this normally harmless bacterium is the cause of Legionnaires' disease. Such a view could lead to erroneous, costly and ineffective action to control this disease through attempts to eliminate this widely distributed organism from water.

The underlying cause of Legionnaires' disease lies in the creation by humans of water systems which permit the organism to thrive and be aerosolized at sufficient concentration to cause human disease. The ageing of the population, the presence of immunocompromised people and of people who impair their lung's defence mechanisms by smoking are also important causal factors. The bacterium, which is not normally a human pathogen, finds itself interacting with humans in this environment. The triangle of causality provides a framework for this type of reasoning, as illustrated in Fig. 5.5. An understanding of the range of causes permits the development of a rational preventive strategy as shown in Fig. 5.6. Before reading on do the exercise in Box 5.3.

In a systematic analysis based on a model as shown in Figs 5.5 and 5.6, attention is deflected from the microorganism as a specific cause, to the environment, host, and agent as interacting causes. This thinking broadens the control strategy. On current thinking the most effective approaches are to design better complex water systems, and to use hygiene and chemical measures to inhibit bacterial growth.

Table 5.5 shows how the epidemiological triangle can be combined with the schema of the levels of prevention to devise a comprehensive framework for thinking about

Box 5.3 Reflection on the value of models

Consider how your thinking on the cause of Legionnaires' disease has changed as a result of the analysis in Figs 5.5 and 5.6.

Table 5.4 Causes of diseases: examples of environmental factors

Home overcrowding
Air composition
Workplace hygiene
Weather
Water composition
Food contamination
Animal/human contact
Cooling tower use

possible preventive actions. Primary prevention is action to prevent the disease or problem from actually arising, secondary prevention is the early detection of the problem to prevent its damaging effects, and tertiary prevention is to contain, and if possible reverse, the damage already done. (As an aside, most clinicians and policy-makers working in clinical settings combine tertiary prevention with the secondary prevention category calling it secondary prevention. Epidemiologists and public health scientists, in this context, usually conform to this simpler schema.) It is worth re-emphasizing that these frameworks are there to aid thinking. Before reading on do the exercise in Box 5.4.

Box 5.4 Combining causal models and the levels of prevention

Think about the control of the three or four health problems you picked and disease X (Chapter 1, Box 1.6) using the triangle and the levels of prevention.

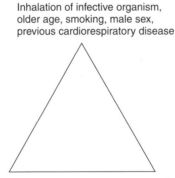

Host:
Inhalation of infective organism, older age, smoking, male sex, previous cardiorespiratory disease

Agent:
Virulent Legionella organisms, e.g. pneumophila serotype

Environment:
Presence of cooling towers and complex hot water systems; aerosols created but not contained; meteorological conditions that take aerosol to humans

Fig. 5.5 Analysis of the causes of Legionnaires' disease: triangle of causation.

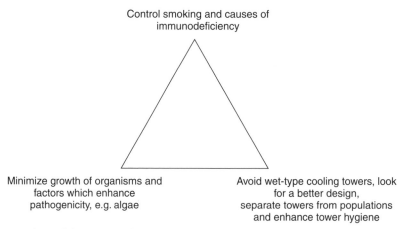

Fig. 5.6 Analysis of the control of Legionnaires' disease: triangle of causation.

Figure 5.7 shows the wheel of causation. The principles behind this model are as for the triangle, but it emphasizes the unity of the interacting factors. The genetic make-up of the individual and its expression in the body (called the phenotype) is shown as the hub of the wheel, but enveloped within an interacting environment. This version of the model emphasizes the fact that the division of the environment into components is somewhat arbitrary.

In Fig. 5.8 the wheel model is applied to phenylketonuria, the classic genetic disorder. Phenylketonuria is an autosomal single gene disease (autosomal means it is not on the sex chromosomes). As a result, an enzyme required to metabolize the dietary amino acid phenylalanine and turn it into tyrosine is deficient, and so phenylalanine accumulates in the blood. Brain damage is the outcome. Early diagnosis, usually through screening, and a diet low in phenylalanine can prevent the disease. The cause of this disease could be said to be a faulty gene. The cause of the disease is combination of a faulty gene, exposure to a diet containing a high amount of phenylalanine (about 15 per cent of the protein of most natural foods), and in the case of failure of diagnosis and dietary advice, a social environment unable to protect the child.

Table 5.5 Control of Legionnaires' disease: triangle and levels of prevention

	Agent	**Host**	**Environment**
Primary	Design and hygiene	Smoking and general health	Use and location of cooling towers
Secondary	Hygiene	Nil	Separate people from source once outbreak has occurred e.g. in a hospital ward
Tertiary	Nil	Medical therapy	Close cooling towers; repair

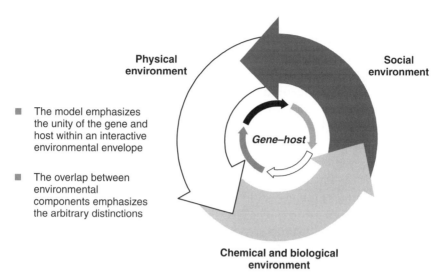

Fig. 5.7 Wheel of causation (Adapted from Mausner and Kramer 1985).

For many disorders such as coronary heart disease, and many cancers, our understanding of the causes is highly complex. Either the causes are truly complex, or equally likely, our understanding is too poor to permit clarity. These disorders are referred to as multifactorial or polyfactorial disorders. As argued earlier, all disorders have several causes and where that is not the case, it is simply a matter of our causal definition. In disorders with multifactorial causation often no specific causes are known, many factors appear to be important, and mechanisms of causation are not apparent.

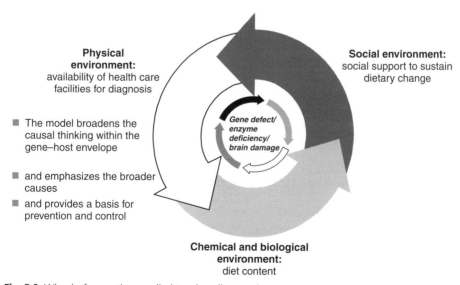

Fig. 5.8 Wheel of causation applied to phenylketonuria.

The complexity of these multifactorial diseases is not adequately captured by the line, wheel, and triangle concepts (which remain useful nonetheless) and is better portrayed by the metaphor of the spider's web. In some portrayals the web is shown as a highly schematized diagram, more like an electronic circuit or an underground transport map. Such portrayals tend to underestimate the complexity and overestimate the state of understanding. The web, as shown in Fig. 5.9, emphasizes the interconnections among the postulated causes. This model, more than the others, indicates the potential for the disease to influence the causes and not just the other way around. For example, lack of exercise may be one of the causes of heart disease and osteoporosis but these diseases can also cause people to stop exercising (called reverse causality). The metaphor of the web permits the still broader causal question: where is the spider that spun the web? (after Krieger 1994). The question can be answered at a number of levels, for example, evolutionary biology, social structures, economics and role of industries. The relatively simple analysis of heart disease causation using the web concept begins to illustrate the great complexity of this disease (see Fig. 5.10).

The purpose of models is to simplify reality and promote understanding. The web permits us to grasp the complexity of multifactorial diseases but the line, triangle and the wheel help us to focus on their essentials. Before reading on do the exercise in Box 5.5.

Box 5.5 Analysing disease using the wheel and web models

Review the health problems or diseases that you picked and disease X (Chapter 1, Box 1.6) using the wheel and web models.

- There is no single cause

- Causes of disease are interacting

- Disentangling causes is almost impossible

- Causality may be two way

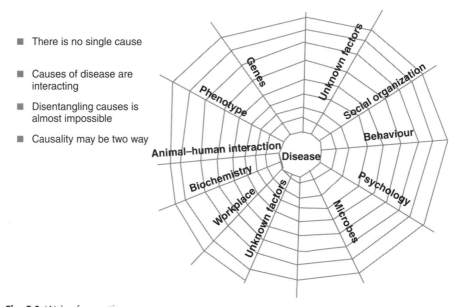

Fig. 5.9 Web of causation.

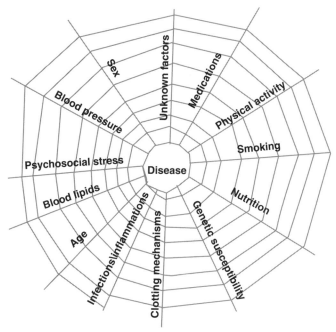

Fig. 5.10 Web of causation and coronary heart disease.

Models provide a means of analysing causal pathways and a foundation for the application of epidemiological knowledge to public health action. Narrow causal thinking based on single causes, in contrast, can mislead epidemiologists into prematurely believing that a problem has been resolved and can seriously distort public health action. Models also help to lay out what is and what is not known and hence to direct research. These causal models also help us to understand the ideas of necessary or sufficient causes.

5.3.2 Necessary and sufficient cause, proximal and distal cause and the interacting component causes, models

Epidemiological thinking on causality has been deeply influenced by the concepts of necessary and sufficient cause, which are easily confused. The fourth (2001) edition of *Last's Dictionary* (p 121) tells us that a necessary cause is 'A causal factor whose presence is required for the occurrence of the effect'. It defines sufficient cause as a 'minimum set of conditions, factors or events needed to produce a given outcome'. A sufficient cause does not require any other determinant for a disease to occur. A factor, or a group of factors, whose presence leads to an effect is a sufficient cause, so some causes of diseases are said to be sufficient in themselves to induce disease while others are said to be necessary components in a larger jigsaw of causes. To take a simple example, the tubercle bacillus is required to cause tuberculosis but, alone, does not always cause it, so it is a necessary, not a sufficient, cause. In other words, a single factor does not cause this disease. This is, of course, the key message of the causal models discussed in the previous section.

The problem is that a cause on its own rarely induces a disease except in the case of extremely serious genetic defects. The necessary and sufficient causes model has theoretical value for analysing causes, but in epidemiology, as Susser (1977) points out, most causal factors are neither necessary nor sufficient, but contributory.

Consider the causes of Down's syndrome (trisomy 21), sickle cell disease, tuberculosis, scurvy, phenylketonuria, and lung cancer. If the cause is sufficient its presence, alone, would induce the disease and if it is necessary, in its absence the disease would not occur. (The reader may wish to reflect on this matter before continuing.)

Down's syndrome is the name given to a disorder where a person has a highly characteristic appearance (leading to the previous name, mongolism), and who will inevitably be mentally retarded because they have three copies of chromosome 21 instead of two (trisomy 21). This genetic feature is a sufficient cause of Down's syndrome. In other words, this chromosome abnormality alone will lead to the characteristics that define Down's syndrome. At present we have no way of influencing this.

Sickle cell disease (two sickle cell gene alleles per cell) is a genetically inherited condition. The position is not quite the same as for Down's syndrome because the word disease leads to an expectation that the person has, or will develop, a health problem. The presence of sickle cell genes is a necessary cause of sickle cell disease. In milder cases especially, external stimuli such as infections are required to cause clinical disease. Here we have another example (phenylketonuria was discussed earlier) of genes being necessary but not always sufficient causes.

Scurvy occurs when there is insufficient vitamin C in the diet to maintain health, usually due to lack of fruit and vegetables. This does not occur in natural circumstances, but does when a restricted diet is taken, as in the past by sailors, and nowadays by food faddists or the mentally disturbed. Vitamin C insufficiency is a necessary and sufficient cause of scurvy. By definition, other diseases, several of which look like scurvy, are not scurvy unless there is a lack of vitamin C. Yet, dietary insufficiency of vitamin C is unnatural, so other factors, in practice, come into play.

For tuberculosis, exposure to the bacillus is necessary but alone it is insufficient in most people to cause disease, and in many people the organism lives harmlessly in the host. For both tuberculosis and scurvy, contributory causes include poor nutritional and socio-economic conditions. These increase both the risk of exposure to the necessary cause and, for tuberculosis, increase the likelihood of the organism actually establishing a clinically important infection.

For phenylketonuria, the necessary cause is a genetic defect and that together with a diet containing normal amounts of phenylalanine is sufficient (Fig. 5.8). For lung cancer tobacco smoke is neither necessary nor sufficient, for there are many other causes. Some smokers do not develop the disease and some non-smokers do.

The above analysis begins to show the strengths and weaknesses of the necessary/sufficient cause concept. When a specific cause of disease is well known it can be incorporated into its definition (as in Down's syndrome, sickle cell disease, and vitamin C deficiency). At that point the specific cause becomes necessary by definition. For complex multifactorial diseases, at least at present, there are no necessary causes. The example of lung cancer illustrates this well. In practice, except for unusual or unhelpful scenarios (e.g. a bolt of lightning, or falling off a cliff), there are no single sufficient factors that inevitably lead to chronic diseases or death. Old age (or perhaps birth!) is probably the only sufficient cause of death. The concept of sufficient causes has, therefore, veered from single causes to group causes.

Rothman's interacting component causes model (Fig. 5.11) has emphasized that the causes of disease comprise a constellation of factors. It has broadened the sufficient cause concept to be a minimal set of conditions which together inevitably produce the disease. Different combinations of these factors may cause the disease. Figure 5.11 is a simplified version of Rothman's ideas. Three combinations of factors (ABC, BED, AEC) are shown here as sufficient causes of the disease. Each of the constituents of the causal 'pie' is necessary, and hence contributes to 100 per cent of the risk of disease attributed to that particular combination of causes. The factors are conceived to act in a biological sequence which determines the period between the beginning of causal action and the initiation of disease. It follows that control of the disease could be achieved by removing one of the components in each 'pie'. If there were a factor common to all 'pies' the disease would be eliminated by removing that factor alone. In this case removing factor A would remove all the disease caused by the first and third constellation of causes. This mode of reasoning, and model, is hard to apply to specific diseases but has considerable theoretical value.

A sequence of causes can be considered in terms of time, and also in terms of space. Causes that are close to the individual—in terms of time or space—are sometimes referred to as proximal causes, in the sense of near to. Those that are distant are called distal causes in the sense of away from. To give an example, proximal causes of lung cancer would be smoking cigarettes and exposure to radiation. Distal causes would be poor diet, poverty, or tobacco farming. Distal causes are sometimes referred to as upstream.

The problem with these complex models, in practice, is that we do not have the knowledge to define even a sufficient constellation of causes i.e. we cannot define the 'pies' in Fig 5.11. The components of the pies, as sufficient causes, must be acting differently

Each of the three components of the interacting constellations of causes (ABC, BED, AEC) are in themselves sufficient and each is necessary

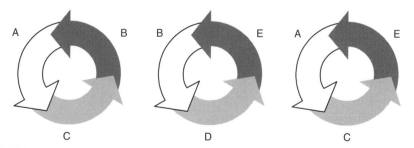

Fig. 5.11 Interacting component causes (Adapted from Rothman and Greenland 1998; see Permissions).

than if they were separate (when they do not cause disease). There is therefore, a modification of the biological effect, i.e. biological interaction that leads to disease. The model is, therefore, useful in thinking about the issues discussed in Chapter 4, Section 4.2.5.

The model is also pertinent to thinking about the strength of the association (Section 5.4.2) and relative and attributable risk (Sections 8.4 and 8.6). Interested readers should consult Rothman's writings.

5.4 Guidelines (elsewhere criteria) for epidemiological reasoning on cause and effect

5.4.1 Comparison of epidemiological and other guidelines for causal reasoning

Turning epidemiological data into an understanding of cause and effect is challenging. To convince colleagues and the public, epidemiologists need an explicit mode of reasoning. There is a myth that there is no subjectivity in science, but in practice scientists, like all other human beings, rely on intuition in evaluating evidence and making judgements. For instance, Einstein intuitively understood the theory of relativity years before he published it and before there was empirical evidence to support the predictions. The theorems of the mathematical genius Srinivasan Ramanujan were intuitive and many have yet to be resolved, though they are generally accepted as correct on the basis of precedent. Subjective judgements on cause and effect in epidemiology should not be dismissed but tested empirically. Epidemiologists place much emphasis on the evaluation of empirical data, and have devised (and adopted from other disciplines) so-called criteria for causality. Criteria is an inappropriate word, as it encourages a checklist approach. Guidelines is better.

The use of such guidelines for reaching causal judgements in epidemiology is controversial. They are not, and must not be used as, a checklist or algorithm for causality. There is no causality score. Rothman (1998) provides a vigorous discussion of the limitations of causal guidelines as stated so clearly by Bradford Hill. Clearly, such guidelines should be seen as a framework for thought about the evidence including from non-epidemiological studies.

The epidemiological mode of causal reasoning comes under frequent attack, particularly from people and organizations who do not agree with particular research findings. The more serious criticisms are that epidemiologists' reasoning lacks a theoretical basis and it falls short of the more rigorous thinking in the experimental sciences. These criticisms are unhelpful and unjustified. Causal thinking in epidemiology draws upon the theories and principles of other disciplines including philosophy, the laboratory sciences, and the social sciences (see Table 5.6 and below) and is theoretically grounded, though this may not be obvious. Epidemiology is predominantly an observational and not experimental science, as are demography, geology, evolutionary biology, palaeontology, and archaeology. Epidemiology is far more complex than most sciences and experimentation in epidemiology is strictly limited by ethical constraints on human research.

Epidemiology has, moreover, contributed new ways of thinking about causality when experiment is not possible. Epidemiological guidelines are, however, designed for thinking about the causes of disease in populations and not in individuals. When applied to the individual, as in the courtroom, they may be wanting.

Table 5.6 summarizes some of the cause and effect thinking in microbiology, health economics, philosophy, and epidemiology. There are commonalities of reasoning. The approach to establishing causality in the experimental medical sciences is illustrated by the Henle–Koch postulates as discussed in detail by Susser (1977) (Table 5.6, column 1). These postulates also have limitations. First, the organism must be present in every case. This is impossible to show for many bacterial diseases including tuberculosis. (In clinical practice a trial of anti-tuberculosis therapy is common when the patient has a clinical picture of tuberculosis but the organism cannot be grown in the laboratory.) Second, the organism must be grown in pure culture. Viral organisms are particularly hard to grow, and so are some bacteria such as the mycobacterium causing leprosy. Third, when inoculated into a susceptible animal (or human) the specific disease should occur. Animal models are sometimes not available, and even when they are the induced disease may be different from the human version. Fourth, the organism must be recovered from the animal (or human).

The Henle–Koch postulates are a counsel of perfection and too stringent. Evans (1978) points out that even when they were developed it was recognized that they were not to be applied rigidly, and that Koch believed that the cholera bacillus caused cholera even though the postulates were not achieved. According to Evans, leprosy, typhoid fever, syphilis, malaria, mycoplasma pneumonia, and *Chlamydia trachomatis* infection are among the microbial diseases which have causes that still do not meet the criteria. Further, with new technologies such as antibody tests and DNA sequencing available the postulates are being superseded. Epidemiologists need to be aware of such criteria, both as a standard to incorporate into their own work, and so they can discuss causality in the context of infectious disease epidemiology.

Philosophers' ideas were considered in Section 5.1. John Stuart Mill (1806–73) was a British philosopher and economist who succinctly offered a practical interpretation of causal thinking in philosophy, the nub of which is now known as Mill's canons (Table 5.6, column 2). Susser (1977) has discussed these in the epidemiological context. The principles are of paramount importance to epidemiology and are essentially incorporated into its own guidelines. The method of concomitant variation corresponds to current ideas on correlation and association (see section 9.11.5); the method of agreement to the search for a factor in common (e.g. in an outbreak of Legionnaires' disease all those sick may have been to a particular air-conditioned hotel); the method of difference is at the core of epidemiological thinking (e.g. why do some people get heart disease and others of the same age and sex do not?); and the method of residues echoes modern ideas of experiments of preventive action, to establish what proportion of disease can be prevented, or where this is not possible, calculations of attributable risk (see Chapter 8). (Readers should note that the order in which the canons are presented in Table 5.6 does not correspond to Mills's numbering of his canons, e.g. the method of concomitant variation is the fifth in his list.)

Table 5.6 A comparison of four modes of thinking about causality

Microbiology: Henle–Koch's postulates	Philosophy: Mill's canons[1]	Economics[2]	Epidemiology: guidelines for causality[3]
The microorganism causing the disease can be demonstrated in every case of the disease	Method of concomitant variation: the phenomenon which varies when another phenomenon varies in a specific way is either a cause, an effect, or connected through some fact of causation	The future cannot predict the present	The cause precedes the effect (temporality)
The organism can be isolated and grown in pure culture	Method of agreement: if there is only one circumstance in common in instances of the phenomenon, then the common circumstance is the cause of effect	The effect (y) can be predicted more accurately by using values of the cause (x) than by not using them	The disease is commoner in those exposed to the cause (strength)
Animals (or humans) exposed to the cultured organism develop the disease	Method of difference: if there is only one difference in the circumstances when a phenomenon occurs compared with when it does not occur, that difference is part of the cause or effect	Instantaneous causation does not exist, since there is a time difference between independent actions. If A, itself, causes B, and A did not exist, B would not have occurred	The amount of exposure relates to the amount of disease (dose–response)
The organism can be grown from the experimentally exposed animal (or human)	The method of residues: remove from the phenomenon any part known to be the effect of known antecedents (causes), and the remainder is the effect of the remaining antecedents	One cause can have many effects and one effect many causes	The causes are linked to diseases in specific and relevant ways (specificity)
		The putative cause A may have an effect by itself or be a part of the cause	Altering the amount of exposure to the cause leads to change in the disease pattern (experiment or natural experiment)
			Different types of studies reach similar conclusions (consistency)

[1] Note: Mill's canons have been paraphrased from original quotations given in Susser (1977, pp. 70–71).

[2] The discussion of causal thinking in economics comes from Charemza and Deadman (1997) and from Hicks (1979).

[3] The guidelines for causality have been reduced to six by the author, for simplicity. Biological plausibility is discussed in the text and is, strictly, not an epidemiological concept.

Economics also evaluates associations in similar ways (Table 5.6, column 3). Even more than epidemiology, health economics relies on observation and modelling, with the scope for experiment being extremely limited. According to Charemza and Deadman (1997), the operational meaning of causality in economics is more on the lines of 'to predict' than 'to produce' (an effect). A scan of the third and fourth columns shows the similarity in concept, if not detail, between economics and epidemiology.

The nub of epidemiological reasoning (Table 5.6, column 4) is that the cause:

◆ must precede the effect

◆ should raise the incidence of the disease in a population

◆ should have a greater effect in greater quantity

◆ be associated with specific and relevant effects

◆ should show consistent effects across a number of studies.

These epidemiological ideas are similar to Mill's canons and to thinking in health economics.

Evidence from experiment, natural or by design, on humans or animals, may show that manipulating exposures changes the disease. Experiment may elucidate the mechanisms by which this happens. The cause–effect relationship should make biological sense. These latter ideas, now integral to epidemiology, are those of the other biological sciences, including the Henle–Koch postulates. The epidemiological guidelines for causality are not an idiosyncratic epidemiological invention. Their validity, as a collective, has not, however, been assessed empirically.

In the modern era an amalgam of epidemiological and basic science criteria are adopted as the standard for causal thinking, as shown in the example in Box 5.6 and in the ensuing examples. Can you see the links between the evidence in Box 5.6 and causal guidelines in Table 5.6? Which of these pieces of evidence match the guidelines for causality? Try this question before reading on.

In the case of Kaposi's sarcoma (Box 5.6) the first and second items of evidence match the ideas underpinning the Henle–Koch postulates. The third and fourth match epidemiological concepts (strength of association) and the data could be converted to a measure of strength such as relative risk (see Chapter 8). The fifth item is a mixture of microbiology (distribution in tissues) and epidemiology (transmission). The sixth item is, again, epidemiology, as is the seventh (temporality).

The emergent principle is this: causation is established by judgement on the basis of evidence from all disciplines. Failure to meet some guidelines (with the exception that the cause must precede the effect, which is not easy to establish conclusively) does not dismiss causality and achievement of some guidelines does not ensure it.

Epidemiology may establish cause in populations unequivocally but this information only applies to individuals in a probabilistic way, which does not prove cause and effect at the individual level. If 90 per cent of all lung cancer in a population is due to smoking, and assuming that is correct, what is the likelihood that in an individual with lung cancer the cause was smoking?

Box 5.6 Aetiology of Kaposi's sarcoma: Evidence cited for a herpesvirus as the cause

1 Viral sequences (DNA) can be detected in sarcoma tissues in most cases.

2 Such sequences are rarely detected in other tissues.

3 Virus is detected in blood cells in 50 per cent of cases but not in controls.

4 HIV positive patients who had the virus in blood cells had a greater risk of developing sarcoma than comparable patients without the virus.

5 The virus is probably sexually transmitted and is found in semen and other genital tissues of healthy adults.

6 Antibody levels in blood correlate with presence of sarcoma.

7 Antibody levels rise before Kaposi's sarcoma appears.

Conclusion: Kaposi's sarcoma is caused by a herpesvirus.

Beiser (1997, p. 581)

The answer is that we do not know. If the person is a non-smoker the cancer may have arisen from passive exposure to tobacco but is more likely to be due to other factors. If the person is a smoker the cause is most likely smoking, but may result from other factors such as exposure to radiation or asbestos. There is no way, at present, to distinguish a lung cancer resulting from smoking from a lung cancer arising from another cause.

A drug or public health intervention may be effective in a population but harmful to an individual. For example, exercise may be good generally but lead to collapse and death in some individuals. Some people are harmed by alcohol and others benefit and the net effect on the health of the population as a whole is unclear. In contrast, the net health effect of tobacco consumption is overwhelmingly negative. This kind of counterintuitive observation lies at the heart of disputes between population scientists and those whose work is based on individuals. Immunization may or may not harm individuals as is so often claimed (MMR and autism, and whopping cough vaccine and neurological disorders), but the benefits far outweigh these harms as population level (epidemiological studies) show. To prove harm in these particular circumstances, i.e. to the individual, is beyond epidemiology (and requires other kinds of sciences). Equally, to prove there is no harm to individuals is also impossible for epidemiology. We can, however, show there is no sizeable harm to the population.

Epidemiological data are difficult to apply in legal cases about individuals. To quote Evans discussing the issue in the USA:

> Legal requirements are concerned with the risk in the *individual*, the plaintiff, and whether the preponderance of evidence supports the conclusion that *that* exposure 'more likely than not' resulted in *that* illness or injury in *that* person.

(1978, p. 194)

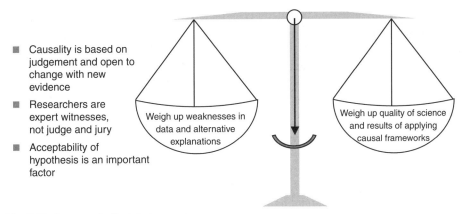

- Causality is based on judgement and open to change with new evidence
- Researchers are expert witnesses, not judge and jury
- Acceptability of hypothesis is an important factor

Weigh up weaknesses in data and alternative explanations

Weigh up quality of science and results of applying causal frameworks

Fig. 5.12 Cause and effect: judgement.

Evans contests that a higher order of proof and specificity is required in legal proof than in epidemiological proof, concluding that epidemiological evidence is often inapplicable in this context. Epidemiology is a science based on studies of groups and cannot be directly applicable to individuals, and this is an inherent limitation. Equally, a factor demonstrated to cause a disease in an individual, by a science of individuals, say toxicology or pathology, may not be demonstrable as harmful in the population, possibly because harmful effects are balanced by beneficial ones. This is an inherent limitation of a science of individuals. The problem lies not with epidemiology itself, but with those who apply epidemiology in these circumstances. (The law too will extrapolate from population data to the individual.) The standard of proof in epidemiology is not of a lower order than in law, it is of a different order. The problem is that so often the best we can offer the individual is average risk derived from the study of groups similar to that individual. That is a limitation of medical sciences collectively. We now consider in detail how epidemiological guidelines for causality help to analyse the causal basis of associations.

5.4.2 **Application of guidelines to associations**

The association (or link or relationship) between disease and postulated causal factors lies at the core of epidemiological thinking. Mostly, such associations are found by observing that disease varies with time, place, or person in observational data. An association rarely reflects a causal relationship, but it may. The preceding chapters on variation and error showed how to separate the probably not causal association from the possibly causal one. Table 5.6 begins and Table 5.7 further develops the questioning and reasoning process used in epidemiology to make the difficult judgement on whether an association may be causal. These six guidelines are a distillation of, or at least echo, the ten Alfred Evans postulates in *Last's Dictionary of Epidemiology* (4th edn) and the nine

Table 5.7 Questions underlying the guidelines for causality and implications of answers for interpretation of associations

Question underlying guideline	Label for guideline	Evidence		
		Unsure	No	Yes
Does the supposed cause precede or coincide with the disease (or other effect)?	Temporality	Judgement premature	Not causal	Causal relation possible
Does exposure to the supposed cause raise the incidence of disease?	Strength of association	Judgement premature	Not causal in the population context but does not rule out causal effects in individuals	Causal relation in populations possible
Does varying exposure to the supposed cause lead to varying amounts of disease?	Dose response	Not critical	Causal relation still possible if there is a threshold effect	Strengthens case for a causal judgement
Is the association between supposed cause and disease(s) limited in range	Specificity	Not critical	Not critical but extra caution— a sign of artefact	Strengthens causal claim
Is the association between supposed cause and outcome consistent across different studies and between subgroups?	Consistency	Defer decision, and await further research unless an immediate judgement is essential	Judgement will require explanation for inconsistent results	Strengthens causal claim
Does manipulating the level of exposure to the supposed cause change disease experience?	Experimental confirmation	Not always possible, so not critical	Caution needed for a causal claim	Strong confirmation of a causal relation
Is the way that the supposed cause exerts its effect on disease understood?	Biological plausibility	Not critical	Not critical but great caution needed for causal claim	Causal judgement strengthened

Bradford Hill criteria. The causal challenge is illustrated by the pyramid of associations and causes in Fig 5.13.

We shall now look at these guidelines in more detail. A visual summary is in figure 5.14.

i. Temporality

Did the cause precede the effect? If the effect is simultaneous with, or precedes, the proposed cause the association is definitely not causal in the direction postulated.

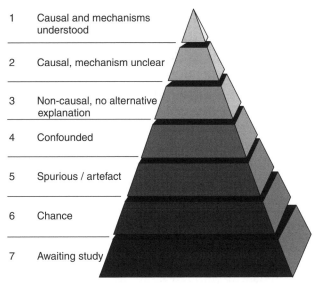

1 Causal and mechanisms understood

2 Causal, mechanism unclear

3 Non-causal, no alternative explanation

4 Confounded

5 Spurious / artefact

6 Chance

7 Awaiting study

Fig. 5.13 Pyramid of associations and causes.

There may be reverse causality. If there is no clear answer the judgement will be tentative, irrespective of other data, no matter how convincing these are. If the effect follows the action of a proposed cause the association may be a causal one and the analysis can proceed. This matter of timing is referred to as temporality. Demonstrating that this guideline is satisfied does not establish causality. Before reading on, do the exercise in Box 5.7.

Thunder follows lightning but is not caused by it. Both are generated simultaneously by an electrical discharge in clouds. The later arrival of the thunder is simply a result of the slower speed of sound than of light. Without an understanding of the nature of thunder and lightning erroneous conclusions about cause and effect are likely. Empirical observation seduces us to err. Generating alternative explanations is an essential discipline in epidemiology. The epidemiological imagination needs to be cultivated for this. Our alternative explanations can be put to the test. It would be hard to test the lightning and thunder association. Earlier, when discussing Hume (section 5.1) we considered the association between flicking a switch and a light going on. If the act of flicking similar switches in other settings turns on a light we are likely to accept a cause and effect relation on empirical grounds. The empirical observation has no explanatory power for exceptions, for example, when the light does not go on because of a break in the wiring, or when it goes on even without the switch being flicked, by water penetration. When there is a deeper understanding of the nature and action of electrical circuits the association may be agreed as causal, especially if it explains exceptions. Just because B follows A does not, of itself, confirm a causal relation. Association is not causation. Deeper understanding, or opening the black box, is essential.

Box 5.7 The deduction of cause and effect from the linkage of events

Reflect on whether the linkage of two events provides convincing evidence on cause and effect. For example thunder follows lightning. Does lightning cause thunder?

If you observe this once or a thousand times does it make a difference? What other explanations might there be?

ii. Strength and dose–response

Does exposure to the cause change disease incidence? If not or we are unsure, there is no epidemiological basis for a conclusion on cause and effect. The failure to demonstrate this does not, however, disprove a causal role. Reflect on Box 5.8 before reading on.

The cause may be so rare that there are insufficient cases available to reach a conclusion. Epidemiology is not good at demonstrating causal links when the rise in disease incidence is low, for example 10–20 per cent excess. Alternatively, there may be some people in the population in whom the cause is operative while in others it has no effect or even an opposite effect, leading to the view that there is no association. It may only be operative in the presence of a cofactor i.e. as part of a package of sufficient causes. The cofactor may be absent in the time, place or population you studied.

It might be reasonable, in some circumstances, to say that the cause studied was operative in raising or reducing disease in individuals but not in the populations. Alternatively, the cause may be operative on everyone. If oxygen is the cause of, say, pancreatic cancer we cannot show this epidemiologically (or even possibly in any other way). The most usual way of measuring the increase in incidence is the relative risk (see Chapter 8). (Other ways of measurement include the correlation coefficient, the regression coefficient, absolute rates, odds ratios and other measures of associations and effects. Some of these and other measures are considered in Chapters 7 and 8. The principle behind this guideline is best illustrated by the relative risk.) The technical name for this guideline is the 'strength of the association'. The greater the relative risk, the greater the strength of the association.

Does the disease incidence vary with the level of exposure? If yes, the case for a causal relation is advanced but, if not, we need to be aware that the effects may be independent of the amount of exposure. It is difficult to find examples to illustrate this. Allergy is one

Box 5.8 Epidemiology fails to uncover a cause

Can you think of circumstances when exposure to a causal factor does not change disease incidence?

example where trivial doses of substances such as peanuts can cause life-threatening reactions. For most exposures the relationship with disease is not linear, but the principle that more exposure leads to more disease tends to hold—dose–response. For high blood pressure there is a threshold above and below which adverse effects arise. Above the threshold the dose–response concept applies. Below the threshold the effects are unclear but some minimal pressure is needed for life. For weight and alcohol consumption, there is an apparent adverse effect at both low values and high values (called a J-shaped distribution). The dose–response relation is also measured using the relative risk (Chapter 8) so this can be considered as a development of the concept of the strength of the association; that is, does the strength of the association vary with the level of exposure? This can also be examined using correlation and regression—see section 9.11.5 for a brief introduction.

Imagine that we had the perfect study. In an imaginary world we can even have the counterfactual data, i.e. what the risk would be in the same population if that population did not have the risk factor. Would these data alone—that tell us the strength of the association—suffice for a cause and effect judgment?

The answer is that, from a population perspective, yes. The closest we come to this, in reality, is the well-designed experiment, in epidemiology this is the trial (Chapter 9). If a trial were free of all errors and biases, the strength of the association would, together with temporality, reflect causality. As yet, all epidemiological trials are imperfect and on highly selected populations. If trials were perfect we would have no need for more than one on any topic and no need for systematic reviews or meta-analysis. In our imperfect but real epidemiological world, the other guidelines are of great importance, for even with meta-analysis usually causality remains obscure.

iii. Specificity

Is the association of the supposed cause specific to relevant diseases and are diseases associated with a limited number of supposed causes? This idea is called specificity. Imagine a factor which was linked to all health effects. Why would that be so? Unless the links to a broad range of diseases can be explained, the case for causality is weakened for non-specificity is characteristic of spurious associations (e.g. underestimating the size of the population denominator; Chapter 7). Some factors do have broad effects, for example poverty and less so smoking. However, even these are not associated with more of every health problem. In the UK, poverty is associated with less malignant melanoma, a skin cancer that includes within its sufficient causes, sunburn and excess exposure to sunlight, an observation which makes sense because these are often a result of holidays in hot climates. Those in poverty are less able to afford to expose themselves to these causes than others. While specificity is not a critically important guideline, epidemiologists should take advantage of the reasoning power it offers.

iv. Consistency

Is the evidence within and between studies consistent? It is wise to be tentative if it is not. Unless the inconsistency can be explained the case for causality is weakened.

Consistency is linked to generalizability of findings. Experience tells us that causal effects tend to be widely applicable, while spurious associations are often local. The systematic review and meta-analysis are ways of assessing consistency in a rigorous way and are considered in the next section.

v. Experiment

Does changing exposure to the supposed cause change disease incidence? This is experimental confirmation. Sometimes there have been natural experiments, with changes over time in exposure to risk factors. For example, a spill of a pollutant into a water supply, the closure of a factory, the availability of a new product, redundancy in a factory, economic collapse of a society, or a change of policy (e.g. putting fluoride into a water supply). Perhaps the greatest of these experiments is the mixing of the genes in Mendelian randomization (see Chapter 3 section 3.3.1). These natural experiments can be vitally important. Often there is no such evidence, and some form of deliberate experimentation will be necessary. The problem is that human experiments or trials are sometimes impossible on ethical grounds and always difficult and expensive to organize. Ethically, the individual involved must have the potential to benefit. For risk factors, as opposed to protective factors, there may be no such benefit. Then the experimental approach requires a valid *in-vitro* or animal model. Causal understanding can be greatly advanced by laboratory and experimental observations. Such data must be integrated with epidemiological observations, to ensure that the theoretically predicted effects do occur in free-living human populations. Experimental methods are introduced in Section 9.7 on trials. The ethics of epidemiology are particularly important to these studies (section 10.10).

vi. Biological plausibility

Is there a biological mechanism by which the supposed cause can induce the effect? This is the guideline of plausibility. If there is plausibility the case for a causal effect will be easier to advance. For truly novel advances, however, the biological plausibility may not be apparent. For example, it is biologically plausible that lying an infant on its back to sleep may lead to it inhaling its own vomit. This biologically plausible theory has been overturned by the biologically implausible observation that lying a child on its back halves the risk of cot death compared to the side or front. The mechanisms are still being worked out. That said, biological plausibility remains important, particularly in confirming causality. The analogy is with the light switch; when there is understanding of the electrical circuit the causal basis of flicking the light switch is confirmed. An understanding of electrical discharges in clouds explains the association between thunder and lightning (see item i above).

Demonstrating biological plausibility is not part of epidemiological methods. This does not, however, mean epidemiologists can forget about it. Epidemiologists need to understand the biology of the diseases they study, explain their hypotheses in biological terms and propose and promote (perhaps even lead) biological research to test hypotheses.

The precedent and inspiration for such work is abundant, as we saw with syndrome X (pellagra) and the work of Joseph Goldberger.

5.4.3 Judging the causal basis of the association

The investigator can now proceed to a conclusion, but the interpretation ought to be tentative for judgements on cause and effect are not universal. An association which meets many or even all of the criteria may, at least theoretically, be non-causal.

George Davey Smith (1992) has shown that the association between cigarette smoking and suicide meets many (but not all) of the guidelines for causality including temporality, strength, and dose–response. Yet, he argues, the association is not causal.

The guidelines are particularly valuable in exposing the lack of evidence for causality, for indicating the need for further research and for avoiding premature conclusions. This said, sometimes firm judgements are possible, and at other times forced upon us, even in the face of limited evidence. A judgement may be essential when policy is to be made. Using a causal framework makes the judgement explicit. Table 5.7 indicates how the questions implicit in causal guidelines can be applied to weigh up evidence.

Three examples of the case for causality (illustrating the need for a systematic mode of analysis) are shown in Table 5.8: diethylstilboestrol as a cause of adenocarcinoma of the vagina (Herbst *et al.* 1971), smoking as a cause of lung cancer (Doll *et al.* 1956), and residential proximity to a coking works as a cause of ill-health (Bhopal *et al.* 1994). Before reading on reflect on the exercise in Box 5.9. Readers are invited to read the original studies (listed in References).

At the time that the key studies referred to in Table 5.8 were published the authors claimed that the smoking–lung cancer association was causal (true but many remained unconvinced), that diethylstilboestrol had caused adenocarcinoma of the vagina (this was accepted), and that residential proximity to a coking works had caused respiratory morbidity but not mortality (the case was not, however, accepted as rock solid, though it was the best that was achievable).

Box 5.9 Reaching a judgement on cause and effect

Reflect on the evidence in Table 5.8 and deliver a verdict on whether the associations between smoking and lung cancer, diethylstilboestrol and adenocarcinoma of the vagina, and living close to a coking works and ill-health are causal.

5.4.4. Reviews, systematic reviews and meta-analysis

Examining the body of work on a topic of research is known by the quaint term literature review, so a request to read the literature is not, in science, a direction to read Shakespeare. The time-honoured approach was to examine past work in chronological order. That is still to be recommended, but, except for the most esoteric of topics, there will be so much

Table 5.8 Three examples of applying the criteria for causality

Question	Smoking and lung cancer	Diethylstilboestrol and adenocarcinoma of the vagina	Living near a coking works and ill-health
Does the supposed cause precede the disease (effect) (temporality)	Yes, clearly so	Yes, maternal exposure to diethylstilboestrol preceded the disease in the offspring	Yes, the coking works was functioning before most people in the study were born
By how much does exposure to the, cause raise the incidence of disease? (strength)	Greatly and as much as 20 to 30-fold in smokers of 20 or more cigarettes per day	Greatly, as estimated from the first case-control study	The excess of disease is modest, varying for each specific cause but is rarely more than 30–50% greater than expected
Does varying exposure lead to varying disease? (dose–response)	Yes, there is a clear relationship and more smoking causes more disease	No clear evidence	The evidence is suggestive that the closer the residence to the coking works the greater the effect on health
Does the cause lead to a rise in a few relevant diseases? (specificity)	No, numerous diseases show an association with smoking	Yes	Yes, the association is restricted mainly to some respiratory diseases
Is the association consistent across different studies and between groups?	Yes, the association is demonstrable in men and women, and across social groups	Yes	There are no directly comparable studies, but it fits with understanding of the role of industrial air pollution
Is the way that the cause exerts its effect on disease understood? (biological plausibility)	Only partly. The tar in cigarettes contains important carcinogens	At the time of the discovery, no	Generally, yes, specifically no. Coking works produce complex mixtures of emissions. Most knowledge is on single components of air pollution, not mixtures
Does manipulating the level of exposure to the cause change disease experience? (experimental confirmation)	Yes. Reducing consumption of cigarettes reduces risk. Persuading people to smoke more would be unethical. Tobacco is carcinogenic to animals	Yes	Don't know. An experiment is not possible, but the plant closed during the research, producing a natural experiment. Closure of the coking plant was not linked to changes in consultation with a general practitioner, but on days when pollution levels were high the consultation rates were high

to read that some selection will be necessary. In standard literature reviews the selection is left to the discretion of the reviewer. The reviewers synthesize the scientific literature that they judge is necessary to answer the questions to be answered. In doing so, reviewers may focus on the work of well-known authorities in the field (particularly themselves!), more recent work, large-scale work, or other people's reviews. More pragmatically, they may choose work that is readily available, in a language they read, or that published in the journals with high reputation. In modern times, work that can be downloaded for free on the Internet is particularly popular. The problem with this traditional form of reviewing is bias, and the resulting erroneous conclusions. This traditional approach is also inefficient, from society's perspective, even though it may conserve the time of the researcher. The researcher's selective approach may miss some important original research work. Since original research work usually costs hundreds of thousands, and even millions, of pounds it is wasteful to miss it.

This is not to say there is no role for such reviews. They are essential for the following:

◆ self-education and education of others, especially on the general principles

◆ as a preliminary way of sketching out the need for research

◆ as the prelude to a systematic review or meta-analysis

◆ where there is sparse information—insufficient to justify a systematic review

◆ as the basis of a commentary on published research

◆ to support a viewpoint, where strict objectivity is not the aim.

The traditional review was in narrative form with an emphasis on the conclusions generated by others' work. The traditional review did not, however, exclude the possibility of extracting the empirical findings of other research. Usually, however, these were presented in text format. The best traditional reviews were analytic and, if necessary, critical but there was no formal way of assessing the quality of the studies.

The traditional review serves those disciplines where generalization is relatively easily or where strict objectivity is not the goal. For example, in describing the action of an enzyme or an eye muscle, a traditional review would probably be enough. Even one definitive article, or even one previous review, might suffice. Equally, a review of the art of Picasso would be subjective—we want the writer's perspective.

What about reviews of topics such as whether salt causes high blood pressure, or whether HIV causes AIDS? The production and marketing of salt is a multi-billion pound endeavour. Every human being's quality of life will be affected by an erroneous review that concluded either that there is no causal link or that there is one. The causal relation between the amount of salt taken and high blood pressure is unlikely to hold, alike, in South African miners, and Ford motor company executives. There are strong, political views against the acceptance of HIV as the fundamental cause of AIDS, at the time of writing most obviously in South Africa. A selective and biased review in the hands of politicians who do not believe in HIV could lead to millions of people dying unnecessarily.

The need for the best possible evidence, especially for making decisions on expensive health service interventions, the need to make reviewing easier so more people can be involved, and the imperative to minimize error and bias have combined to lead to an explosion in the methods and outputs of systematic reviews. A systematic review has the following characteristics:

1 It is managed in the manner of a research project with a clear, written plan (protocol) stating the context (usually by a traditional review), goals, questions, methods, analysis and outputs. This is a systematic approach.

2 It is aiming to review everything published that is relevant to the goals. If it does not review everything then it reviews a sample, with the selection of the sample being unbiased. Mostly, the sample is based on defining timeframes. The search for relevant data is systematic.

3 The information from original research is usually extracted (often into a form) and entered into a database or tables in a systematic way, and presented in some logical way.

4 The data extracted above are the focus of the review rather than the text of the original articles. The findings are the results of this systematic review and are synthesised and discussed collectively.

The author of the systematic review has the dual challenge of pinpointing and dealing with the errors and biases in the original papers, and those that arise from compiling the results in this way. Many of the biases and errors occurring in primary research are mirrored in these synthesised data sets.

In our example of salt and high blood pressure, we are likely to find tens of thousands of articles on the subject. Thousands of others may be difficult to find. It may need a working lifetime to find and read them. Yet the results may be required in a year, to assist in a forthcoming health policy.

The usual solution is to clarify and narrow the research questions, and hence the goals and scope of the review. We may, say, narrow it to—does salt cause high blood pressure in warm climate countries (or specify the countries), and specify a timescale for the field-work of the research (say, 1965 onwards). It is common (but not usually good) practice to restrict the review to English language publications. In this example, we may also restrict to case–control and cohort studies and trials in human populations. We would start our search of publications using electronic search engines and databases, before looking at reference lists in publications, and consulting experts. By this time, we should have a good idea of the resources needed to complete the review. If it is still beyond the resources available, further inclusion and exclusion criteria will be needed.

One logical solution, when there is a great deal of material, is to restrict studies to the best possible study design for that question. For a question such as how much type 2 diabetes there is in society, we may restrict to cross-sectional studies. For the question, what is the association between obesity and type 2 diabetes, we may restrict to cohort studies.

The evidence that is now at hand can be interpreted using the frameworks in Chapters 4 and 5. While we can search for evidence to support the guidelines for causality, it is clear that the systematic review is, in itself, the basis of a judgement on consistency. Consistency is particularly powerful when the evidence comes from a range of study designs, so there is a case for either including several designs within the one systematic review or doing a series of systematic reviews e.g. salt/blood pressure reviews of case–control and cohort studies separately. Other types of evidence e.g. laboratory research, can be considered in the discussion.

Imagine now that we find 10 cohort studies all showing that people eating more salt, say X grams more, have about 50 per cent more hypertension than those who eat less salt, with the results of individual studies ranging from 35–65 per cent excess. Assume we have checked out these studies and there are no imperfections of note and that everything points to a causal relation. What else can we do? What other additional analysis is possible?

Every estimate of risk has a random error and this can be estimated by calculating confidence intervals (CI) around it. The narrower the CI, the greater the precision. In one of the studies one may find the excess is 40 per cent with a CI of 25–55 per cent. The range of the CI is narrower when the sample size is larger. A larger sample size can be mimicked by combining the 10 studies. Ideally, we would obtain the original data from the 10 studies and re-analyse them together. In practice, that is often not feasible. There are statistical techniques for combining the studies even without obtaining the original data. Either approach to combining data is known as meta-analysis.

In epidemiology it is most unusual for studies either to be done in similar ways, or to give similar results. The differences in the methods between the studies might give rise to different results. Alternatively, differences in the populations might do so. It is not easy to disentangle these possibilities. It is not at all improbable that of our 10 studies, 2 show that high salt is associated with lower blood pressure, 3 show no association and 5 show higher blood pressure. What are we to do now? Is there some rigorous way of summarizing or synthesizing these results?

The epidemiologist foresees this need and adopts in the previously stated protocol an approach to extract value from this muddled picture:

1 Are some of these studies too unreliable to include in the meta-analysis? These will be sifted out early.

2 Are studies of different sizes (almost certainly)? If so, the larger studies will be given more weight (both judgementally and statistically)?

3 Are some studies of higher quality than others? These will be given more weight.

4 Is it reliable to combine data? This will be judged on: (a) methods being sufficiently similar and; (b) a statistical test (of heterogeneity) to see whether the effects are too different for them, reasonably, to be explained by random errors.

5 If the variation in findings is too great to explain by methodological or random variation, then, until shown otherwise, the best explanation is that the differences reflect the real population differences in the relation of salt to blood pressure. It would be misleading to combine all the studies, but it might be possible to aggregate some on the basis of some prior or coherent approach, e.g. those in countries with warm climates separately from those in cold climates.

In adopting the meta-analytic method we are getting better understanding of the effect size, thus contributing to a more precise knowledge of the strength and dose-response of the association.

So systematic reviews and meta-analyses provide direct input into two causal guidelines—consistency and strength of associations. In applied epidemiology they provide more precise data on the burden of disease, and the effect of interventions.

This account is of the principles of systematic reviews, but there is a vast pool of technical knowledge and technical solutions. There are many websites and books for the interested reader—some of them, including the Cochrane and Campbell Collaboration websites, are listed in the bibliography.

5.4.5 Interpretation of data, paradigms, study design, and causal criteria

Causal knowledge is born in the imagination and understanding of the disease process; data fuels the investigator's imagination and understanding. Scientific data do not, in themselves, offer knowledge. Indeed, the same data can be interpreted in quite different ways depending on the way of thought of the investigator. For example, as detailed in Gould, data that one scientist, Samuel Morton, interpreted as showing clear differences by 'race' in cranial capacity and hence brain size (and ultimately intelligence—see Gould, 1984), was interpreted by another, Stephen Gould (1984), as showing no noteworthy differences. The opposite conclusions drawn from the same data set arose because of differences in the way of seeing the world (including the research world) of the two investigators. This way of seeing the world is often referred to as the paradigm. The paradigm within which epidemiologists work will determine the nature of the causal links they see and emphasize. There is a strong case for researchers to make explicit in their writings their guiding research philosophy and paradigm (see also Chapter 10).

Causal thinking and study design (discussed in Chapter 9) are distinct, though interlinked, issues. No epidemiological design confirms causality and no design is incapable of adding important evidence. In all studies there are limitations and pitfalls. There are differences among the various study designs in both the type of pitfalls and their likelihood (see Chapter 9). While a single observation may spark off causal understanding, it would be wise to exercise great caution until further observations confirm or refute the idea. Exceptionally, however, there may be no time to delay.

Table 5.9 indicates the potential contributions of various study designs to the epidemiological criteria for causality. Note that with the exception of consistency, to which all designs contribute, and biological plausibility, to which no epidemiological designs contribute directly, all epidemiological studies contribute to some but not all criteria. This must not be confused with the hierarchy of evidence that has emerged in relation to the effectiveness and cost-effectiveness of interventions, or even of measuring the burden of disease. Each purpose requires its own hierarchy.

5.5 Epidemiological theory illustrated by this chapter

Several theories underpin epidemiological causal thinking. First and foremost is the theory that diseases arise from a complex interaction of genetic and environmental factors. Second, there is a theory that causes of disease in individuals may not necessarily be

Table 5.9 Potential contributions of study design (see Chapter 9) to causal guidelines

Guideline	Case series	Cross-sectional	Case–control	Cohort	Trial
Temporality	Sometimes	Sometimes	Sometimes	Often	Usually
Strength or dose–response	Sometimes	Sometimes	Often	Always	Always
Experimental confirmation	Sometimes, in the case of natural experiment	Sometimes, in case of repeated studies, following an intervention	Seldom	Sometimes, following natural changes	Always
Specificity	Sometimes	Sometimes	Yes, for disease	Yes for the risk factor(s)	Yes for the risk or preventive factor
Biological plausibility	Not directly	Not directly	Not directly	Not directly	Not directly
Consistency	Yes	Yes	Yes	Yes	Yes

demonstrable as causes of disease in populations and vice versa. The third (and pragmatic) epidemiological theory of causation is that reliable cause and effect judgements are achievable through hypothesis generation and testing, with data interpreted using a logical framework of analysis, which draws on multidisciplinary perspectives.

5.6 **Conclusion**

The most important aim of epidemiology is to generate and use cause and effect theories to break the links between disease and its causes and to improve public health. The misapplication of theory may have serious repercussions including deaths on a mass scale, while the proper application of theory can transform the control of disease.

It is difficult to achieve trustworthy causal knowledge because of the complexity of diseases, the long timescales over which many human diseases develop, and ethical restraints on human experimentation. Nonetheless, there is an imperative to act, even when our knowledge is incomplete, for lives depend on our science. In the words of Bradford Hill (1965):

> All scientific work is incomplete—whether it be observational or experimental. That does not confer upon us a freedom to ignore the knowledge we already have, or to postpone the action that it appears to demand at a given time.
>
> Bradford Hill (1965, p. 300)

A rigorous analysis of all the scientific data available is essential, though to quote Bradford Hill again, 'this does not imply crossing every 't', and swords with every critic, before we act'.

Epidemiology engages with health policy-makers and planners who are the users of much of the work. Rothman (1986) has helped to open up the prickly question, posed by

Lanes, of whether epidemiologists (as scientists) ought to be engaged in choosing between theories of causation or whether they should simply present the evidence and the theory options to policy-makers and leave the choices to them. Clearly, the latter approach would go counter to current practice. Readers need to ponder on this question and form their own views. The debate continues in the scientific journals. Whatever viewpoint prevails, epidemiology has a responsibility to understand the theories of causation used by other disciplines, and to educate others about the mode of thought in epidemiology.

Simplistic notions of epidemiology about causality, for example that a cause is something which raises the incidence of disease, are not particularly helpful in persuading sceptical people of the strength of the epidemiological evidence. Demonstrating to the sceptics' satisfaction that a cause raises the disease incidence is complex and requires detailed understanding by both parties of causal reasoning in epidemiology. Developing effective actions, a difficult challenge usually achieved in cross-disciplinary partnerships, is also demanding in epidemiological knowledge.

Epidemiology provides a broad perspective on the causes of disease which contrasts with the narrower one of the physical and most biological sciences. This complementary perspective is a great strength. The causal models reinforce this perspective and provide a framework to organize ideas.

The prevailing attitude in epidemiology, that all judgements of cause and effect are tentative, is both pragmatic and in line with modern thinking about the nature of scientific advances. The increasing understanding that the data do not hold an unequivocal answer, and that the answers derived are dependent on human judgement (symbolized in Fig. 5.12, on p 145), though apparently common sense,is harder to accept because it gives space for subjectivity where science prefers objectivity.

Epidemiologists should be alert for error, the play of chance, and the constant presence of bias, and should apply guidelines for causality as an aid to thinking and not as a checklist. Only rarely will causal mechanisms be understood, as symbolized by the pyramid of associations in Figure 5.13. Epidemiologists need to utilize the power of reviews for generating causal hypotheses, and of systematic reviews and meta-analyses for powerful portrayal of the evidence. Finally, epidemiology should seek corroboration from other scientific disciplines in terms of both data and scientific frameworks for cause and effect.

Seeking causal associations is like panning for gold, for it usually yields nothing but grit and mud (error and bias). Often we find gold flakes and specks (risk factors, relating to the causal pathway). Sometimes we get a nugget (causal factor). Rarely a gold mine is discovered. Like panning for gold, a great deal of hard work is required to find a gold mine. When it is discovered, panning alone will not be enough, and much sophisticated equipment and skills will be needed to take full advantage of the discovery. In epidemiology, this implies working with other laboratory and population-based scientific disciplines (including social sciences) to gain understanding of the mechanisms by which the cause operates. Epidemiology needs an international council to assess evidence to establish the causal credentials of the multiplicity of associations being generated.

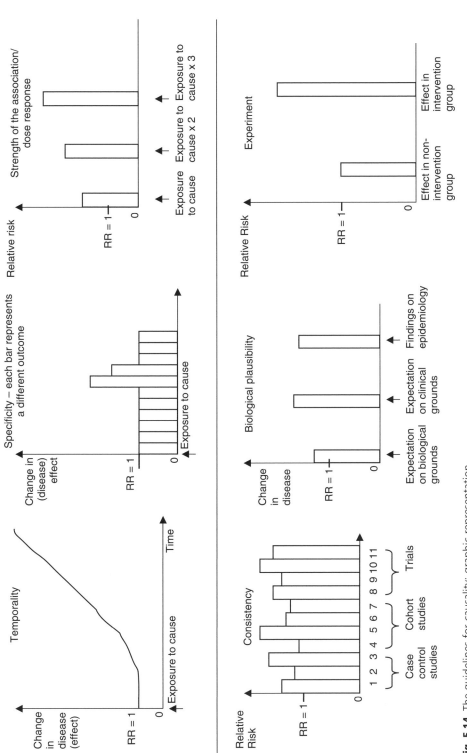

Fig. 5.14 The guidelines for causality: graphic representation.

Associations would then be categorised according to the pyramid of associations and causes, to help guide both future research and public health action.

Summary

Cause and effect understanding is the highest form of scientific knowledge, for it permits prediction and generalization, one of the main purposes of science. Understanding of cause and effect has also been a preoccupation of philosophy. A comparison of epidemiological and other forms of causal thinking shows similarity, which reflects the debt which epidemiologists owe to other, older disciplines. Epidemiology is increasingly influencing thinking in other sciences.

An association between disease and the postulated causal factors lies at the core of epidemiology. Causal knowledge can be greatly advanced by experimental observations on what happens to disease incidence when the causal factors are manipulated. The ultimate aim of epidemiology is to use cause and effect knowledge to break links between disease and its causes and to improve public health. The application of erroneous knowledge has serious repercussions.

In epidemiology demonstrating causality is difficult because of the long and complex natural history of many human diseases and because of ethical restraints on human experimentation. Epidemiologists should: hold the attitude that all judgements of cause and effect are tentative; understand that causal thinking demands a judgement; be alert for error, the play of chance, and bias; utilize the power of causal models that broaden causal perspectives; use the power of reviews and data synthesis; apply guidelines for causality as an aid to thinking and not as a checklist; and look for corroboration of causality from other scientific frameworks for assessment of cause and effect.

Sample examination questions

Give yourself 10 minutes for every 25% of marks.

Many of the questions at the end of Chapter 9 are highly relevant to this chapter, and you may need to read that chapter before doing some of the questions here.

Question 1 The phrase 'association is not causation' is often used in epidemiology. List five non-causal factors that can lead to association. (25%)
Answer Associations that are non-causal can be generated by chance, errors, bias in the selection of study populations, bias in the quality of information, failing to compare like with like (confounding), fraud, etc.

Question 2 Which of the guidelines (also known as criteria) for causal reasoning can clinical trials make a contribution to? Which do they not contribute to? (25%)
Answer Trials can contribute to the following causal guidelines:

- Temporality-intervention comes first, outcome is observed
- Strength of the association (dose–response may be possible if varying levels of the intervention are studied)

- Consistency—if they support other studies
- Specificity of the disease outcome, but not exposure (usually only one exposure is changed)
- Experimental confirmation—trials are experiments
- Trials do not contribute, at least directly, to biological plausibility unless specific effort is made to collect data on the biological mechanisms within the trial.

Question 3 Which of the guidelines (also known as criteria) for causal reasoning can cohort studies make a contribution to? Which do they not contribute to? (25%)

Answer Cohort studies can contribute to temporality by showing that the exposure precedes disease; to strength of the association by measuring the relative risk; to dose–response by measuring the association as the exposure increases; to consistency either by comparison with other kinds of studies or with other cohort studies; and to specificity, i.e. the range of outcomes that exposures lead to. They cannot contribute directly to biological plausibility though they can test a biologically derived hypothesis. They cannot give experimental confirmation though (a) they can be used to study natural experiments and (b) to find people to do trials on.

Question 4 What is the value of the concept of 'consistency' in helping you assess an association? (25%)

Answer (b) 'Consistency' of an association is linked to generalizability of findings. For example, causal effects tend to be widely applicable, while spurious associations are often local. Unless the lack of consistency in findings can be explained the case for an association is weakened.

Chapter 6

Interrelated concepts in the epidemiology of disease
Natural history, spectrum, iceberg, population patterns, and screening

Objectives

On completion of this chapter you should understand:

- that the natural history of disease is the unchecked progression of disease in an individual;
- that natural history ranks alongside causal understanding in importance for the prevention and control of disease;
- that the technical and ethical challenges in describing the natural history of disease are great, particularly where the time between exposure to the causal agents and the onset of disease is long;
- that the changing pattern of disease in populations over time, and the spectrum of the presentation of disease, are related to natural history;
- that the 'iceberg of disease' is a metaphor emphasizing that the number of cases ascertained (those visible) is outweighed by those not discovered (those invisible);
- how the iceberg of disease phenomenon thwarts assessment of the true burden of disease, the need for services and the selection of representative cases for epidemiological study;
- that screening is the application of tests to diagnose disease (or its precursors) in an earlier phase of the natural history of disease than is achieved in routine medical practice;
- that the key to successful screening is a simple test, which can be applied to large populations with minimum harm and has a high degree of accuracy in separating those who need more detailed investigation from those who don't;
- that the potential of screening is vast but there are important limitations such as the inability to influence the natural history of many diseases, and the need to balance the costs and benefits of earlier diagnosis.

Box 6.1 Potential effects of an exposure to a causal agent

Reflect on the possible outcomes in an individual of exposure to a causal agent. The causal agents to consider include microbes (say those causing Legionnaires' disease or tuberculosis) and inanimate exposures (say particulate air pollution or tobacco smoke).

6.1 Natural history of disease, the incubation period and acute/chronic diseases

The natural history of disease is the uninterrupted progression in an individual of the development of disease from the moment that it is initiated by exposure to the causal agents. Do the exercise in Box 6.1 before reading on.

There are four main types of response. First, the exposure may have no effect. The exposure may have had no effect because the dose was too low or the recipient was not susceptible. Alternatively, as a cofactor was missing so there was no package of sufficient causes. There may, however, have been an effect but one too small to notice. Strictly speaking, then, for such individuals there is no 'history of disease' or even precursors of disease. Nonetheless, from an epidemiological and public health perspective this type of response is important, because we may learn how to protect those individuals who do develop disease with this level of exposure.

Second, there may be some demonstrable damaging effect of the exposure which may be repaired. Microbiological, immunological, biochemical, or pathological studies may be able to demonstrate inflammation, tissue change, and repair. This type of response is likely to lead to some illness, possibly non-specific symptoms and signs such as tiredness and fever.

Third, the effect may be an illness that is rapidly contained by the body's defence mechanism. In this case there will usually be a short illness. In the case of tuberculosis there may be a fever which subsides. The tuberculosis bacilli are contained, though they remain alive. Fourth, the illness may progress until it leads to continuing long-term problems, irreversible damage, or death. This progression may be curtailed by treatment (but then it no longer represents the natural history of disease).

The outcome of the exposure will depend on the interactions of host, agent, and environmental factors. For example, an elderly person with cardiorespiratory diseases may die on exposure to smog on a cold wintry day, when similar exposure of a younger person (with the same amount of smog) would have no important adverse effect. The natural history, as outlined in these four responses to exposure, is a biological and clinical concept of great importance to all medical sciences, including epidemiology.

Figure 6.1 provides an idealized view of the concept. The idea is that individuals start life healthy or at least disease free. As they age they are exposed to disease-causing agents which, cumulatively, increase their susceptibility to disease, some of it chronic. In the early years,

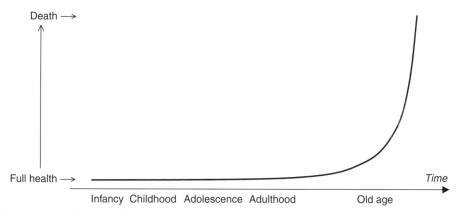

Fig. 6.1 Natural history of disease, idealized.

exposure to disease agents causes little lasting harm. This cumulative burden eventually leads to death. With the exception of the period *in utero* and early infancy, which are perilous times in terms of health risks, this idealized picture is becoming true in the affluent parts of the world, where the pattern of health, ill-health, and death generally follows that shown in Figure 6.1. The burden of serious ill-health is being 'compressed' into the later part of life. The same concept can be applied to individual diseases.

Tuberculosis provides an excellent example, illustrated in Fig. 6.2, which shows the natural history in one hypothetical individual in a simple way. This person was exposed to the tubercle bacillus in early childhood but the primary tuberculosis which followed hardly impaired his health. He harboured this illness through childhood but it recurred in adolescence (possibly because of other health problems at that time) with recovery. Then a second recurrence in early old age led to death. Figure 6.3 shows a typical path for the natural history of coronary heart disease (CHD). The causes exert their effect in early life

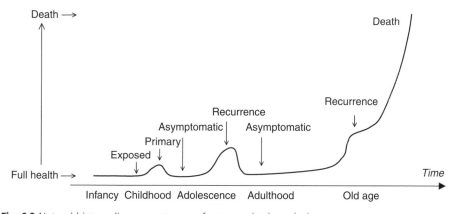

Fig. 6.2 Natural history disease: outcome of untreated tuberculosis.

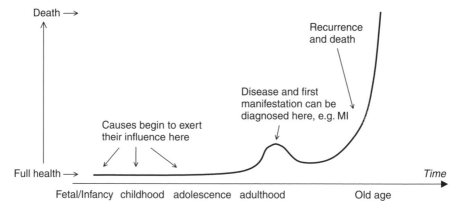

Fig. 6.3 Natural history of CHD.

and the development of atheroma usually begins in adolescence (or earlier). Disease may not be manifest until adulthood (often middle age). The first clinical occurrence may be angina or heart attack, with partial recovery, until recurrence and death in later life.

While it is of vital importance, information on natural history is very hard to obtain. Reflect on the questions in Box 6.2 before reading on.

In practice, the natural history of diseases such as tuberculosis is interrupted as soon as possible either by treatment or by immunization with BCG. It would be ethically unacceptable *anywhere in the world* to observe the natural history of tuberculosis. Treatment is curative and cheap. As a medical diagnosis is essential to define the natural history of disease, the truth about it is seldom known for two major reasons. First, the act of diagnosis and follow-up by a physician may initiate changes in the disease process, for example, through the placebo effect, or by changing the behaviour of the person observed. This principle is clear in the case of psychological disorders, say depression or anxiety, but probably applies to all diseases in a more subtle form. For example, the observation of the natural history of CHD by repeat electrocardiogram or Rose Angina Questionnaire in people is likely to raise awareness of the disease and induce some modifications of lifestyle. Second, the scientific objective of observing the natural history of disease clashes with the ethical medical imperative to act to alleviate, contain, or treat the disease.

Box 6.2 Obstacles to studying the natural history of disease

- What difficulties can you see in studying the true natural history of disease?
- Would you be willing to participate in a natural history study?
- What might be the effect on you of being in such a study?

For medically qualified epidemiologists the ethical imperative is clear, but it is less so for non-medical ones, for there is no widely agreed and enforced ethical code for science (see Chapter 10.11). In cases of doubt, all epidemiologists should ensure that their work is cleared by an ethical committee. Defining the natural history of most diseases in the modern world is, therefore, problematic.

Studies of the natural history of disease are potentially ethically explosive. One infamous example was the US Public Health Service's Tuskegee Syphilis Study (see Jones 1993), where 600 'negro' men, many with active syphilis, in the state of Alabama in the USA were followed up for a period of about 40 years. They were actively shielded from treatment by the investigators. The investigators believed that the scientific value of their observations exceeded the right of their subjects to therapy. There was no informed consent by the subjects. Even if there had been, the study would still be unethical, because it clashes with the medical ethical imperative to do good and not harm (this example is also discussed in Chapter 4 and in Chapter 10 because it is one of the defining chapters in the modern history of the ethics of medical science).

The ethical principles for epidemiological studies of natural history are that:

◆ these studies can only be done on informed individuals;

◆ studies are only permissible when there is no known effective therapy;

◆ if an effective therapy becomes available (after the study starts) then the study will need to be modified or abandoned.

The placebo group in some clinical trials is, potentially, an important source of information on the natural history (see Chapter 9). The emerging principle for trials is that the control group should receive the best available therapy, and not placebo, so this source of data on the natural history of disease may dry up.

Follow-up, or cohort, studies are needed to define accurately the natural history of disease (see Chapter 9 for a discussion of cohort studies). Repeated observation of the same individuals over long time periods is usually necessary in chronic diseases. Ideally, a disease-free population would be observed closely and repeatedly, until either the population is no longer at any risk of the disease or until death. For example, in an ideal study of the natural history of gestational diabetes a representative sample of pregnant women would be followed, with observations to include tests of blood sugar levels. For those who did not develop diabetes in pregnancy, the observations could stop until the next pregnancy. For those who did develop diabetes, follow-up would continue after pregnancy, to assess whether it resolves and whether there are long-term adverse outcomes. In the latter case the follow-up may be measured in decades, and in those with continuing diabetes and complications, until death. With this information we can decide whether gestational diabetes is a harmful phenomenon, and develop appropriate health services, on appropriate timescales. To take one simple question: does gestational diabetes herald type 2 diabetes in later life? If not, after pregnancy the woman need not be followed up, at least in relation to diabetes. If yes, such women may need to be followed up. In practice such cohort studies are rare, and long-term observations may prove costly or impossible. The natural history is usually pieced together from a mixture of observations, including those from single individuals (case reports) or from case series observed by clinicians, rather than in formal epidemiological studies. In Chapter 9 I show how each study design links to natural history.

The time between exposure to the agent and the development of disease is called the incubation period. It varies greatly in individuals but in populations the pattern can be defined both for broad categories of disease and for specific diagnoses. Diseases that have long incubation periods, usually measured in years and sometimes decades, generally have a long clinical course and, if so, by convention they are called chronic diseases (the label is embedded in medicine, even though it is problematic). An example of a chronic disease is chronic bronchitis. This disease is likely to have been caused by prolonged exposure to a mixture of agents including respiratory infections in childhood and adulthood, air pollution, and tobacco smoke. Chronic bronchitis is likely to run a clinical course measured in decades and the damage is usually irreversible. Other examples of chronic diseases include rheumatoid arthritis, CHD, diabetes, and most cancers.

Some chronic diseases, paradoxically, lead to sudden and unexpected death (e.g. a stroke or heart attack); the diagnosis is then made at a post-mortem. The label chronic disease is based on the natural history as defined in many individuals, not the clinical course in an individual. The opportunity to control and treat a chronic disease may be short, but the opportunity to prevent it will be prolonged.

Diseases with a short incubation period (days, weeks, and sometimes months) usually have a short course (say, less than a year), and by convention are known as acute diseases. These include most infections and many toxic disorders e.g. influenza, food poisoning, and carbon monoxide poisoning. Paradoxically, the effects of acute disease may also be severe and prolonged, such as post-viral syndromes. Clearly, an acute disease can leave permanent (chronic) sequelae; for example, meningitis can lead to chronic deafness. The incubation period, together with minimal clinical information on the nature of the illness (e.g. a rash and fever), may be sufficient to identify the disease. This is particularly the case with infectious diseases. For example, vomiting within a few hours of eating a meal in a group of people is much more likely to be due to *Staphlyococcus aureas* food poisoning than salmonella.

Knowledge of the natural history is vital for disease prevention policies, particularly for secondary prevention based on screening, and provides the underlying rationale for all medical practice. Indeed, the whole purpose of medicine is to influence the natural history of disease by reducing and delaying ill-health. Figure 6.4 illustrates this. When this is achieved through deliberate actions by societies the collective endeavour is public health.

The natural history concept applies to individuals but it has implications for thinking about disease in populations. First, changes in the natural history of disease in individuals do, of course, affect the population pattern. Improved general nutrition, for example, reduces the likelihood of an individual developing secondary tuberculosis. In turn this reduces the risk of person-to-person transmission, and hence the incidence of clinical tuberculosis and death. Second, the various paths to progression in individuals can be aggregated to produce a portrait of what alternatives may happen in a population. This is shown in Fig. 6.5 and will be discussed in Section 6.3.

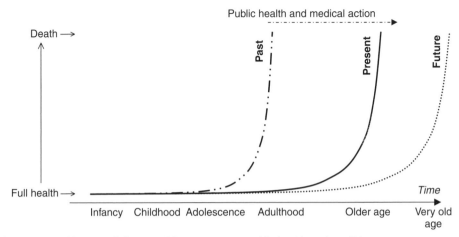

Fig. 6.4 Natural history of disease: giving purpose to public health and medicine.

6.2 **The population pattern of disease: changes over time (secular trends)**

The concept of the natural history of disease should not be (but is) confused with the changing pattern of disease in populations over time, for example, the decline in recent decades of gastric cancer, stroke, heart disease, and tuberculosis, or the rise of AIDS, asthma and childhood leukaemia. It is commonplace to hear or read that the natural history of stroke has changed in the past hundred years. Such trends should not be referred to in this way. There is no widely agreed word or phrase to capture this concept, though the

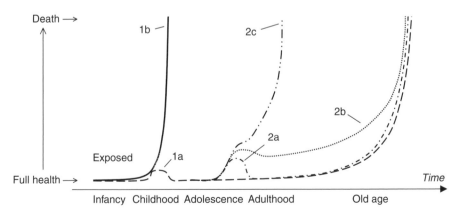

Fig. 6.5 Natural history of disease: pathways in tuberculosis. 1a: Primary infection with complete remission (death from other causes); 1b: fatal tuberculous meningitis; 2a: recurrence with successful treatment (death from other causes); 2b: TB with residual disability (and TB contributory or actual cause of death); 2c: recurrence with fatal outcome.

'secular trend' in disease (secular in the sense of long term) is sometimes used. The secular trend is, however, a limited concept; it does not capture the point that the incidence of the disease may not change much but the population pattern of disease occurrence may be radically altered. For example, the distribution of a disease across socio-economic groups may change, as it has for CHD which has become less common in wealthy, and more common in poor, populations. The pattern of AIDS, for example, is becoming commoner in heterosexuals. An appropriate phrase that captures this broader concept is the 'population pattern of disease' (PPOD), yet it is more specific than a phrase that is often used – the epidemiology of disease. The main measure of PPOD is the disease incidence given over time, place and person (see Chapter 7).

Clearly, changes in the natural history of disease and in the population pattern are linked. Before reading on consider the exercise in Box 6.3.

Reducing the population's susceptibility would diminish the number of cases of overt, diagnosed disease, while enhanced susceptibility would have the opposite effect. The secular trend would change. If the changes in susceptibility are uneven across a population, there will be other changes in the PPOD too, for example the change in inequalities in CHD referred to above.

The duration of an episode of disease is likely to be linked to susceptibility, and hence the capacity to fight against the disease. A shorter course is also likely to have a better outcome, with less long-term morbidity or mortality. While the disease incidence will not be affected, the prevalence and case fatality is likely to be (Chapters 7 and 8). These changes will be reflected in the PPOD.

The length of the incubation period can affect disease patterns. If the incubation period lengthens in a chronic disease from 20 to 30 years, then the disease burden will decline, at least for some time. The severity of the disease can also change either as a result of changed virulence of the disease agent or changed susceptibility of the host. This will alter the balance between diagnosed and undiagnosed cases and change the measured incidence and prevalence and hence PPOD.

Box 6.3 Interrelationship between natural history and population pattern of disease

Assuming there are no changes to exposure to the causal agent, what effect would changing the natural history have on the population pattern? Consider, for example, the effect of:

◆ Reduced and enhanced susceptibility;

◆ A shorter or longer course of disease;

◆ A longer and shorter incubation period;

◆ A more severe or less severe disease.

The idea that an exposure can lead to variants (and varying severity) of the same disease is the spectrum of disease (also an idea that is understandably confused with the natural history of disease).

6.3 Spectrum of disease: a clinical concept fundamental to epidemiology

The spectrum of disease captures the idea that diseases present with varying signs, symptoms, and severity. For example if a hundred people are exposed simultaneously to an aerosol contaminated with the Legionnaires' disease bacillus, most (about 98 per cent) will have no perceptible problems. The remainder will have disease which varies from a mild influenza-like illness to a fulminating pneumonia. Of those who become ill about 10–15 per cent will die unless effective treatment is given. The mortality rate will be higher in some settings and population groups, such as in nursing homes or hospital outbreaks where the frail or elderly are. The period of time between exposure and first symptoms will vary from as little as 2 days in some people to as much as 10 days in others. The symptoms and signs of illness will vary greatly; some people have an illness dominated by neurological problems, others by chest problems. Among survivors, some will recover fully and others will be left with disability. This principle of variability of outcome applies to nearly all diseases whether infections, toxic problems, or cancers.

Tuberculosis is a particularly good example and is illustrated in Table 6.1 and Fig. 6.5, which combines the natural history and spectrum of disease concepts. Figure 6.5 develops this idea from a population perspective where the collective observations on a number of individuals are summarized as possible pathways in the natural history. With some exceptions children develop a mild illness (or a subclinical problem) from which they recover. This illness is not usually recognized as primary tuberculosis, but as a febrile illness of childhood. This progression is shown by line 1a in Fig. 6.5 on p 169. Rarely, this first exposure will lead to a serious infection which may be systemic (i.e. affects the whole body). Tuberculous meningitis is one of the rare, potentially fatal outcomes of such infection (line 1b). More usually, the primary tuberculosis is followed by a lifetime of cohabitation by the agent and host with living organisms sealed off in the lymph glands

Table 6.1 Spectrum of disease: tuberculosis

Primary tuberculosis	Secondary tuberculosis
No symptoms	Fever and weight loss
Minor self-limiting illness	Enlarged lymph glands
Grumbling illness with fevers	Persistent cough
Overwhelming illness such as tuberculous meningitis	Skin rashes
	Septicaemia (miliary tuberculosis)

of the patient (line 1a). In some cases, particularly when the natural defence mechanisms of the patient are weakened by other illnesses (e.g. AIDS, age, or other factors), the bacillus overcomes the defence mechanisms to cause secondary tuberculosis (line 2). The commonest form of this disease is respiratory, or lymphatic, but it may be a more general illness with fevers and weight loss. In most instances the disease will respond to therapy (after which we are not observing the natural history but the prognosis) or heal spontaneously (line 2a). Some people will be left with permanent disability (line 2b) while others will die (line 2c).

The spectrum of disease is, primarily, a population concept with obvious and important implications for clinical medicine. Doctors who are not aware of the full spectrum of disease, particularly the less severe or rare forms, are likely to be misled. The variants within the spectrum of disease may differ in different population groups. For example, while pulmonary tuberculosis is the dominant mode of clinical presentation in European-origin residents in the UK, lymph node tuberculosis is the commonest form in UK residents of Indian subcontinent origin. Coronary heart disease is more likely to present as angina in women, and as a heart attack in men. In the elderly and in people with diabetes, in particular, coronary heart disease may present as a silent myocardial infarction, that is, a heart attack without chest pain.

Some diseases occur more than once. Presentation of the same disease may differ at different times. The first occurrence of malaria is likely to be far more severe than subsequent episodes. In chronic diseases, however, recurrences may be characteristic; for example, if a person develops pain in the tongue in one occurrence of angina, then that person is likely to have a similar pattern at recurrence, rather than, say, pain in the left arm.

The fact that diseases may be mild or even 'silent' are among the many explanations for undiagnosed disease in the community, even when people are served by an excellent health service, a phenomenon described by the metaphor of the iceberg of disease (see Last 1963).

6.4 The unmeasured burden of disease: the metaphors of the iceberg and the pyramid

Surprisingly, for most health problems and within all health-care systems, there are large numbers of undiscovered or misdiagnosed cases of disease. The exceptions to this generalization are the serious diseases which have obvious symptoms which lead to a rapid and accurate diagnosis. Lung cancer is an excellent example of an exception, while prostate cancer is illustrative of the generalization. Lung cancer has characteristic symptoms e.g. cough, weight loss, blood in the sputum, and, if untreated, spreads and is invariably fatal. Prostate cancer may remain localized, with no signs or symptoms and in these circumstances poses little threat to health. Yet prostate cancer also may kill, and be diagnosed too late to cure. Serious and killing disorders such as diabetes, atrial fibrillation and hypertension are other good examples of this iceberg phenomenon. This principle applies alike to populations served by comprehensive, publicly funded health-care systems and to those with private services only available to those who can pay. Obviously, the number of undiagnosed cases in relation to those diagnosed will be bigger where the health-care system is poor.

The metaphor for this phenomenon is the iceberg of disease and symptoms. Cases that have been correctly diagnosed are the tip of the iceberg, visible and easily measured. In most diseases, as with the iceberg, the larger amount lurks unseen, unmeasured and easily forgotten with potentially catastrophic consequences. Figure 6.6 illustrates this and develops the iceberg concept as a pyramid by using its clearer structure and shape. At the tip of the pyramid are the cases which are diseased, diagnosed, treated, and controlled. The next block is the diagnosed but uncontrolled cases. The failure to control the disease arises from either technical or organizational factors or from the patient's preferences not to participate in therapy (so-called non-compliance or non-adherence). The third block comprises the patients with undiagnosed disease, which may be a reflection of the difficulties of making the diagnosis or the failure to access health care. The fourth block is the population that harbours the causal factors for disease, but remains disease free. The final block is the population free of both disease and causal factors. Blocks 1 and 2 correspond to the iceberg above sea level and 3 and 4 to below sea level. The pyramid comprises both the diseased population and those potentially diseased (i.e. it is a whole population concept), while the iceberg relates only to the diseased population.

There is a specific and minimal level of health care need at each level (Fig. 6.7). For block 1 the need is for vigilance and perhaps follow-up. For block 2 there is a need for review and effective and acceptable care. For block 3 there is a need for screening for people with early disease. For block 4 there is a need for health education. For block 5 there is a need for health promotion to maintain this desirable state.

Epidemiology that forgets the iceberg phenomenon, and merely counts the number of cases actually seen by clinicians and diagnosed, is misleading. Both for applied and causal research, epidemiology on statistics obtained from routine systems like hospital admissions is likely to be compromised. The missing cases thwart efforts to assess the

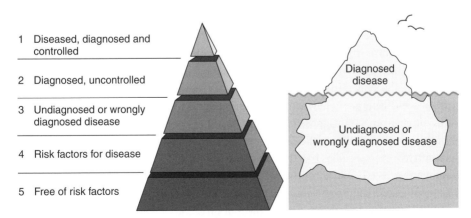

Fig. 6.6 Pyramid of health and disease: building on the iceberg of disease.

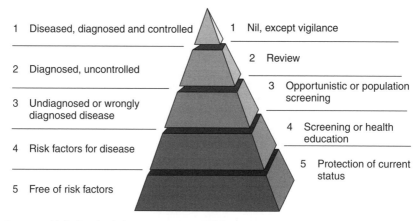

1 Diseased, diagnosed and controlled   1 Nil, except vigilance

2 Diagnosed, uncontrolled

2 Review

3 Opportunistic or population screening

3 Undiagnosed or wrongly diagnosed disease

4 Screening or health education

4 Risk factors for disease

5 Protection of current status

5 Free of risk factors

Fig. 6.7 Pyramid (iceberg) of disease: potential health and health care need.

true burden of disease. This creates difficulties in judging priorities and assessing the need for health services. There are no easy rules or formulae to apply to judge the true burden of disease using data on those diagnosed. However, experience with diabetes indicates that, in the absence of opportunistic or systematic screening, about 50 per cent of the cases in the community are diagnosed at any point in time. The findings for hypertension are about the same. For less serious diseases (migraine, eczema, back pain) or those which tend to get less attention (thyroid disorders, chronic bronchitis, peptic ulcer, and osteoarthritis) the proportion diagnosed would be lower. It is reasonable for researchers and health planners to assume that the true burden of disease is much higher than their data show, and unreasonable to reach conclusions without reference to the iceberg phenomenon (as is too often the case).

Unidentified cases may be different from identified ones, in terms of both the natural history and the spectrum of disease. For example, people with undiagnosed prostate cancer are less likely to have urinary symptoms or pain compared with those diagnosed. Where symptoms and disease progression and outcome are related, the undiagnosed cases are likely to be less severe. For this reason a screening programme (see next section) may uncover not just cases of disease at an earlier stage of the natural history but also less aggressive and severe cases. This may mislead the evaluation of screening programmes. In contrast, when symptoms and signs are not evident in the early stages of disease, as in high blood pressure or chronic glaucoma, undiagnosed cases may be just as severe as diagnosed ones.

Epidemiological studies of the causes and consequences of disease should, ideally, be of representative cases. Studies based on selected cases from the tip of the iceberg may give an erroneous view. The study of the outcome of prostate cancer based on cases diagnosed in hospital would lead to the view that the disease is usually, if not always, progressive. Studies of unselected cases, however, show that prostatic cancer can be a static, or slowly progressive phenomenon.

Patients who are at the tip of the iceberg are more likely to have multiple health problems than others because these diseases bring them to medical attention, which in turn increases the diagnostic activity. Their susceptibilities to various diseases, the causal pathway, and their outcomes may differ too. For example, people with cardiorespiratory problems and diabetes, and those living alone or in poverty, are more likely to be admitted to hospital. False and misleading associations may be generated. This is the basis of the bias known as Berkson's bias (Chapter 4).

6.5 Screening: picking up disease or disease susceptibility early

6.5.1 Introduction: definition, purposes, and ethics

The dictionary provides many meanings of the word screen, but the two that correspond to the epidemiological one are: to sift coarsely, and to sort out by tests.

Screening is the use of tests to help diagnose diseases (or their precursor conditions) in an earlier phase of their natural history or at the less severe end of the spectrum than usual. In so doing, screening uncovers the iceberg of disease. On the pyramid model in Fig. 6.7, screening is applied to block 3 and, less commonly, to block 4. The main aim is to reverse, halt, or slow the progression of disease more effectively than would normally happen. This is the only aim of screening that is unequivocally ethically justifiable. Providing knowledge about the diagnosis, whether to the patient or professional, is, on its own, insufficient reason for screening.

There are, however, some more controversial purposes of screening. Screening is also done to protect society, even though the individual may not benefit, or might even be harmed. Screening potential immigrants at the point at which a visa is issued or at the port of entry (for both contagious and chronic diseases) is an example. To measure prevalence of HIV infection there has been anonymous screening of pregnant women attending antenatal clinics. Screening may be done to select out unhealthy people, for example, for a job. The police, fire brigade, armed forces, and airlines are employers that screen potential employees in detail. Screening is sometimes done to help to allocate health care resources that are limited. The most extreme example is the practice of triage in wartime, when those unlikely to survive war wounds are left untreated so saving resources for those likely to survive. Screening may be done to identify disease at an early stage to help understand the natural history. In these circumstances, when the screening is not primarily for the benefit of individuals being screened, there are difficult ethical issues, the stage of useful particularly in genetic screening.

The ethical viewpoint, that the natural history of disease must be influenced favourably, sets limits on the scope of screening, and poses important challenges to epidemiology and public health. This means that the natural history of the disease needs to be understood, there need to be effective interventions for treating or controlling the disease, and the screening test needs to detect the problem at a stage when the disease is not advanced beyond the stage of useful therapy. These aims of screening are summarized in Box 6.4.

Screening applies tests to people who have not actively sought clinical care or advice for the disease to be tested for. At best they have been invited and have consented

Box 6.4 Aims of screening

- Better prognosis/outcome for individuals
- Protect society from contagious disease
- Rational, more efficient allocation of resources
- Selection of healthy individuals
- Research (e.g. on natural history of disease)

to be screened, and at worst they may have been screened without their informed consent. This is the feature that distinguishes screening from normal clinical practice where the patient has initiated the contact. The ethical basis of screening is fundamentally different from testing in clinical settings because who initiates the test and why is all-important.

6.5.2 Choosing what to screen for: criteria of Wilson and Jungner

Potentially, screening could be done for every disease for which there is a diagnostic test or diagnostic signs and symptoms. To guide the rational development of screening programmes there are several sets of criteria, usually variants of those of Wilson and Jungner (1968), as listed in Table 6.2.

Table 6.2 The criteria of Wilson and Junger

1 The condition sought should be an important health problem
2 There should be an accepted treatment for patients with recognized disease
3 Facilities for diagnosis and treatment should be available
4 There should be a recognizable latent or early symptomatic stage
5 There should be a suitable test or examination
6 The test should be acceptable to the population
7 The natural history of the disease, including latent disease, should be adequately understood
8 There should be an agreed policy on whom to treat
9 The cost of case-finding (including diagnosis and treatment of patients diagnosed) should be economically balanced in relation to possible expenditure on medical care as a whole
10 Case-finding should be a continuing process and not a 'once for all' project

Adapted from Holland and Stewart (1990, pp. 12–13) with permission (see Permissions).

These can be crystallized as six questions:

1 Is there an effective intervention?

2 Does intervention earlier than usual improve outcome?

3 Is there an effective screening test that recognizes disease earlier than usual?

4 Is the test available, affordable, and acceptable to the target population?

5 Is the disease one that commands priority?

6 Do the benefits of screening exceed the costs in this society?

If the answer to these six questions is yes then the case for screening is sound. The final decision will, as ever, depend on availability of resources and the priority of this programme in relation to others.

Screening programmes need more careful evaluation than clinical care. The reasons for this include: the fact that screening is a professionally initiated activity; the outcomes of screening are not easily measured for they accumulate over long time periods; the acceptability of a programme may change with time; the performance of the test may change over time, particularly if the frequency of disease changes; and screening is an expensive and difficult process which is hard both to put in place and to withdraw.

Screening for hypertension illustrates the issues well. Hypertension is a major causal factor in stroke, coronary heart disease, cardiac hypertrophy, heart failure, and in disorders of other organs, particularly the kidney. Mostly the cause of high blood pressure in an individual cannot be found, and this type of disease is called essential hypertension, where essential means 'of unknown cause'. In perhaps 5–10 per cent of cases there is an identifiable cause (e.g. severe kidney diseases leading to hypertension), and this form is known as secondary hypertension. Hypertension is not, strictly, a disease but a precursor of disease. Nonetheless, its importance and close association with diseases has led to it being considered, in practice, as a disease.

Hypertension usually occurs without symptoms and may first present as a stroke or heart attack. The challenge is to prevent this. As some of the changes induced by hypertension occur at an early stage of the natural history and may quickly become irreversible, this is best done through screening. Before reading on, do the exercise in Box 6.5.

Wilson and Jungner's criteria are met and the answer to the six questions above is, more or less, yes. The problem is a priority. Effective, acceptable treatments that improve long-term health outcomes are available. A screening test is widely available and

Box 6.5 Screening for hypertension

Even if your knowledge of high blood pressure is limited, assess this condition against the criteria in Table 6.2 (perhaps after a little extra reading). Now, apply the six questions on the previous page.

acceptable though it has some problems. The benefits of screening for hypertension far exceed the costs. The screening test is measurement of the blood pressure, usually using a sphygmomanometer, on one or a small number of occasions. Sometimes two readings may be made, 5 to 30 minutes apart. The diagnostic test is, effectively, repetition of the same test on several occasions combined with a clinical history, examination, and other tests to check for other diseases, particularly those that cause specific forms of hypertension. A check is also made on whether the adverse consequences of high blood pressure have occurred e.g. on the eyes, or kidneys. Additional tests of high blood pressure are possible but are used infrequently, at least in screening, including 24-hour readings using equipment that permits measurement while the person is ambulatory. Blood pressure screening based on the sphygmomanometer is done in many settings: in routine clinical practice in primary care and hospital settings; in pre-employment physical examinations; in workplace health programmes, as part of a periodic check up; in well-woman/well-man clinics; in antenatal clinics; and even in pharmacies and supermarkets. As the equipment and expertise to do the test is so widespread there is little need for a specially designed population-based screening programme.

6.5.3 Sensitivity, specificity and predictive powers of screening tests

Screening will make blocks 1 and 2 in the pyramid of disease (Fig. 6.6) grow and block 3 shrink. The danger is that through false positive tests, people in blocks 4 and 5 are wrongly placed in blocks 1 and 2, and through false negative tests people in blocks 1 and 2 are placed in blocks 4 and 5.

The ideal test would pick up all or most cases of hypertension in the population tested. This attribute of the test is known as high sensitivity (or, alternatively, as the true positive rate). To help remember this, such a test would be sensitive to the presence of disease. Clearly, the ideal test would also correctly identify all people who do not have the disease. Think of this as the test being specific to those who have the disease. This attribute of the test is the specificity (or, alternatively, as the true negative rate). The ideal test would, therefore, correctly identify both cases and non-cases.

In the ideal test, therefore, when cases go for more detailed clinical examination, the screening test result is confirmed, i.e. a screening test predicts the final result. A positive test in ideal circumstances predicts with 100 per cent accuracy the presence of hypertension and, similarly, a negative test predicts its absence. These attributes are known as the predictive powers.

There is, of course, no such perfect test, whether for screening or for diagnosis. As 100 per cent accuracy is not attainable with any diagnostic procedures, we apply the best available means of diagnosis as the gold standard against which the screening test is compared. The accuracy of a test is assessed in population groups and this places evaluation of screening tests in the domain of epidemiology.

These four measures, sensitivity, specificity and predictive power of a positive and negative test, are the main way to assess the performance of a screening or diagnostic test. These and other measures of test performance can be calculated from the 2 × 2 table

Table 6.3 The 2 × 2 table: assessing the performance of the screening test

Screening test	Disease (true/definitive test)		
	Present	Absent	Total
+ve	a	b	a + b
−ve	c	d	c + d
Total	a + c	b + d	a + b + c + d

Sensitivity or true positive rate = $a/(a + c)$. Predictive power of a +ve test = $a/(a + b)$.
Specificity or true negative rate = $d/(b + d)$. Predictive power of a -ve test = $d/(c + d)$.

as shown in Table 6.3. The rows of Table 6.3 show the results of the screening test, the columns the disease status. The disease status is said to be the true status of the person based either on a definitive (gold standard) series of tests or on clinical observation, often made over long time periods (possibly checked post-mortem). As even the definitive test is never 100 per cent accurate, a screening test is being evaluated against another imperfect, albeit better, test.

Table 6.3 uses a standard notation and layout: the letter 'a' represents true positive results on the screening test, 'b' false positives, 'c' false negatives, and 'd' true negatives. The formulae for the four measures are in the table. The best way to understand these formulae and to interpret the data is through practice. Try the exercise in Box 6.6, before reading on.

The sensitivity (93.4%) and specificity (98.2%) of the test are very high, as shown in Table 6.4. (This level of accuracy is unusual in clinical practice.) In other words, in these circumstances the test will correctly identify most people who have the disease (a), and also correctly identify most people who are disease free (d). Nonetheless, about one person in twenty who does have the disease will be misclassified as disease free (c), and hence wrongly reassured. Far fewer people without disease will be misclassified as having

Box 6.6 Calculating sensitivity and specificity

Five hundred patients known to have a particular disease were screened with a new test. Five hundred controls without this disease were also screened. Of the 500 patients 467 had a positive test. Of the healthy group without the disease 9 had a positive test. Create a 2 × 2 table based on Table 6.3 and reflect on the interpretation of the data.

Calculate sensitivity and specificity of the test. Is this a good performance? What are the implications for those wrongly classified by the test?

Table 6.4 Calculation of sensitivity and specificity based on data in Box 6.5

Screening test	Diseased (true/definitive test)		
	+ve	−ve	
+ve	467 (a)	9 (b)	476 (a + b)
−ve	33 (c)	491 (d)	524 (c + d)
	500 (a + c)	500 (b + d)	1000 (a + b + c + d)

Sensitivity = $a/(a + c)$ = 473/500 = 93.4%.
Specificity = $d/(b + d)$ = 491/500 = 98.2%.

the disease (b). This is reassuring from a population perspective, but it is not the information of direct interest to individuals and their doctors who want to know the implications of their individual results. This is given by predictive powers. Reflect on Box 6.7 before reading on.

The predictive power of a positive test is $a/(a + b)$ = 467/476 = 98.1%; and of a negative test is $d/(c + d)$ = 491/524 = 93.7%. In other words, only 1 or 2 per cent of those testing positive will have this result overturned by the definitive test. More of those with a negative test, however, will have this result overturned. This excellent performance is, however, a result of the artificial nature of the population, in which 50 per cent have the disease. That is, of course, unusual. Usually we consider a disease as common if 1 per cent or more of the population has it. Before reading on, imagine that you take this test to a country where no one has the disease i.e. the prevalence of the disease is 0 per cent. What will happen to the predictive powers of a positive and negative test? Now imagine the same for a population where 100 per cent have the disease.

The prevalence of the disease has a profound effect on the predictive power (but not on sensitivity and specificity). Imagine that the prevalence of a disease is actually zero. Then all screening test positive cases must, of necessity, be false positives (i.e. b in the notation in Table 6.4) and all screen negatives will be correct (i.e. d in the notation in Table 6.4). The predictive power of a positive test is zero since a is zero (and the predictive power of a negative test is 100 per cent).

If the prevalence of a condition is 100 per cent then, logically, all screen positive cases will have the condition (and screen negatives will all be false), so the predictive power of

Box 6.7 Predictive powers

If a man is positive on the screening test and asks what is his chance of having the disease eventually, i.e. once all the definitive tests are done, what can we advise? Similarly, what do we advise if the test is negative on the screening test? From Table 6.4 calculate predictive powers.

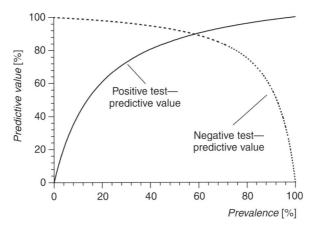

Fig. 6.8 Changes of predictive values with the prevalence of a disease (this example is calculated with a test sensitivity of 0.93 and a specificity of 0.85) (Source: Mausner and Kramer 1985; see Permissions).

a positive test is 100 per cent (and of a negative test zero). Predictive powers vary with disease/outcome prevalence, as shown in your exercise of the imagination and in Fig. 6.8. You can examine the effect of varying prevalence on predictive powers by doing the exercise in Box 6.8. In practice most diseases are uncommon, so the predictive power of a positive screening test tends to be low.

As the prevalence declines, as Table 6.5(a) and (b) shows, the predictive power of a positive test declines, and the opposite is true for a negative test. When the prevalence is 1 per cent—a figure which actually represents a disease that is considered common in the community—the predictive power of this same test is 34.2 per cent, in other words, in 6.5 of 10 cases the screening test will be wrong, and the person will be subjected to unnecessary anxiety and tests.

It is generally the case, in theory, that the sensitivity and specificity of a test are independent of prevalence but in practice they may not be. As the prevalence of the

Box 6.8 Varying prevalence: impact on predictive power

Assume that the test in Table 6.4 is applied to a population of (a) patients attending general practice, and that there the prevalence of the disease is 10 per cent; and (b) in a community setting where the prevalence is 1 per cent. Your populations are 1000 in each of these circumstances. The sensitivity and specificity is as in Table 6.4. Prepare two 2 × 2 tables, complete the cells starting with $(a + c)$, $(b + d)$, and $(a + b + c + d)$, and calculate the predictive powers. Now compare your answers with Tables 6.5(a) and 6.5(b).

Table 6.5(a) Predictive power (prevalence of disease = 10%)

Screening test	Disease (definitive test)		
	+ve	−ve	
+ve	93.4	16.2	109.6
−ve	6.6	883.8	890.4
	100	900	1000

Predictive power of positive test = $a/(a + b)$ = 93.4/109.6 = 85.2%.
Predictive power of negative test = $d/(d + c)$ = 883.8/890.4 = 99.3%.

disease declines the accuracy of observers is diminished, reducing the sensitivity (Fowkes 1986). This is, of course, due to misclassification error.

6.5.4 Setting the cut-off point for a positive screening test: introducing the relation between sensitivity and specificity and the ROC curve

The sensitivity and specificity are profoundly affected by the 'cut-off', i.e. the value of the measure at which a test is defined as positive. This is a very difficult decision. How do we make it? How would you make this decision? Continue with the example of high blood pressure. What would be the consequences of choosing a low and high cut-off?

We could observe the disease outcomes over some years and see whether organ damage occurs. For blood pressure, for example, we could take any cut-off value that is associated with a higher risk of disease. Because, by and large, low blood pressures are better, this could mean a cut-off value less than 120/80 mmHg, the average in most industrialized populations. The problem is that about half of the population would thereby be defined as hypertensive, and for most people so defined the true additional risk of disease outcome would be very low.

Based on a low cut-off point, say 120/80 mmHg, and knowing that the frequency of disease outcome is low, the sensitivity of the test for true adverse hypertensive disease would be very high, the specificity low, the predictive power of a positive test low, and the predictive power of a negative test high. If we took the hypertensive cut-off value as

Table 6.5(b) Predictive power (prevalence of disease = 1%)

Screening test	Disease (definitive test)		
	+ve	−ve	
+ve	9.3	17.8	27.2
−ve	0.7	972.2	972.8
	10	990	1000

Predictive power of a positive test = $a/(a + b)$ = 9.3/27.2 = 34.2%.
Predictive power of a negative test = $d/(c + d)$ = 972.2/972.8 = 99.9%.

180/120 mmHg few people would be defined as hypertensive and for those that were the frequency of adverse disease outcome would be high. Sensitivity for hypertensive disease outcomes would be low, specificity high, predictive power of a positive test high and of a negative test low.

There is a price to be paid for each choice. The lower cut-off picks up nearly all cases, but creates unnecessary anxiety and the risk of unnecessary treatment among those who were not destined to develop hypertensive disease outcomes (false positives). The higher cut-off, however, misses such cases (false negatives). Setting the cut-off point is a matter of difficult judgement, balancing the costs and benefits of false positives and false negatives. For blood pressure the clinically agreed cut-off point has been reducing over the years from about 160/100 mmHg to 140/90 mmHg. This is partly to do with the availability of better therapies and better services and partly to reducing professional tolerance of the adverse effects of high blood pressure.

The reason why sensitivity and specificity vary is, primarily, that we are using different cut-off points for a positive test. As the cut-off is relaxed, sensitivity approaches 100 per cent and specificity approaches 0 per cent. There are methods that can help to visualize and hence make these difficult judgements on cut-off points, but they do not provide an automatic answer. Figure 6.9 shows simple diagrams of sensitivity and specificity, symbolizing the fact that as one goes up the other comes down. In Fig. 6.9 (a) showing sensitivity and specificity in relation to cut-off points, we see that as one rises the other falls. We can use this picture to make decisions. If we are content with picking up 50 per cent of cases (sensitivity) we can see that specificity will be 50 per cent. If we want to pick up 90 per cent of cases (sensitivity), we get 10 per cent specificity. There is a cross-over point. At this point we seem to have a point of balance. Imagine the relationship looked more like 6.9 (b). Here, we can pick up 70 per cent of cases (sensitivity) with 30 per cent specificity. We might want to maximize sensitivity and specificity. The sum of sensitivity and specificity is 100. If we accept sensitivity of 10 per cent (specificity about 98 per cent) then we have a sum of about 110.

We can also refine this kind of decision by plotting sensitivity against specificity, or more commonly 1 minus specificity, or 100-specificity when using percentages. This creates a graph with one line. For historical reasons a graph of sensitivity in relation to 1 minus specificity is known as a receiver operating curve or ROC for short.

Now try the exercise in Box 6.9 (p. 184).

Now graph your results of sensitivity, specificity, and 100-specificity using the figures in Table 6.6. Compare your results with Figure 6.10 a and b.

If we are assessing ECG as a screening test for LVH, we might wish to compare that with something else, e.g. high blood pressure. This graph-based approach is particularly helpful for comparing several different screening tests for the same outcome, say, BMI compared with waist circumference as a screening test for type 2 diabetes mellitus. The layout as shown in Fig. 6.10b (ROC curve) permits the easy calculation of the area under the curve (AUC), which gives a summary number. This number can be compared for several tests. The straight line across the diagonal in Figure 6.10b is the ROC curve

Box 6.9 Calculating sensitivity, specificity and I00-specificity—blood pressure and LVH

In a study of 500 people, examining blood pressure and disease, the outcome was an enlarged heart (left ventricular hypertrophy, or LVH for short). The outcome was, let us assume, based on a perfect measure. The results were as follows:

Blood pressure	True outcome		
	LVH	No LVH	Totals
< 120	5	95	100
≥ 120–129	10	90	100
≥ 130–139	15	85	100
≥ 140–149	30	70	100
> 150	40	60	100
Totals	100	400	500

   What proportion of all the cases is correctly defined as LVH if we set the blood pressure cut-off at ≥120 mmHg i.e. what is the sensitivity? Do the calculations for each potential cut-off i.e. ≥120, ≥130 etc. To do this prepare 2 × 2 tables for each cut-off point. Now, what proportion of no-LVH people are correctly assigned i.e. specificity, at each cut-off. Calculate 100-specificity also. Compare your results with Table 6.6 and the appendix, which shows the 2 × 2 tables underlying the results.

achieved when the test results are no better than chance. The area under the straight line is 0.5 (50%). A value above 0.5 indicates the test can usefully distinguish between individuals with and without disease. If the test was perfect the area would be 1 (or 100%). For our fictitious example BP can be seen to be discriminative. The curve does not tell us the 'right' cut-off, but helps us choose.

Table 6.6 Sensitivity, specificity and I-specificity at varying cut-off points for blood pressure (see appendix for 2 × 2 tables)

Cut-off	Sensitivity (base 100)	Specificity (base 400)	100-Specificity
Any blood pressure (mmHg)	All 100 cases picked up = 100%	None of 400 no LVH group declared negative = 0%	100%
≥120–	95 cases = 95% (5 in < 120 range missed)	95 –ve = 24%	76%
≥130	85 cases = 85%	185 –ve = 46%	54%
≥140	70 cases = 70%	270 –ve = 77%	23%
≥150	40 cases = 40%	340 –ve = 85%	15%

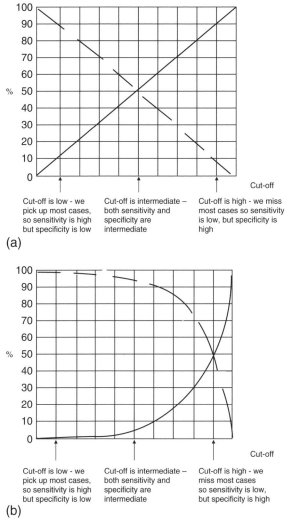

Fig. 6.9 Stylized relationship between sensitivity and specificity. (a) Simplified relationship between sensitivity (broken line) and specificity (solid line) and cut-off point. (b) Simplified but more realistic relationship between sensitivity (broken line) and specificity (solid line).

6.5.5 Distributions of the factors we are screening for—explaining the relations between sensitivity and specificity

You may wish to reflect on why sensitivity and specificity have this relationship where one rises while the other falls. There is a fundamental reason that means it is, more or less, one of the axioms of screening and diagnostic tests.

The underlying reason for the reciprocal nature of the sensitivity and specificity is that, for most diseases, and for many causes of disease, cases and non-cases belong to one,

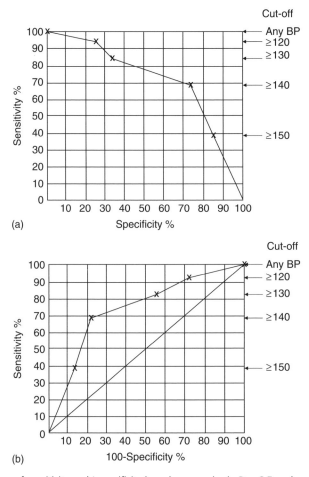

Fig. 6.10 Relation of sensitivity and l-specificity based on exercise in Box 6.5 and results in Table 6.6.
(a) Relationship of sensitivity and specificity based on exercise in Box 6.9 and results in Table 6.6.
(b) Relationship of sensitivity and 1-specificity based on exercise in Box 6.9 and Table 6.6.

not separate, distributions of values. This is illustrated in Fig. 6.11. In Fig. 6.11(a) there are three distributions which could be described as low, medium, and high blood pressure with varying levels of risk of hypertensive end-organ disease. The risk is indicated by the shading, with darker shading meaning higher risk. If the objective were to separate Group A from C cut-off points are comparatively easy to set. A value of 155 mmHg systolic blood pressure would clearly separate the high (Group C) and low risk (Group A) groups. Misclassification would be uncommon in distributions like Fig. 6.11 (a) and, importantly, the classification of people in Group A as Group C, and vice versa, would be rare. At a cut-off of 155 mmHg one can see that a few people at highest risk of disease (shaded as grey) are missed; mostly they belong to Group B. Extremely few people who belong to Group A will be wrongly judged as at high risk of hypertensive disease

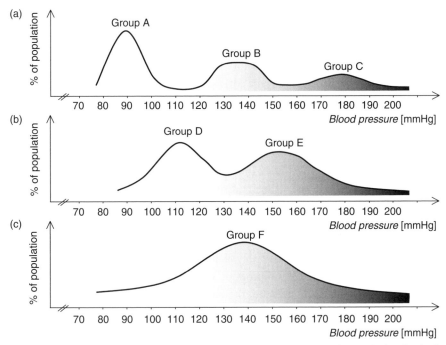

Fig. 6.11 Blood pressure: three distributions of values. Darker shading indicates higher level of risk of adverse outcome.

(by being placed in Group B or rarely in Group C). Even with this artificial distribution—the screener's ideal—there is some misclassification error.

Figure 6.11(b) shows a more realistic, but rarely seen, so-called bimodal (two peak), distribution. The distribution implies there are two groups of people—one with high blood pressure and high risk of disease (Group E) and one with low blood pressure and low risk of disease (Group D)—with overlap between them. Setting the cut-off point to separate the two groups here is more problematic. Setting it at 155 mmHg will lead to many people at high risk of disease being missed, and setting it at 120 mmHg to many people who are actually at low risk being screened positive. This type of distribution is not common but it illustrates the idea behind screening. There is a natural, though not necessarily correct, cut-off value which divides groups D and E at about 130 mmHg.

Figure 6.11(c), however, is the picture portraying the distribution of the risk factors for many common disorders including stroke and CHD (risk factor: hypertension), diabetes (risk factor: blood sugar), and glaucoma (risk factor: intraocular pressure). There is no natural separation between people at risk of disease and not at risk. The cut-off point is set solely on a judgement balancing the importance of avoiding false positives (achieving high specificity), versus avoiding missing true positives (achieving high sensitivity). For hypertension the judgement is not clear, for neither a false positive nor a false negative result is a trivial matter. Looking at Figure 6.11(c), where would you set the cut-off point? What would you like to know to help you in the task?

Three types of information are essential to help to define the cut-off point. First, we need a clear understanding of the natural history of the disease (untreated) at each level of the risk factor. Second, we need to know the adverse and beneficial consequences of treatment. Third, we need to know the sensitivity, specificity, and predictive powers of the screening test in the population to be screened.

A fourth action is desirable. This is the definition of subgroups of the population according to their level of risk by screening for interacting risk factors. For example, it is unlikely that a blood pressure of 150/100 has the same consequence for everyone. It is likely to pose a greater risk of heart disease for a smoker, a person with diabetes, someone with high cholesterol, and someone who is genetically susceptible to coronary heart disease. In the future, when the screening programme includes a scan of the genome for disease susceptibility genes, prediction of risk will be improved. A person's risk of adverse outcomes, shown as grey shading on the distribution curve (Fig. 6.11) is likely to be determined by a combination of environmental and genetic factors and not just the blood pressure level. So, the cut-off may well be different for different populations or subpopulations.

Unfortunately, there are errors in measurement and true variations in the environment and the biology of the person. Errors also occur in the recording and interpretation of the result. Even when these problems are resolved the relation between a screening test result and the disease outcome may differ between populations. Some of these problems are illustrated in relation to hypertension, but these principles can be generalized to most screening tests.

Some of the problems with screening for hypertension based on sphygmomanometry are these:

- Hypertensive disease is a consequence of long-term raised pressure of blood inside a complex vascular system. In screening we measure the pressure at one or a few time points, using an indirect measure of the true intra-arterial pressure, usually at one place in the vasculature, i.e. the arm.

- Individuals and groups are differentially susceptible to the consequences of a particular level of blood pressure. We generally ignore this.

- Blood pressure is variable, changing from minute to minute in response to stimuli including smoking, external temperature, exercise, emotional stress, and posture. Blood pressure also shows a 24-hour (circadian) rhythm, and is much lower at night than during working hours. Finally, in most populations blood pressure rises with age. A measure at one time (or even two or three times) is no more than a snapshot of highly variable factors.

- The measurement of blood pressure by manual sphygmomanometry requires some skill, including the ability to choose and apply the right cuff in the right way, release the pressure in the cuff and coordinate what is heard (Korotkoff sounds) while watching a falling column of mercury (or a digital display) and taking the readings at the appropriate moment. Observer errors are common, ranging from crude ones such as those caused by deafness to the more subtle ones such as preference for particular numbers, usually those ending in 5 or 0, so causing rounding errors. Automated methods also have problems. Automation only removes the problem of observer error, but machines can also go wrong.

- Poorly maintained equipment is a common cause of measurement errors. Sphygmomanometers are robust instruments but they do go wrong, and need regular calibration and occasional repair.

These sorts of problems, which arise in many screening programmes and research projects using a variety of tests (from questionnaires to blood tests), can be partially solved by following these principles:

- Study and quantify the relationship between the screening test (here blood pressure by sphygmomanometer) and the underlying measure of interest (here intra-arterial blood pressure). In this way you confirm whether, in principle, the screening measure is a good indicator of the underlying phenomenon to be measured.

- Study and quantify the relationship between the screening test and disease outcome in the population as a whole and in population subgroups.

- Standardize the measurement. For blood pressure, as a minimum in clinical practice, the person must be sitting, at rest for 5 minutes, and the cuff needs to be of specified and appropriate size for the body build of the person screened. Ideally, the blood pressures would be taken at the same time of day, in a controlled physical environment, and the subject should not have smoked for at least 20 minutes. In a research context still more stringent criteria are necessary.

- Training needs to be provided to those doing the screening in a standard way, and skills need to be regularly updated and checked.

- Equipment needs rigorous quality checks.

Imagine that all this is in place for blood pressure screening. How good in practice is a population-based blood pressure screening programme? This question requires careful evaluation: a complex subject beyond the scope of this book. Table 6.7, however, gives a sketch of the main ways that screening programmes are evaluated, the study designs usually used, and some of the potential problems. This table provides a foundation for further reading.

There are three important biases (Table 6.8) that are vitally important in interpreting data from non-trial-based evaluations. The solutions given are only partial ones.

Screening programmes are often implemented before there is good evidence of benefit. The reason why this happens is not wholly clear but screening often seems good on common-sense grounds. Clinical practice, with screening on an ad hoc basis (so-called opportunistic screening), may long precede the implementation of a formal screening programme. This may make rigorous evaluation based on a randomized controlled trial

Table 6.7 Evaluation of screening programmes: in practice

Option	Design	Problem
Examination of trends in morbidity/mortality	Before/after screening programme comparisons	Natural fluctuations in disease occur over time making interpretation difficult
Geographical comparisons in trends in mortality and morbidity	Regional/international comparisons of places with and without screening	Variation in diagnostic and treatment practices between places makes interpretation difficult
Audit/surveillance of cases to assess the stage of disease when diagnosis is made	Case series analysis over time (see Chapter 9)	Screened cases are probably self-selected volunteers, higher social class, at an earlier stage of disease (lead time bias) and may have less severe disease
Comparison of incidence, case fatality, and mortality in screened vs unscreened populations within the same population at a particular time or time period	Population case series, case–control and cohort studies (see Chapter 9)	Differences between screened and unscreened groups are many; apparent benefits may be due to these. Unscreened cases are those missed by screening, refused uptake, lost to follow-up and cases picked up between screenings
Experimental implementation of screening	Trials (see Chapter 9)	The ethical, practical, and financial constraints of organizing effective, large trials

(Chapter 9) impossible. Figure 6.12 illustrates why rigorous evaluation is essential. A vast amount of costly work is entailed in screening. There are side-effects.

6.6 Applications of the concepts of natural history, spectrum, population pattern, and screening

These concepts are directly applicable to health care. Health policies can be formulated and evaluated in terms of their expected influence on the natural history, spectrum and population pattern of diseases. Simply put, the purpose of all health policy would be to

Table 6.8 Three biases and their solutions

Bias	Solution
Self-selection i.e. those accepting screening are different from those declining it	Match comparison populations for all the important characteristics
'Lead time' bias, i.e. screened cases are picked up at an earlier stage	(a) Adjust survival data for estimated lead time (b) Stage disease and compare morbidity/mortality within stages
Speed of disease progression i.e. 'length bias': cases picked up by a screening may be less severe, and slowly progressive compared with others	Awareness

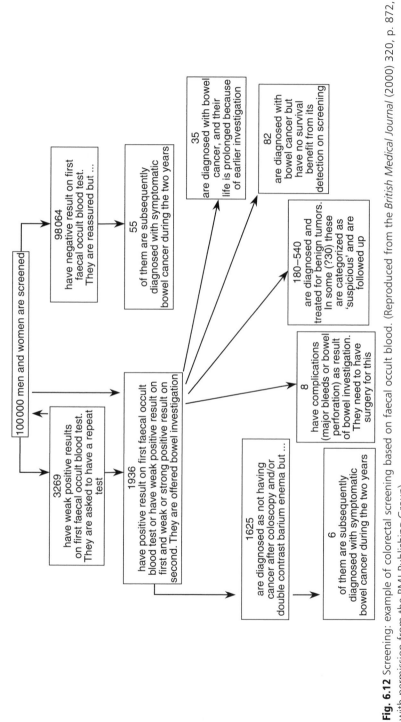

100 000 men and women are screened

3269
have weak positive results
on first faecal occult blood test.
They are asked to have a repeat
test

98 064
have negative result on first
faecal occult blood test.
They are reassured but …

1936
have positive result on first faecal occult
blood test or have weak positive result on
first and weak or strong positive result on
second. They are offered bowel investigation

55
of them are subsequently
diagnosed with symptomatic
bowel cancer during the two years

35
are diagnosed with bowel
cancer, and their
life is prolonged because
of earlier investigation

82
are diagnosed with
bowel cancer but
have no survival
benefit from its
detection on screening

180–540
are diagnosed and
treated for benign tumors.
In some (?30) these
are categorized as
'suspicious' and are
followed up

8
have complications
(major bleeds or bowel
perforation) as result
of bowel investigation.
They need to have
surgery for this

1625
are diagnosed as not having
cancer after coloscopy and/or
double contrast barium enema but …

6
of them are subsequently
diagnosed with symptomatic
bowel cancer during the two years

Fig. 6.12 Screening: example of colorectal screening based on faecal occult blood. (Reproduced from the *British Medical Journal* (2000) 320, p. 872, with permission from the BMJ Publishing Group).

shift the natural history of disease to the right and alter the spectrum so disease is less severe (Figs 6.4 and 6.5). This will alter the population pattern, with reduced disease compressed into the later stages of life. In the UK the idea of health gain, closely related to this concept, was popular in the 1990s, and is now called health improvement. Public health and medical action can be seen as the forces spearheading the attack against ill-health and disease (Fig. 6.4). The natural history of disease concept focuses attention to the long timescales in disease causation and prevention and hence the potential for screening.

Figure 6.3 illustrates the challenge in relation to coronary heart disease. The main adverse outcomes are angina and heart attack in middle and old age. However, as the causes exert their influence from conception onwards, a policy for heart disease control should work across the life course and would therefore need to be seen as a 50–75-year plan. One surprising, and yet predictable, consequence of the decline in heart disease mortality is a rising prevalence of angina. The spectrum of this disease has changed; as fewer people die from heart attack mainly because of better treatment, more develop the less serious consequences. Instead of being a disease of late middle age, often ending in death, it is becoming one of old age. Both circumstances enhance the prospects for effective screening.

Knowing the natural history of disease can radically alter the organization of health care. With this knowledge care can be proactive, in relation to disease control, screening, rehabilitation and long-term surveillance. It may also provide the scientific rationale for health care agencies to seek partnership with other agencies such as education, housing, and social services. For example, knowing the role of early life events in the genesis of heart disease and diabetes alters fundamentally our approach to these problems. Suddenly, these diseases are not seen as a matter for adult health care alone. The rationale for cross-disciplinary working within health care (primary health care, paediatrics, obstetrics, nutrition, and adult medicine) is clear. The need to influence the policies which foster good education and health of mothers and their infants unites people in health care, housing, employment, agriculture, and nutrition.

The discovery that the period between exposure, pathogenic effect, and disease may be decades (indeed, sometimes the disease never occurs because of death from other causes) makes the process of discovery of disease processes fraught with problems. Scientists studying people with disease now may need to obtain information about the life circumstances of the patient in childhood and even *in utero* (the fetal origins hypothesis), as for coronary heart disease (Fig. 6.3). Information may be needed for the period even before the conception of the patient or even the patient's parents' conception! This strains most scientific methods. Epidemiological methods which require people to recall information on causal factors are severely limited by lack of quality data. How can we ask, reliably, a 60-year-old patient with a heart attack about her life circumstances in infancy (e.g. birthweight) and in the teenage years, say on diet? This challenge is leading to the development and testing of new methods such as the life-grid approach where questioning is linked to memorable life events. e.g. smoking habits at the time of marriage or at the birth of the first child. It also spurs the development of birth cohort studies.

Prospective epidemiological methods entail delay, measured in the same order of time as the natural history of the disease. A cohort study (Chapter 9) to study the full range of known and postulated risk factors for coronary heart disease would need to last for about 70 years, and even then would not provide information about the causes and course of the disease in very old age. Furthermore, the ethical basis of research that observes people without intervening is increasingly questioned. For these reasons the natural history of most human diseases is patchily understood, and that of coronary heart disease will probably never be fully grasped.

Prevention of disease is dependent on understanding the natural history of disease. The timing of prevention interventions is critically important, for in some diseases the pathogenic effects are irreversible. Natural history of disease is also essential to diagnosis, therapeutics, and prognosis. For example, in managing the care of a child presenting for the first time with an epileptic fit, the physician needs to understand what the likely course of events is and whether this child is likely to have epilepsy long term or whether this episode is likely to be a single one. This knowledge will affect both therapy (are preventive drugs necessary?) and general care (can the patient be discharged from specialist care or does the patient need long-term review?). The parents and child will put great emphasis on the long-term outcome, which cannot be easily or accurately predicted for the individual but is usually based on the aggregated natural history in past patients, i.e. epidemiological data.

The level of need for health services is often underestimated. New services designed to meet demands commonly find that new demands emerge to again outstrip supply. This may perplex and frustrate health planners, who conclude that the demand for health care is infinite when the simple explanation is that some of the previously unidentified cases (the iceberg below the sea) are coming to light as a result of the extra service, or cases are being identified at an earlier point in their natural history.

The iceberg of disease phenomenon underpins the idea that health policy should be based on a realistic estimate of the size of the unidentified population of cases and those at risk. This principle is easy to state but hard to implement. First, estimating the true size of the disease iceberg is not easy, and requires representative population-based surveys, which have their own limitations and costs. Some diseases, especially rare ones such as multiple sclerosis, or those with a very short natural history such as transient ischaemic attacks, are not suitable for study using survey methods, and rely on disease registers which can only list diagnosed cases. Second, not all those with identifiable disease in the context of an epidemiological survey will, in practice, ever be identifiable by a routine service. Services based on the true numbers of cases could be wasteful. An example of this would be the number of people who have diabetes.

The WHO definition of diabetes includes a glucose tolerance test in standardized conditions. Such a test can be done in research conditions but is not easy in routine practice. The results for an individual may change over relatively short periods of time, so a single test is insufficient. Some people with diabetes would not wish to avail themselves of the services even once the diagnosis was made in this way. Basing services for diabetes on epidemiological surveys of the true size of the iceberg could, therefore, lead to over-provision. Population-based surveys are, therefore, complementary to information on service utilization.

By combining health utilization statistics, epidemiological survey data, and their own experience, clinical staff can assess the level of service needed. Clinicians need to take an active approach to identifying cases in the submerged part of the iceberg and work both with epidemiologists in assessing the true population burden of the disease, and with primary care staff to understand the specific clinical requirements of these cases. Health promotion's primary role is to attack the submerged parts of the iceberg of disease. This is done by organizing society and the environment to protect the whole population, by a combination of education and early detection of disease through screening targeted at blocks 3, 4 and 5 as conceptualized in the pyramid of disease (Fig. 6.7).

6.7 **Epidemiological theory: symbiosis with clinical medicine and social sciences**

In pointing to epidemiological theories underpinning this chapter, it would be futile to seek to disentangle them from other clinical sciences. Epidemiology has been pre-eminent in promoting the theory that many diseases are initiated by events acting years, or decades, before any clinical manifestation. This has created a subspecialty of life-course epidemiology. Epidemiology has emphasized, and contributed greatly to, building the picture of both the natural history of disease, and the spectrum of disease. The spectrum concept has illustrated that diseases may manifest themselves in many ways, including asymptomatic yet damaging forms. Shifts in diseases' natural history and the spectrum partly underlie changes in population patterns of disease and help to explain the iceberg concept of disease. In trying to understand why some people with symptoms and signs of disease seek care, and hence are diagnosed, while others do not, epidemiology crosses to the social sciences, linking into theories of illness-seeking behaviour. These theoretical constructs have immense practical significance, both in terms of prevention, early detection, and management of disease, and in terms of managing health services, for example explaining why demand rises as health service capacity increases. Screening is an application of epidemiology, but it rests on other theoretical concepts, particularly the natural history of disease. Epidemiology has shown, irrefutably, that disease patterns are consistently shifting in populations. Epidemiology will never finish its work.

6.8 **Conclusion**

Understanding the interrelated concepts of the natural history, spectrum, population pattern and iceberg of disease and their relation to screening is crucial to the epidemiological endeavour. Natural history is usually pieced together from an understanding of causes and their effects, and outcomes of disease, and hence lies at the heart of epidemiology. Rational health policy, health care, and health promotion require a knowledge of the natural history. The ethical and technical difficulties of studying natural history is a deterrent, however, and the necessary work is too rarely done.

The model of the natural history of disease provides a unifying common purpose for all the medical sciences, and all branches of the healing and caring health profession: to influence the natural history of disease by reducing or delaying exposure to the causal agents; to promote resistance to these agents; to detect the pathogenic effects early while disease onset can be prevented or delayed (often through screening), and to manage disease onset to minimize complications and long-term effects including delaying death. This is a mission which engages everyone in the health professions.

Summary

The natural history of disease is the uninterrupted progression of disease from its initiation by exposure to the causal agents to either spontaneous resolution, containment by the body's repair mechanisms, or to a clinically detectable problem. Natural history includes the long-term course of that problem, but without treatment. The natural history is seldom known, for the act of diagnosis and treatment influences it. Studies of natural history impose profound ethical difficulties. The pattern of disease progression may be distinctive. As the causes of some diseases act decades before the disease is diagnosed, often the only way of studying the natural history of disease is to do follow-up (cohort) studies. The impact of knowledge about the natural history of disease is often profound. For example, understanding that coronary heart disease, a killer in middle and old age, is influenced by factors acting in the uterine and early childhood environment significantly alters the strategy of prevention. The primary purpose of public health and medicine is to influence favourably the natural history of disease.

The natural history of disease is related to (and influences), but is not synonymous with, the changing pattern of disease in populations or the different levels of severity with which a disease may present (spectrum of disease).

For many health problems the number of cases identified is exceeded by those not discovered. An illustrative metaphor is the iceberg. Correctly diagnosed cases are represented by the tip of the iceberg visible above sea level, and undiagnosed ones by the larger presence below sea level. An alternative metaphor of the pyramid of disease develops this into a population concept. The iceberg phenomenon thwarts epidemiological efforts to assess the true burden of disease and creates difficulties in accurately judging the need and demand for services. Since unidentified cases are different from identified ones it is often impossible to identify truly unselected and representative cases for epidemiological studies.

Screening is the application of tests to diagnose disease (or its precursors) in an earlier phase of the natural history of disease (often in well people) or in a less severe part of the disease spectrum than is achieved in routine medical practice. Screening uncovers the iceberg of disease. Screening tests are not usually diagnostic but they may be, usually by repetition of the test for example in screening for high blood pressure. The key to successful screening is a simple test that can be applied to large populations with minimum harm and a high degree of accuracy in separating those who need more detailed investigation from those who do not. The ideal test would have high sensitivity (i.e. it picks up cases) and specificity (i.e. it correctly identifies non-cases). A person positive on the screening test would have a high probability of being confirmed as a case. A person negative on the screening test would have high probability of being confirmed as problem free. The potential of screening is vast but there are important limitations such as the inability to influence the natural history of many diseases, either because of lack of effective interventions or lack of services to deliver them. There is a need to balance the benefits of earlier diagnosis against penalties such as engendering anxiety and the danger of both further tests and treatments. These concepts are highly interrelated.

Exercises from the first edition

Do the exercises in Boxes 6.7 and 6.8 based on the data in the table below, which is slightly different from that in the text.

The answer to the exercise in Box 6.7 is that the predictive power of a positive test is $a/(a + b) = 473/480 = 98.5\%$; and of a negative test is $d/(c + d) = 493/520 = 94.8\%$. The answers to the questions in Box 6.8 are in the tables below.

Data for calculation of predictive powers

Screening test	Diseased (true/definitive test)		
	+ve	−ve	
+ve	473 (a)	7 (b)	480 (a + b)
−ve	27 (c)	493 (d)	520 (c + d)
	500 (a + c)	500 (b + d)	1000 (a + b + c + d)

Sensitivity = $a/(a + c)$ = 473/500 = 94.6%.
Specificity = $d/(b + d)$ = 493/500 = 98.6%.

Answer Predictive power (prevalence of disease = 10%).

Screening test	Disease (definitive test)		
	+ve	−ve	
+ve	94.6	12.6	107.2
−ve	5.4	887.4	892.8
	100	900	1000

Predictive power of positive test = $a/(a + b)$ = 94.6/107.2 = 88.2%.
Predictive power of negative test = $d/(d + c)$ = 887.4/892.8 = 99.4%.

Answer Predictive power (prevalence of disease = 1%).

Screening test	Disease (definitive test)		
	+ve	−ve	
+ve	9.46	13.86	23.32
−ve	0.54	976.14	976.68
	10	990	1000

Predictive power of a positive test = $a/(a + b)$ = 9.46/23.32 = 40.6%.

Predictive power of a negative test = $d/(c + d)$ = 976.14/976.68 = 99.9%.

Sample examination questions

Give yourself 10 minutes for every 25% of marks.

Question 1 Define what is meant by natural history of disease and explain why this is difficult to study in epidemiology. (25%)

Answer The natural history of disease is the processes and outcomes that arise following the event that triggers the onset of disease and leads to either resolution or death. The concept implies that there has been no interference with this process. The ideal in public health is that disease occurs only at the end of life so people live long lives without disability.

Natural history is difficult to study because of ethical, policy and legal requirements to treat people whenever possible, or at the least to alleviate their problems when there is no treatment. So human studies of the natural history of disease are extremely difficult.

Question 2 Define screening and briefly outline its principal benefits. (25%)

Answer Screening is the use of tests to help diagnose diseases (or their precursor conditions) in an earlier phase of their natural history or at the less severe end of the spectrum than is achieved in routine clinical practice. In so doing, screening attempts to uncover the iceberg of disease. The main aim is to reverse, halt or slow the progression of disease more effectively than would normally happen.

Screening is also done to protect society, even though the individual may not benefit, or might even be harmed.

Screening may be done to select out unhealthy people e.g. for a job.

Screening is sometimes done to help allocate health care resources that are limited.

Screening may be done simply for research, for example, to identify disease at an early stage to help understand the natural history.

Potential benefits of screening

- Better prognosis/outcome for individuals
- Protect society from contagious disease

Answer 1

	Actual glucose status		Total
Laboratory results	Present	Absent	
Present	90 (a)	40 (b)	130 (a+b)
Absent	10 (c)	60 (d)	70 (c+d)
Total	100 (a+c)	100 (b+d)	200 (a+b+c+d)

◆ Rational allocation of resources

◆ Selection of healthy individuals

◆ Research (natural history of disease)

Question 3 A hospital laboratory is asked to test 200 specimens of urine, of which 100 are known to contain glucose; the remaining 100 being free of glucose. The laboratory reports 130 with glucose, 90 of which were known to contain glucose.

1 Create a 2 × 2 table for the above data (10 %)

2 Calculate sensitivity and specificity for the laboratory's test results (10 %)

3 What can be said about the test's performance? What are the onsequences of using this test for a screening programme to detect glycosuria, i.e. glucose in the urine, which may be seen in diabetes in (a) hospital settings and (b) community settings, where prevalence of glycosuria will be lower? (30 %)

Answer 2 Sensitivity = a/a+c = 90/100 = 90.0 %; specificity = d/b+d = 60/100 = 60.0 %.

Answer 3 The performance of this test is poor. The laboratory's glycosuria test shows a sensitivity of 90.0% and specificity of only 60.0%. These results suggest that about 1 in 10 true cases will be misidentified as not having glycosuria which is worrying as patients are falsely reassured. On the other hand, the relatively low specificity rate suggests the laboratory will mislabel as positive a large number (4 out of 10 cases) of true negatives, and therefore overestimate the number of cases. This creates much unnecessary anxiety to people.

The prevalence of disease influences the yield or number of cases detected by a screening programme.

◆ In a high-prevalence population such as in a hospital, the percentage of test positive found to be positive (assessed using the positive predictive value) is likely to be high.

◆ In a low-prevalence population, the positive predictive value will be lower, and a much higher proportion of those with positive screening results will not be found to have the disease upon further diagnostic investigation. The test will be even less effective in the community.

Question 4 Why is the concept of the iceberg of disease important for epidemiological research describing the burden and distribution of disease? And health care planning?

Answer The iceberg of disease is important because:

- Epidemiological research describing the burden of disease will underestimate the problem, sometimes by a great amount. For common disorders such as headache the true burden may be 10 times or more that which is recorded or noted in records. For serious disorders such as diabetes mellitus the true burden may be double that known. Studies of the distribution of disease by time, place or person (the epidemiological triad) may reach wrong conclusions, e.g. investigators may conclude that disease incidence is rising over time, but in reality the incidence is stable, but the iceberg of disease is being uncovered by more doctors more able to diagnose disease, especially in community settings.

- If a service is planned for the known amount of disease there will be insufficient resource. If additional resources are made available e.g. an additional doctor, more of the iceberg of disease will be uncovered. The service to the community is likely to be improved but again there may be pressure for additional resources, as the number of patients rises.

Appendix

2 × 2 tables for ROC curve data in Table 6.8

		Cases		
	Test	+	–	
Cut off	+	95	305	
≥ 120	–	5	95	
		100	400	500

Sens = 95% Spec 24% 1-spec = 76%.

		Cases		
	Test	+	–	
Cut off	+	80	215	
≥ 130	–	15	185	
		100	400	

Sens = 85% Spec 46% 1-spec = 54%.

		Cases		
	Test	+	–	
Cut off	+	70	130	
≥ 140	–	30	270	
		100	400	

Sens = 70% Spec 68% 1-spec = 32%.

Continued

2 × 2 tables for ROC curve data in Table 6.8

		Cases		
	Test	+	−	
Cut off	+	40	60	100
≥ 150	−	60	340	400
		100	400	500

Sens = 40% Spec 85% 1-spec = 15%.

Chapter 7

The concept of risk and fundamental measures of disease frequency
Incidence and prevalence

Objectives

On completion of the chapter you should understand:

+ that risk is the likelihood in a defined population of developing a disease or risk factor;

+ that epidemiology measures the quantity of disease in populations (absolute or actual measure of risk) and how this quantity compares between populations (relative measure of risk);

+ that a risk factor is a characteristic that is associated with disease or precursor of disease (usually the exposure variable);

+ the meaning and application of the words rate, ratio and proportion in everyday and epidemiological language;

+ that the fundamental measures of disease frequency in epidemiology are the incidence and prevalence rates;

+ the differences and similarities between the incidence rate estimated using a person–time denominator and using a population denominator;

+ that there are great challenges in accurately measuring the events (numerator) and populations at risk (denominator) needed to calculate incidence and prevalence;

+ the interrelationship between incidence and prevalence;

+ the advantages of using subgroup-specific, as opposed to overall, rates.

7.1 Introduction: risks, risk factors, and causes

In everyday language, risk is the possibility of suffering harm or danger. A person at risk from an environmental or behavioural factor is someone endangered. This everyday concept of risk factors is clearly a causal one, that is, a risk increases a person's chances of harm, or danger, or indeed, of contracting a disease.

Risk in epidemiology also usually refers to the likelihood (probability) of dying or developing a disease, or its precursors, so the word is used similarly to everyday language. In epidemiology our prime interest is in the association between the probability

Box 7.1 Risk factors and causes

Reflect on the phrases 'risk factor' and 'cause of disease'. What is the difference between them?

of disease, or risk, and those environmental, individual, and social characteristics which influence the risk. The influencing characteristics are called risk factors. Reflect on the question in Box 7.1 before reading on.

In epidemiology the phrase 'risk factor' does not necessarily imply that the characteristic has a causal effect (association is not causation). The problem is that this is too often forgotten. The phrase 'risk marker' is sometimes used in preference to risk factor, simply to emphasize that no causal relationship is presumed. This has no logical advantages and it wrongly implies that a risk factor (rather than marker) is causal. Some risk factors may be agreed to have more than a statistical association with disease. When a causal relationship is agreed the phrase causal factor, or simply cause, is used. For example, we say smoking is a cause of coronary heart disease (CHD). For most CHD risk factors (e.g. hyperhomocystinaemia, low levels of high-density lipoprotein cholesterol (HDL), high C-reactive protein, job strain) we may imply, but rarely claim, a causal role. Much of epidemiology concerns the search for causal risk factors as covered in Chapters 3–5.

In contemporary epidemiology there is imprecision in the interpretation and use of these vital phrases. The confusion leads to attribution of cause where it is merely association, and alternatively the failure to speak of an association as causal when it is. Such confusion has led to much criticism of epidemiology. Chapters 3, 4 and 5 explain the difficulties involved in achieving causal understanding, and the reader will appreciate that a cautious approach is usually to be applauded rather than criticized.

As already discussed, associations are rarely causal, but their analysis is the starting point of causal understanding in epidemiology. This chapter and the next two consider the basic epidemiological tools needed to supply the information for this task.

7.2 Quantifying disease frequency, risk factors, and their relationships: issues of terminology

Epidemiological studies measure, present, and interpret data on the frequency of death, illness, and disease and of risk factors. The epidemiological question is, in what quantity does the disease occur in a population (absolute measures) and how does this compare with other populations (relative measures)? Table 7.1 lists the main measures that answer these questions and that are to be discussed in this and the next chapter. The epidemiological strategy for working out causes of disease works best by using the comparative (relative) approach, while that for assessing a population's health needs works best by examining that population's actual health pattern (absolute approach).

Table 7.1 Some epidemiological measures in relation to whether they provide absolute (actual) or relative frequency

Numbers of cases	Absolute
Proportional mortality	Absolute
Proportional mortality ratio	Relative
Overall (crude) prevalence and incidence rates	Absolute
Specific prevalence and incidence rates	Absolute
Standardized rates	Absolute/relative mix
Standardized ratios	Relative
Relative risk	Relative
Odds ratio	Relative
Attributable risks	Absolute
Numbers needed to treat and prevent	Absolute
Life years lost	Absolute
Disability-adjusted life year (DALY)	Absolute
Quality-adjusted life year (QALY)	Absolute

While there are many measures, two underpin virtually all epidemiology: incidence and prevalence rates. These are discussed in detail in this chapter. Table 7.2, which is the same as Table 1.4, gives brief definitions of incidence and prevalence rates and indicates the type of studies (discussed in Chapter 9) from which such data are derived.

For their interpretation epidemiological studies need to provide accurate information on the timing and location of measurements. It is truly remarkable how many published reports and papers omit this information. They also need to give the number and characteristics of disease cases, and of the population from which they come. Numbers of cases, or people with the risk factors, usually comprise the numerator, the population from which they come is usually the denominator.

Table 7.2 Introduction to incidence and prevalence rates

Measure	Key features	Type of study	Formulae
Incidence	Count of new cases over a period of time in a population of known size defined by characteristics (age, sex, etc.), and place and time boundaries	Disease register Cohort Trial	New cases ÷ population at risk or New cases ÷ time spent by the study population at risk
Prevalence	Count of cases (new and old) at a point in time in a population of known size defined by characteristics (age, sex, etc.) and place	Cross-sectional Disease register	All cases ÷ population at risk

Box 7.2 Terminology

Define the following terms, using a dictionary if necessary.

ratio

rate

proportion

The numerator is the upper number of a fraction and the denominator is the lower number i.e. as in $^a/_b$ where a is the numerator and b the denominator. From this simple arithmetic we construct virtually the entirety of quantitative epidemiology. Epidemiology has developed a terminology based on, but not corresponding exactly to, everyday and mathematical words for similar ideas. This is a potential cause of difficulty, for which there is no easy remedy. Indeed, there has been a great deal of heated debate over the last 20–30 years that readers may wish to access (see references). I refer to it briefly here.

Before reading on, try the exercise in Box 7.2.

A ratio is any number in relation to another. A rate comprising the numerator in relation to the denominator is, therefore, a type of ratio. The word ratio is commonly used in epidemiology, but is usually reserved for summarizing the division of one ratio by another. This is explained in Chapter 8 in the discussion of the proportional mortality and morbidity ratios, standardized mortality ratio, and odds ratio.

In epidemiology the word rate is usually, but not always, used for a ratio where the numerator and denominator have different qualities, for example, deaths/population. The fraction, numerator divided by the denominator, is in common practice called the rate in epidemiology, public health and medicine. The dictionary meaning of the word rate, which corresponds best to its use in epidemiology, is a quantity measured with respect to another quantity. This is the way the word rate is used in this book, largely because this reflects its use in most journals (including those specialising in epidemiology), books, the media, and verbal discourse. It is also in line with its use in allied disciplines e.g. sociology, economics, and demography. Some writers, basing their views on sciences such as physics and chemistry, which are sciences distant in concepts, methods, and applications from epidemiology, advise that all rates must have a time dimension. This has caused a rift between such definitions and day-to-day practice, a confusion in terminology, and quarrels about semantics. Some flexibility, and awareness of the issues, are recommended to readers. I refer to this debate later in the chapter.

A proportion in epidemiology is usually a ratio where the numerator is a part of the denominator, so both must have the same qualities. For example, deaths due to one cause/deaths due to all causes. This corresponds to the dictionary definition of one part in relation to another, though the word has many other meanings that overlap with rate and ratio.

Disease frequency is usually measured by the incidence rate and/or the prevalence rate. From basic data on disease, death, risk factors, and population counts many summary measures of health status and risk, some of which are listed in Table 7.1, can be calculated as shown in this and the next chapter. Different ways of presenting the same data have a major impact on the perception of risk and, in particular, relative and actual (or, absolute) measures of frequency portray dramatically different priorities. Epidemiological data should be presented, wherever possible, to indicate both relative and actual frequency as discussed in Chapter 8.

The patterns of diseases (and of their risk factors) are constantly changing, mainly because the environment within which populations live is changing. Frequency data must, therefore, be described in the context of the population, the place, and the time of the study. Readers should search for these crucial contextual details, which are too often missing in reports (Chapter 10).

The following principles in the analysis of differences and changes in disease frequency apply to all epidemiological measures but are explained and emphasized for incidence rates. However, the likelihood of artefacts explaining differences and changes in disease frequency is greater with prevalence measures than with incidence rates, simply because prevalence rates are more complex, being influenced not only by disease occurrence but also by death and recovery.

7.3 Incidence and incidence rate: the concepts of person-time incidence, and cumulative incidence

The meanings of the word incidence in epidemiology that correspond to its dictionary definition are: the act of happening and the extent or frequency of occurrence. The meaning of incidence in everyday English is broad, which explains why this word is so commonly used to mean different things, even in epidemiology. In epidemiology incidence rate is the frequency of *new* occurrences of an event in a population at risk of the event, in a period of time (Table 7.2). The word *new* is the key defining feature. The meaningful interpretation of disease incidence requires the number of new cases (the numerator), the population at risk (denominator), the time period, and the place of study. For simplicity, the discussion here assumes the event is a disease but it could be some other outcome. To avoid the controversy around the word rate some writers say, for example, incidence instead of incidence rate. I have done this sometimes. Strictly, however, the incidence (without the ward rate) of a disease is a count of new cases unrelated to a denominator, and therefore it is not a rate.

The incidence rate is a fundamental measure in epidemiology and yet the concept underlying it has evolved in recent decades. It is difficult to grasp and to convey. Presently there are two main variants, sometimes, but often not, differentiated as the person-time incidence rate and cumulative incidence rate, which are easily confused (Table 7.3 summarizes some of their qualities). One reason for confusion is the use of several terms that convey the same underlying concept. Person-time incidence is also known simply as incidence rate. Person-time incidence rate ranges from zero to infinity, as a number of deaths might occur over a short period of time.

Cumulative incidence is also usually simply referred to as incidence rate, so causing confusion with person-time incidence rate. It is also known as incidence proportion,

Table 7.3 Qualities of the incidence rate obtained using the person and person-time denominator (numerator is identical)

Person denominator (cumulative incidence rate or simply incidence rate)	Person-time denominator (or incidence rate)
Ranges from 0 to 1* Measures absolute risk (probability) of new disease* e.g. cases/10 000 people = 5%	Ranges from zero to infinity Not clearly interpreted as a measure of absolute risk, e.g. 50 cases per 1000 person-years
Can be used to construct relative risks	Can be used to construct relative risks
Incidence rates can be calculated with population estimates, e.g. from a census, and disease from a register	Person-time incidence rates usually cannot be calculated in population estimates
Can only be used directly in cohort studies where study participants are enrolled at about the same time	Can be used either when enrolment is at about the same time or when enrolment is spread over time

* When the denominator is the population at the beginning of the study.

cumulative incidence and cumulative proportion. Cumulative incidence rate is also often used synonymously with risk. The cumulative incidence rate varies from 0 to 1 (or 0–100 per cent). Readers will need to become accustomed, and alert to, these two related concepts underlying incidence rates and their synonyms. For simplicity I will use one word—incidence rate—to capture two conceptual approaches, one based on a population denominator, the other on a person-time denominator. When readers are examining incidence data they should seek out which of these concepts is in use.

The need for these two approaches is best understood by an example. Assume the rate of a disease is 20 per cent per year and we follow up 100 people. After 6 months, on average, 10 people will develop the disease. If there are no deaths from this disease, and the disease does recur and there is no immunity then the denominator remains 100. We would expect, on average, another 10 cases in the next 6 months. There might, however, be deaths or some immunity in cases. After one year, we might assume that even in these circumstances, 20 new cases will occur. Do you agree? How many new cases occur by the first 6 months, on average? Then, how many new cases will occur in the second 6 months?

On average we'd expect about 10 cases at the 6-month point. For diseases that occur only once these 10 people are no longer at risk after 6 months. This would certainly be true for many infectious diseases that are followed by life-long immunity. This would also apply to those chronic diseases that only occur once. When the outcome of interest is death, then these 10 are no longer at risk.

The denominator is, we now see, 100 only at the beginning of the study. In theory, for first-event only studies e.g. death, as each case occurs it should be subtracted from the denominator. So, in our example, the denominator would be approximately 95 at the 3-month stage, 90.25 (not 90) at 6 months, 85.7 (not 85) at 9 months and 81.5 (not 80) at 12 months.

In a large population, and a common disease, the denominator would be diminishing almost continuously. To take this fully into account we would need to measure incidence rate in very small increments of time. There are theoretical measures of the occurrence of disease over a period of time approaching zero. Figure 7.1 illustrates this point. The formula for one such measure, force of morbidity (adapted from the first edition of the *Dictionary of Epidemiology* by Last) is reproduced in the appendix. Most readers of this book will not need such formulae but they will come across these ideas.

A number of closely linked concepts relating to the incidence rate at a point in time are described by these effectively synonymous phrases—forces of morbidity and mortality, hazard rate, instantaneous incidence density, instantaneous incidence rate, disease intensity, and person-time incidence rate. In practice epidemiologists mainly work with the last of these. The person-time denominator is simply the amount of time that the study population as a whole has spent at risk (disease-free, or alive, in the case of mortality studies).

The formula for this is:

$$\text{Person-time incidence rate} = \frac{\text{New occurrences of outcome over a period of time}}{\text{Time spent by the study population at risk over this period of time (person-years of observations)}} \quad (7.1)$$

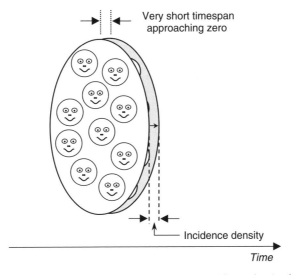

Fig. 7.1 Incidence rate in a period of time approaching zero—incidence density, forces of mortality/morbidity, hazard rates, disease intensity: a pictorial representation.

$$\text{Or more simply (after Rothman)} = \frac{\text{Disease occurrences}}{\text{Sum of time periods}} \tag{7.2}$$

Figure 7.2 illustrates this. In Fig. 7.2 we start with a population of 10 people in the denominator (smiling faces) and none in the numerator. In the first year there are no cases so the incidence rate is $^0/_{10}$ years of observation. In the second year 1 case occurs. We assume that cases are occurring evenly over time. On average, therefore, each case contributes 0.5 years of observation. So in this second year, the 10 people have contributed 9.5 years of observation, 19.5 in total. So the incidence rate is $^1/_{19.5} = 0.0512$ per year of observation = 51.2 cases per 1000 years of observation. This procedure continues until the end of the study, here 3 cases and 35.5 years of observation = $3 \div 35.5 = 0.0845$ per year of observation or 84.5 cases per 1000 years of observation. This formula provides investigators with great flexibility, particularly in cohort studies where investigators know, for each person, the exact date of entry into the study and the date of onset of disease or death. Its flexibility also allows study subjects to enter the study at different times, and it makes handling losses to follow-up and death easy (for these simply contribute less time to the denominator).

It does have some disadvantages. First, it does not give an easily interpreted direct measure of risk, i.e. probability; the incidence rate will be expressed, for example, as 102/10 000 years. This is not a problem for relative measures but it is for actual/absolute ones.

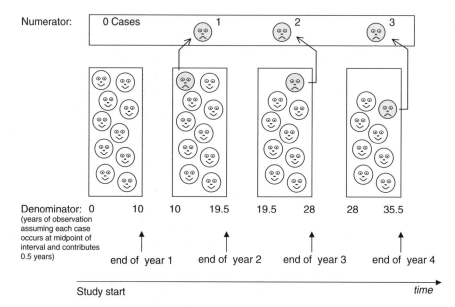

Fig. 7.2 Incidence rate—3 cases per 35.5 person-years—estimated using the person-time denominator: a pictorial representation.

Secondly, there is an assumption underlying this estimate that the incidence rate in those entering and leaving the study at different times, and those lost to follow-up, is the same as in others in the study population. Neither of these assumptions are self-evidently true. Most diseases, however, present different risk at different ages and calendar periods. Thirdly, the formula assumes that the disease occurs evenly over time, for the time periods contributed by those in the study for a short time are given the same weight as those contributed by people in the study for a long time. This gives the person contributing 50 years to a study five times the weight of a person contributing 10 years, and 50 times the weight of those contributing one year. A study with a large number of people with small time contributions may, if the assumption does not hold, come to a conclusion different from that of a study comprising mostly people with large time contributions.

The number of people in the person-time denominator can be judged only from a knowledge of the average time period of observation, which is only a reasonable estimate if there is no skew in the distribution (so investigators need to give this information).

In historical, and much current, epidemiological practice, this problem of the diminishing denominator has been sidestepped. The standard, and time-honoured, formula for incidence rate is:

$$\frac{\text{New occurrences of outcome over a period of time}}{\text{Population at risk over that period of time}} \tag{7.3}$$

The resulting fraction is usually multiplied by an appropriate number; for example, by 100 to give a rate per hundred which is a percentage, or by 1000 to give a rate per thousand.

When the baseline population is the denominator this measure is commonly referred to as cumulative incidence rate. It is a direct measure of the probability of a new event occurring in a population, and hence the risk of that event.

In this formula the person-based denominator is fixed at one point in time, usually at the beginning or middle of the time period; for example, if the study is 1 year long, the denominator might be the baseline population. If the disease is recurrent, and the investigator is interested in all, and not just new occurrences, then using a baseline denominator is correct, for the whole population remains at risk of the event of interest. Deaths should, however, be subtracted from the denominator if possible. When the person denominator is so adjusted, the cumulative incidence and person-time rates converge.

Particularly in studies of the causes of disease, investigators often choose to study only first occurrences. If so, when the disease is common, adjusting the denominator is usually advised. If the incidence of the disease or death was only 0.5 per cent per year then on practical (but not theoretical) grounds the investigator might argue that adjusting the denominator is unnecessary, for it would only decrease from 100 to about 99.75 at the 6 months stage, and have no important effect on the calculation.

In many studies the denominator is not adjusted because the information is not available to do this, the investigators have not thought to do so, the outcome is too rare for it to matter, or because investigators are interested in all events.

Box 7.3 Two approaches for measuring incidence rate

(a) Imagine a cohort study with follow-up over 5 years to answer the question: What is the incidence of coronary heart disease in 45–74 year old people? Consider the advantages and disadvantages of the two approaches for measuring incidence rate.

(b) Imagine a study of the incidence of coronary heart disease or mortality based on a register of diseases (or deaths) compiled for 5 years. Again, consider the advantages and disadvantages of the two approaches for measuring incidence.

Do the exercise in Box 7.3 before reading on. To prepare you may wish to read the relevant sections on case series (section 9.3) and on cohort studies in Chapter 9 (section 9.6) first.

In the cohort study—(a) in Box 7.3—the decision on which formula to use will, in theory, depend on the design of the study. If the cohort is assembled at one point of time—say all people born on one day, or army personnel retiring in a particular month of the year—then there is an open choice. In the case of CHD in 45–74 year olds, we could enrol all people of this age from a general practice or other population registers providing age. The participants would then be followed up over time to observe the outcome. The denominator could be the study population at the beginning or the midpoint of the interval of time in question. This will be apt, particularly when absolute/actual rates are the prime output of the analysis, i.e. risk data are needed. If the study sample in the cohort is recruited over a prolonged period of time, say over 3 years, then a person denominator is not appropriate and a person-time approach is much better. When relative measures are the prime output the elegant choice, in both instances, is the person-time denominator.

Mostly, incidence rates are calculated by setting up registers of deaths or disease—as in (b) in Box 7.3—and using census or other estimates of the size of the population from which the cases arose for the denominator. Information on migration, and other means by which a person is effectively lost from the system capturing data for the register, is not usually available on all the individuals making up the denominator. The assumption is made that the population is fairly stable and usually the midpoint of the time period is used. If the disease is uncommon, as is usually the case, adjusting the denominator to remove the new cases would make little difference to the incidence rate. If the disease is common, the denominator could be adjusted by assuming that the cases occur evenly through the year so reducing the denominator by 50 per cent of the number of cases. In this kind of study, with no information on each of the individuals in the denominator, there is no added value to a person-time based denominator. Table 7.4 summarizes the advantages and disadvantages of the two types of denominator.

The concepts and algebraic formulae for incidence rates require reflection, but putting the concepts into practice in measuring the incidence of disease accurately is a still

Table 7.4 Main advantages and disadvantages of person and person-time denominators in the context of (a) cohort and (b) register-based studies of incidence rates

	Advantages	Disadvantages
(a) Cohort study		
Person denominator	Measures risk directly	Requires everyone in the study to be enrolled at about the same time
	Choices of time periods to present incidence data on e.g. over 1 year, over 5 years	Not easy to account for losses to follow-up
		Baseline population becomes an inaccurate estimate of the population at risk for common diseases
Person-time denominator	Very flexible in coping with people entering and leaving study at different times	No easily interpreted direct measure of risk
	Study population can be enrolled over long periods of time	Assumes disease occurrence is evenly spread across time
		Ideally, requires information on date of onset of disease
(b) Register-based study		
Person denominator	Can use population size data from census and other sources if necessary	Accurate census based estimates of denominator are required
	Can use population at midpoint of interval as estimate	Routine population data may give inexact denominator size
	Otherwise as for cohort studies	Otherwise as for cohort studies
Person-time denominator	Not usually applicable, but when it is, then as for cohort studies	Information to calculate person-years is not usually available

greater challenge. The following discussion of measuring events (numerators) and population (denominators) is applicable to all rates in epidemiology.

7.4 Numerator: defining, diagnosing, and coding disease accurately

In contemporary epidemiology the greatest challenge is accurate data collection. The difficulties start with the numerator, that is, the upper number in a vulgar fraction as in the formula for incidence rate, e.g. number of new cases. Epidemiological studies are usually based on diagnoses made by someone else, not the investigator. There have been some notable exceptions, mainly work by solo clinical investigators such as the general practitioner William Pickles who described the pattern of occurrence and natural history of several diseases in his own patients (Pickles 1939). With the advent of the multidisciplinary, team-based approach of modern health care, the specialization of medical practice, and the need for large studies, epidemiologists rarely make their own diagnoses. Herein lies a difficulty. How can epidemiologists ensure that the diagnoses are accurate? After all, in their studies epidemiologists must take responsibility for the validity of the data, including diagnosis. Clearly, they cannot be sure, but their confidence will be increased by a valid case definition, information on symptoms, signs and tests relevant to the case definition, and health care staff who have been trained well in diagnosis.

An information system is needed to hold the clinical data. Since neither the basic clinical information, nor the diagnosis, is likely to be recorded in unambiguous and consistent words, a means of judging the evidence to make or confirm a diagnosis is needed. A patient may have several diseases in the course of one illness. Imagine, for example, a person who has a feverish illness diagnosed on laboratory tests as influenza, who develops cough and shortness of breath shown to be pneumonia, followed by a deep venous thrombosis (a blood clot in the veins). The doctors suspect that pulmonary embolus (a blood clot in the lungs) has occurred but before it can be confirmed by tests, the patient collapses and dies unexpectedly. Assume that there is no post-mortem because the relatives refuse permission. These diagnoses will need to be extracted from a complex set of medical records, traditionally handwritten, though increasingly typed and held electronically. Which diagnoses will go on the death certificate (and ultimately our research database) and in what order? Do the exercise in Box 7.4 now.

Imagine that you are an epidemiologist who acquires 600 000 such death certificates on all causes of death and that you wish to study the incidence of mortality from pulmonary embolus. The task of extracting a list of cases of death due to pulmonary embolus is not a trivial one. One problem will be differences in writing style and words, with some doctors using pulmonary thrombosis, some lung embolus, some omitting it altogether from the death certificate. Compare your completed certificate with mine below.

1a Pulmonary embolus

 b Pneumonia

 c Influenza

11 Deep venous thrombosis

If you disagreed, then your experience is true to life.

One solution, which makes both the choosing of diagnoses and the handling of data easier, is a list of codes for disease. There are several such sets of codes but the most important one is the International Classification of Diseases (ICD) of the WHO.

Box 7.4 Entering diagnosis on a death certificate

Complete the specimen death certificate in Table 7.5 for the above person (as described above in para 2, section 7.4). Take care to order the causes as instructed.

Table 7.5 Specimen death certificate

CAUSE OF DEATH
The condition thought to be the 'Underlying Cause of Death' should appear in the lowest completed line of Part 1.
I (a) Disease or condition directly leading to death
(b) Other disease or condition, if any, leading to I(a)
(c) Other disease or condition, if any, leading to I(b)
II Other significant conditions CONTRIBUTING TO THE DEATH but not related to the disease or condition causing it

The order of the causes of death on the certificate of death is important, for there is a long tradition that only the underlying cause of death is coded, entered into computer, analysed and published. This tradition has been overturned recently in the UK and the USA, and all the causes are now coded and available for analysis. Before reading on do the exercise in Box 7.5.

My codes are I26, J18, J10, I80.1. In studies of disease incidence there is the complication, which does not apply to death, that a decision needs to be made on whether the case is a new case or an old one and whether the person is at risk. The investigator with 600 000 death certificates (or hospital records) has to turn these into useful epidemiological information, including the accurate count of cases. Epidemiologists commonly use such existing data sets, particularly if the coding and computer entry has already been done. This is efficient as the costs of collecting anew such data are high. It is a common mistake, however, to analyse such data sets as if they consisted of valid, complete data. Epidemiologists have a duty to understand the weaknesses and limitations of such data sets, for they are responsible for data accuracy and interpretation of everything they publish.

Two examples, lower limb amputation and Legionnaires' disease, provide contrasting perspectives on the problem of achieving accuracy in the numerator. The words 'lower limb amputation' convey the essence of the case definition, and it is a small step to define it further in terms of anatomy, that is, what part of the limb is amputated. There is no great need for the diagnosis to be confirmed by a doctor or by checking medical records. The amputee will almost certainly have been treated by the health service and probably hospitalized.

Box 7.5 Coding of diagnosis

- Based on your completed death certificate code the causes of death (see Table 7.6).
- Reconsider your choice of order of causes of death after reading the coding rule from the ICD (see footnotes of Table 7.6).

Table 7.6 Selected codes from ICD-10, with brief notes on coding rules

Chapter IX	Diseases of circulatory system	I00–I99	
	Hypertension	I10–I5	
	Ischaemic heart disease	I20–25	
	Cerebrovascular	I60–69	
	Phlebitis and thrombophlebitis	I80	I80.0 of superficial vessels of lower extremities I80.1 of femoral vein of other lower extremities (deep vein thrombosis)
	Other venous embolism and thrombosis	I82	
	Varicose veins of lower extremities	I83	
	Pulmonary embolism	I26	
Chapter X	**Disease of respiratory system**	**J00–J99**	
	Influenza due to influenza virus	J10	(J10 with pneumonia)
	Influenza, virus not identified	J11	(J11 with pneumonia)
	Viral pneumonia, not elsewhere classified	J12	
	Bacterial pneumonia, not elsewhere classified	J15	
	Pneumonia, organism unspecified	J18	
	Respiratory failure, not elsewhere classified	J96	
Chapter XVII Symptoms, signs, etc. not elsewhere classified			
Respiratory arrest (cardiorespiratory failure)		R00–R99	
		R09.2	

Note: The causes of death to be recorded are all those that resulted in or contributed to death, and the circumstances of accident or violence which produced injury.

The underlying cause of death is (a) the disease or injury which initiated the train of events leading directly to death or (b) the circumstances of the accident or violence which produced the fatal injury.

Adapted from the *International Classification of Diseases*, tenth edition (see Permissions).

The obvious place to look for data is the hospital admissions or discharges information system, or the operating theatre records or the limb-fitting centre. It seems straightforward. Figure 7.3 shows the result of a study. Of the 291 cases identified, only 17 were recorded in all three information systems. If the authors had relied on operation records alone, which seems a reasonable strategy, 192/291 (66 per cent) of cases would have been identified. Even for such a straightforward diagnosis, the difficulty in defining the numerator accurately is extreme.

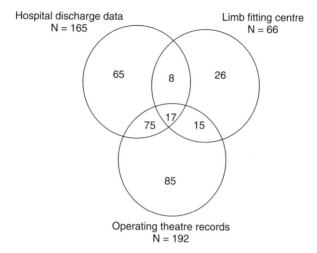

Hospital discharge data
N = 165

Limb fitting centre
N = 66

65

8

26

75

17

15

85

Operating theatre records
N = 192

Fig. 7.3 Use of routine information to measure the number of people with limb amputation: ascertainment based on three data sources. Data from Leeds Health Authority (England), July 1992 to December 1993. Total number of cases of LEA = 291. (Source of data, Bodansky 1997; unpublished figure from Williams et al., see Permissions).

There is a worldwide movement for health care to be planned rationally based on data from routine sources. The resources for a 'needs'-based service for amputees planned using 'routine' information from the hospital discharge data would have been depleted rapidly. It is best to incorporate information on past resource requirement in planning the health service. When information is available from several independent sources, the capture–recapture technique, originally designed for measuring the size of animal populations, can sometimes be used. Discussion of this technique is beyond the scope of this book (see references).

In contrast with lower limb amputation Legionnaires' disease is complex. This pneumonia cannot be differentiated from other forms of pneumonia clinically and has a wide spectrum of presentation (see Chapter 6); some patients have minimal illness and others a wide variety of signs and symptoms. Most patients are likely to be cared for in the community (as a flu-like illness or pneumonia) rather than be admitted to hospital. The challenge is for the physician to consider this diagnosis and order the necessary laboratory tests. The tests are often difficult to interpret, especially as culture of the organism is only successful in a minority of cases. There was, until the publication of ICD 10 very recently, no specific ICD code for this pneumonia so information about cases could not be extracted by searching in routine information systems, including those for hospital inpatients. This meant that for epidemiological studies a specific register of cases had to be maintained. Since the diagnosis requires both clinical and laboratory information a register cannot be maintained from laboratory records alone. As it is a rare disease, incidence studies require the participation of a large number of physicians in supplying information to a registry. Add to this the need to protect the confidentiality of clinical information and it is not surprising that there is a huge 'iceberg' effect for this (and similar) diseases. Fewer than 10 per cent of all cases are counted in most registers. The reader should ponder on the difficulties of measuring the incidence rate of this and similar diseases.

To calculate the incidence rate of disease the procedures for registration of cases will need to include rules to judge whether a case is new or old and decide whether to include recurrences. For example, in a study of the incidence of bronchiolitis, the common cold or acute myocardial infarction, the investigator needs to decide whether only the first occurrence is included as a new case or whether each occurrence is to be included. As there is no general rule, each study will need to make this decision in the light of its aims. These decisions are not always easy except for the incidence of mortality, diseases which are irreversible (e.g. amputation of a limb), diseases which usually occur only once (e.g. measles), or diseases agreed by definition or convention to be lifelong diseases (e.g. diabetes).

Where the prime purpose of the study is to measure the frequency of disease to assess its importance or assess need for services, all cases must be included. Where the aim is to make comparisons between populations to develop or test causal hypotheses there is a choice. In measuring the incidence of stroke, for example, all new and recurrent cases will probably be included if we are doing the study to measure the need for services or evaluating interventions. In a study of whether cholesterol is a causal risk factor for stroke, possibly based on studying groups of subjects with low and high cholesterol, there is a choice. Interpretation of the findings of such a study is usually easier if first occurrences only are included. The simplified rule is this: for burden of disease and health needs—all cases, for causes of disease new cases.

There is a truism that epidemiology is the science of denominators but that is simplistic. The accurate collection of numerator data is an enormous, underestimated problem in epidemiology.

7.5 Denominator

The quality of the data in the denominator (the lower number in a fraction) is crucial. Our primary need, for incidence rates, is to know the number of people at risk of disease. As a simple rule, if people are at risk of being in the numerator, the population from which they came should be in the denominator. Clearly, women are not endangered from testicular cancer, or men from cancer of the cervix. In these cases the denominator would be sex-specific. It is common and good practice in epidemiology to consider men and women separately for most analysis, for their disease patterns are often different. If their patterns are demonstrably not different, data can be combined. Often, the choice of denominator is common sense but sometimes it is not. Try the exercise in Box 7.6 now.

The key step is to understand the definition of the health problem under study. The infant mortality rate is by definition the number of deaths within the first year of life. The word infant, actually meaning a very young child, has been given a more precise

Box 7.6 Defining the denominator

◆ What might be your denominator for a study defining the incidence rate of

   (a) infant mortality;

   (b) the sudden infant death syndrome (cot death); and

   (c) myocardial infarction?

◆ What information would you need to make a rational choice?

meaning here. The logical denominator would be the population of 0–1 year olds, or the person-years of observation of a cohort of newborns (which is less than the population because of deaths, migrations and losses to follow-up). By definition, however, the denominator for infant mortality rate is the number of live births. The reason is a practical one, for this information is easy to obtain, accurate and up to date. Effectively, this defines a cohort for which outcomes are obtained from mortality data. In contrast, to know the size of the population of 0–1 year olds would require a more regular census or only occasional data analysis (the population census is mostly done every 10 years). To measure person-years of observation would need follow-up of members of our cohort individually. Since infant mortality rates are less than 1 per cent in industrialized countries, to follow up individuals to collect 100 deaths would need a study of more than 10 000 infants. The formula for infant mortality rate in a particular year can now be seen as a pragmatic compromise, and is:

$$\frac{\text{Number of dealths in infants under one year in year X}}{\text{Number of liveborn in year X}} \quad (7.4)$$

To choose a denominator for sudden infant death syndrome (SIDS) we need to know the definition of the disease, for example:

> Sudden death of an infant under one year of age, which remains unexplained after a thorough case investigation, including performance of a complete autopsy, examination of the death scene, and review of the clinical history.
>
> US National Institute of Child Health (1991)

The denominator is infants less than 1-year old. The denominator choice here is driven by the definition of the disease, for identical deaths after the first year would not be called SIDS or 'cot' deaths. Older children are not at risk of SIDS by definition.

For the incidence rate of myocardial infarction the denominator would be those at risk. It would be reasonable to exclude children and adolescents, for myocardial infarction is extremely rare in these groups. There is no scientific rationale for excluding the elderly, one sex (sometimes women are excluded), or particular ethnic groups. If the numerator comprises only selected cases based on age, sex, or ethnic group then the denominator will need to reflect this. In research focusing on the causes of disease those who have already had a heart attack before, and are therefore no longer at risk of having a *first* attack, might reasonably be excluded. The cause of a recurrent myocardial infarction may be different from a first one, and hence deserve separate study. If the information is to be used for priority setting or health needs assessment the study should measure the incidence of first, recurrent and total infarcts.

The principles in terms of establishing the numerator and the denominator, discussed in the context of disease incidence studies, are similar but more complex in relation to prevalence.

7.6 Prevalence and prevalence rate

Prevalence is the extent to which something exists. In epidemiology (Table 7.2) prevalence is the count of all instances of the factor of interest in the study population. The key features of prevalence are given in Table 7.2. For simplicity, let us assume the factor of interest is a disease, but it could be something else, such as a behaviour or an abnormal value in a blood test. As with incidence rate, prevalence rate is usually expressed in relation to a population at risk, but sometimes another type of denominator may be chosen. For example, the prevalence rate of congenital abnormalities is usually expressed in relation to the number of live births.

The term prevalence rate, as used here, reflects its continuing widespread usage but, as discussed earlier, some authorities contend that a rate must have a time dimension. The argument has led to confusion that is not clarified by *Last's Dictionary of Epidemiology* (2001). Readers are advised to be aware of these arguments. I use either the traditional, widespread, and continuing approach of saying prevalence rate or the emergent (but, strictly speaking, inaccurate) trend simply to say prevalence.

There are three types of prevalence rates: point, period, and lifetime.

The point prevalence rate, as the phrase implies, comprises all the cases of a disease that exist in a place at a point in time. The denominator is chosen to represent those at risk. The population at risk is often specifically recruited into the study so this number is known. In studies where the investigators have not recruited the population at risk, the denominator is usually derived from population estimates. It is unlikely that such estimates will exist for a point in time (e.g. they are usually mid-year estimates, from the census). Inaccuracy in estimating prevalence is, therefore, likely. In a study of the prevalence of, say, menstrual irregularity, the denominator would be women who are menstruating, and a choice of the age group 15–45 years of age might be reasonable. For prevalence rate, unlike incidence rate, there is no requirement to exclude from the denominator those people who already have the disease. As the denominator includes the numerator the prevalence is, mathematically, a proportion and ranges from 0 to 1 (or, 0–100 per cent). The formula is simple:

$$\text{Point prevalence rate} = \frac{\text{All cases of the factor of interest at time X}}{\text{Population at risk at time X}} \qquad (7.5)$$

Period prevalence is a way of recognizing and overcoming the limitations of prevalence studies done at a point in time. All cases whether old, new, or recurrent, arising over a defined period, say a year, are counted. The denominator is the average population over the period (or midpoint estimate). Period prevalence, which combines the concept of incidence and point prevalence, is particularly useful in gauging the burden of episodic, recurrent diseases such as depression, anxiety, or migraine. Both point prevalence and incidence, alone, tend to underestimate the size of such problems so a combination is desirable. The formula is:

$$\text{Period prevalence rate} = \frac{\text{All cases (old and new) of the factor of interest during time period}}{\text{Average population at risk during time period}} \quad (7.6)$$

Lifetime prevalence is the ultimate extension of the idea of period prevalence, and is the proportion of the population who have ever had the disease. This can be derived systematically from a birth cohort study (where people are followed up from birth). We can derive the proportion of the population who have ever had asthma, for example, by the age of 5, 10, 15, 30, and 45 years or more until all are dead. Lifetime prevalence has value for drawing attention to how common some disorders are. For example, over a lifetime mental health problems are extremely common. The formula is:

$$\text{Lifetime prevalence} = \frac{\text{No. who ever had the factor of interest during lifetime}}{\text{Population at risk (at the beginning of the time period)}} \quad (7.7)$$

The algebraic formulae for prevalence rates are simple but, as with incidence, their measurement accurately is problematic. Most of the principles discussed in relation to incidence apply to prevalence; for example, the need for a valid case definition and information to judge whether a case qualifies, a system for collection of information on the numerator, and defining and measuring an appropriate denominator. Imagine we are interested in measuring the prevalence of type 2 diabetes. Now try the exercise in Box 7.7 before reading on.

The first and crucial step is to decide on the definition. The usual choices are:

◆ The WHO definition of a plasma glucose of or more than 11.1 mmol/L 2 hours after a standard oral glucose tolerance test. To meet this definition your study population will need to undergo this test which involves fasting overnight, then drinking the standard 75g glucose drink and having blood taken 120 minutes later. This will require a special study, for such information does not exist in routine information systems. Since such a test is potentially dangerous or inadvisable in those with diabetes, not everyone will be able to do it.

◆ The definition of the American Diabetes Association, now adopted by WHO, of a fasting plasma blood glucose level of more than 7mmol/L. Again this information

Box 7.7 Defining the numerator and denominator for the prevalence of diabetes

In general terms consider the steps you will need to take to count the numerator and denominator to measure the population prevalence of type 2 diabetes.

does not exist in routine records so a special study will be needed. This test is simpler than the glucose tolerance test but will lead to a different list of people diagnosed and a different prevalence rate than the definition above. In both of these definitions, the denominator will be the people who undergo the test.

♦ Definitions based on a mixture of symptoms, signs, and of a variety of diagnostic strategies used in normal clinical practice. This approach is relatively easy, for the cases can be identified from medical records or registers, but is likely to underestimate the prevalence greatly. Sometimes access to medical records will not be possible, leaving the investigators to rely on self-report of doctors' diagnosis by the study participants at interview or by questionnaire. This will underestimate the prevalence even more, for some participants will fail to report such a diagnosis.

The second step is to select an appropriate population at risk. Identifying unbiased sample populations, and enlisting their cooperation in prevalence (cross-sectional) studies is a formidable task which will be discussed more fully in Chapter 9. Unlike incidence studies, which are concerned with events including death, point prevalence studies are usually of survivors. With the exception of autopsy-based prevalence studies deaths are not included. This causes survivor bias. In our studies of type 2 diabetes mellitus (as above), the reason for underestimating the burden and severity of the point prevalence of the disease in a community-based study is that people have either died or are in institutions (hospitals, nursing homes).

The duration of the prevalence study depends on what it measures: point, period, or lifetime prevalence. Point prevalence studies should take place on a particular day or narrow time interval. In practice, observations on hundreds, sometimes thousands, of people cannot be made in this way and measurements take place over months or even years. Figures 7.4 and 7.5 are simple illustrations of the effects this can have.

Figure 7.4 is a study of a common permanent condition in 20 people, divided into four groups to make fieldwork easier, and spread over the year. The lines show the onset of the disease. The shading in the figure, which shows the fieldwork periods, is simply to help the counting. Do the exercise in Box 7.8 before reading on.

The point prevalence (denominator of 20) is 10 per cent in January (two cases exist, numbers 1 and 15), 20 per cent in July (four cases, numbers 1, 3, 15, 18), and 25 per cent in December (numbers 1, 3, 12, 15, 18). The (cumulative) incidence is 16.6 per cent (3 new cases/18 at risk; two already had the disease). Of course, the incident cases (especially case 12) may not be recognized in the field. Assume there is a registration system

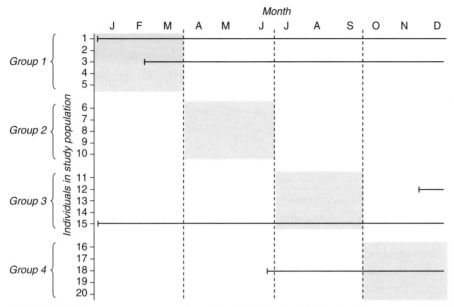

Fig. 7.4 Study of a common permanent problem. Each horizontal line denotes a case and shading the fieldwork order.

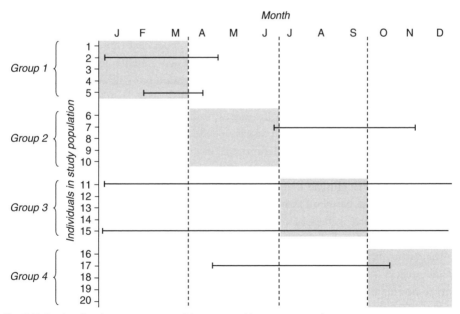

Fig. 7.5 Study of an impermanent problem, e.g. taking up an exercise programme.

Box 7.8 Measuring prevalence and incidence rates in a permanent condition

In Fig. 7.4 what is the point prevalence rate in January, July, and December? What is the cumulative annual incidence rate? What is the period prevalence rate? What is the lifetime prevalence rate? Have the fieldwork team identified all cases? What would be the effect of doing the study in a different order, say group 4 went first, group 3 followed, etc.

to pick them up. The period prevalence is the sum of initial prevalent cases(2) plus incident cases(3) divided by the denominator (20) 25 per cent. Here the denominator is again 20, the entire population under study. We cannot calculate lifetime prevalence on these data; we need to know what will happen to our study population until they die. Of these cases only one (no. 12) will be missed by the fieldwork team; the fieldwork is before the date of onset. If the fieldwork order was changed, for example, group 4 first (January–March), group 3 second (April–June), group 2 third (January–September), and group 1 last (October–December), case no. 18 would also be missed (in addition to case 12). In the study, as actually conducted, one case is missed and the prevalence is underestimated.

Figure 7.5 represents a study of a changeable condition, say, taking up an exercise programme. Do the exercise in Box 7.9 before reading on.

The point prevalence is 15 per cent in January (3/20, numbers 2, 11, 15), 20 per cent in July (numbers 7, 11, 15, 17), and 10 per cent in December (numbers 11 and 15). The cumulative incidence of exercise uptake is 3/17 which is 17.6 per cent (numbers 5, 7, 17)-note that the 3 already taking exercise are excluded from the denominator here as they are not at risk. The period prevalence is 30 per cent. On this occasion our fieldwork team misses no cases. If the fieldwork order had been group 4 (January–March), 3, 2, 1 then cases 2, 5 and 17 would have been missed. Now try the exercise in Box 7.10 before reading on.

The first and surprisingly difficult task is to define and measure angina. The diagnosis of angina is a clinical one with no definitive signs or symptoms and no specific diagnostic test. The sensitivity and specificity of the main approaches to diagnosis in the community, that is, clinical history or ECG, are low. The health authority could be advised to use data based on numbers of people seen by the service in previous years. As there is a massive iceberg of angina in the community, many people, often with the severest disease and destined for sudden death or heart attack, will be missed.

The second difficult task is to differentiate those people with angina who would benefit from surgery from those who would do as well on medical therapy. The usual way to do this is coronary angiogram, an invasive procedure whereby the narrowing of the coronary arteries is displayed using X-ray techniques. The dangers of this procedure are sufficient to preclude its use in epidemiological surveys of apparently healthy populations. For this reason a preliminary test—the exercise ECG—is often done, and those positive on this get the angiogram.

Box 7.9 Measuring incidence and prevalence rates in a changeable condition

- What is the point prevalence rate of exercise uptake in January, July, and December?
- What is the cumulative incidence rate and period prevalence rate of exercise uptake by end-December?
- Have the fieldwork teams identified all the cases?
- What would be the effect of a different order of field work, say group 4 went first, group 3 second, etc.?

The investigator needs to define angina for the purpose of this task and design a study to estimate the fraction of cases that will require surgery. Since angina is rarely a problem in the young, it could be reasonable to limit the investigation to adults, perhaps 35 years or more. The incidence rate is not helpful for planning here because it hugely underestimates the burden of the problem. The point prevalence estimate is the number of people with angina in the community. Period prevalence (say over a year) is probably the most useful measure, for it informs the planner of the number of people in the community that will require service in that year. Lifetime prevalence is of no immediate value here. The period prevalence could be measured by a combination of clinical examinations and tests, and a register of cases. Once the population of angina patients has been identified, further tests, including exercise ECGs and angiography, will help to identify the need for surgery or medical management. Incidence and prevalence are clearly related. This is discussed below.

Box 7.10 Incidence and prevalence rates in the context of planning a service

A health authority (or an equivalent body such as an insurance agency or a managed care organization) serving 500 000 people wishes to cost and plan a service for the medical and surgical management of angina in the population, with particular emphasis on the numbers of cases requiring surgery. Angina is a typical symptom of coronary heart disease characterized by chest pain on exertion.

You are invited to assist. Consider the general principles that you would apply to the task.

Consider the relative merits of measuring incidence, point prevalence, period prevalence, and lifetime prevalence rates.

7.7 **Relationship of incidence and prevalence**

There is a close relationship between incidence and prevalence. The relationship is shown in simple form in Fig. 7.6, as the bath model. The inflow is the incidence, the bath water the prevalence (pool of cases). The prevalence pool is changed by death, recovery, or migration (the outflow). Figure 7.7 develops this simple idea in relation to a population. The population is enhanced by births and immigration, and diminished by deaths and emigration. This population is the water supply to the bath. Some incident cases die before reaching the prevalence pool, such as sudden infant death syndrome cases. The recovered cases may rejoin the main population.

There is a mathematical relationship between incidence and prevalence which only works in fixed populations, whereas we live in dynamic ones. Imagine a fixed population of 100 newborn infants all of whom survive for the duration of the study, say 5 years. The number of new cases over 5 years (5-year cumulative incidence) of a chronic, but non-fatal disease, and the total number of cases at the end of the study (5-year period prevalence) are identical. So if 2 new cases occur per year we will have 10 at the end of the study. The cumulative incidence rate, and the period prevalence rate will be 10 per cent. The point prevalence rate at the end of 5 years will also be 10 per cent.

If the duration of the disease is less than 5 years or death occurs, then the point prevalence at the end of 5 years will be smaller than the 5-year cumulative incidence.

In fixed populations, when the prevalence is low, the prevalence is approximately equal to the incidence rate × average duration of disease. It follows that incidence rate is approximately = point prevalence rate ÷ duration; and duration is approximately = point prevalence rate ÷ incidence rate.

In a dynamic population, however, the prevalence of a disease cannot be predicted from knowledge of the incidence (or vice versa) because of migration into and out of the

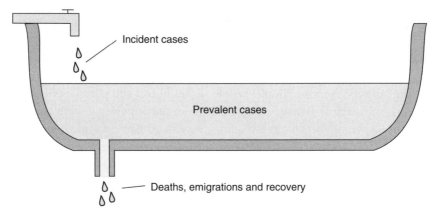

Fig. 7.6 Incidence, prevalence, and the bath model of disease. (Adapted from a figure provided by Howel, see Permissions).

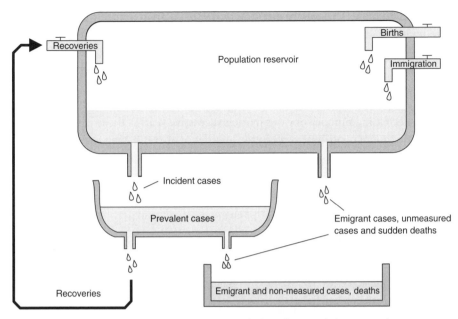

Fig. 7.7 Incidence and prevalence in a natural population: the population reservoir.

population, deaths, changing disease rates, changes in prognosis, and error in measuring the incidence (or prevalence) accurately. In practice, either both the prevalence and incidence are measured or a choice of one is made. The formula linking incidence and prevalence can be used, at best, as an approximation. The exercise in Box 7.11 provides a simple example to permit you to develop your understanding. Do this exercise before reading on. You will find the answers in Table 7.7.

The incidence rate (cumulative) of myopia, based on the denominator at the beginning of the study, is 100/10 000 per year = 1 per cent. The alternative is to take the population at risk at the midpoint of the time interval, at 6 months. By then 50 people will be myopic and hence no longer at risk. The incidence rate then is 100/9950 = 1.005%. The incidence rate estimated by the person-time denominator of myopia is identical but expressed differently, i.e. per person years of observation. The total person-years of observation is 9950 (9900 given by those not myopic, and 50 by those 100 people who are myopic for they give, on average, 0.5 years). The result is 1000/9950 person years, that is, 1005 per 100 000 person-years.

The point prevalence at the beginning is zero, and at 6 months, on average, half of all cases will have occurred, so it is 50/10 000 (0.5%) and by the end of the year it is 100/10 000 (1%). The period prevalence at one year is also 100/10 000 (1%).

The actual duration of myopia among cases is, on average, half of the time of follow-up. The prevalence is low and the population is fixed so our simple formula on p. 224 will give a good estimate. The average duration of myopia is approximately point prevalence at the midpoint of the interval ÷ incidence =250 ÷ 100 = 2.5 years. The predicted approximate point prevalence at 5 years = annual incidence rate × average duration × years of observation = 100 per 10 thousand × 2.5 years = 250 per 10 000. The incidence rate based on the formula is, approximately point prevalence ÷ duration = 250/2.5 = 100.

The prevalence rate as calculated above slightly overestimates the reality because there will be a decreasing number of cases in each successive year, as those who have already had myopia cannot contribute twice to the prevalence of ever having had this.

A better estimate of the period prevalence at 5 years is 490.1/10 000 (or 4.9%) as follows:

◆ 1st year incident cases = 100, leaving 9900 at risk

◆ 2nd year incident cases = 1 per cent of 9900 = 99, leaving 9801

Box 7.11 Incidence and prevalence of myopia – short-sightedness

Imagine a population of 10 000 new school children, aged 5 years. Your interest is in the incidence and prevalence of short-sightedness (myopia). Assume myopia is permanent. You follow the children for one year. All of the study population survive, all medical and eye test records are available, and all are available for interview and examination. Assume that the occurrence of myopia is spread evenly through the year, and that at recruitment none had myopia. Over the year you find that 100 recruits had myopia.

◆ What is the 1-year cumulative incidence rate of myopia? Calculate this with the baseline denominator of the children at risk. Also, do this with the estimated at risk population at the midpoint of the time interval of the study.

◆ What is the 1-year incidence rate per 100 000 years of observation based on the person-time denominator?

◆ What is the point prevalence rate of having had myopia at the beginning, middle, and end of the year?

◆ What is the period prevalence rate over the year?

◆ If the cumulative incidence rate remains the same over time, and assuming a fixed denominator of 10 000 what is the period prevalence rate of myopia by the end of five years? (In practice it will be lower as the denominator will diminish as children develop myopia so the number of cases will decline each year.)

◆ What is the estimate of the point prevalence of myopia over the 5-year period?

◆ What is the estimated average duration of myopia by the end of the 5 years?

◆ What is the estimated point prevalence using the formula approach?

◆ What is the estimated incidence rate based on the formula approach.

- 3rd year incident cases = 1 per cent of 9801 = 98.01, leaving 9702.99
- 4th year incident cases = 1 per cent of 9702.99 = 97.03, leaving 9605.96
- 5th year incident cases = 1 per cent of 9605.99 = 96.06, leaving 9509.9 cases

The total number of cases is 490.1 compared with 500 in Table 7.7. The period prevalence then was 490.1/10 000 = 4.9% rather than 5%.

The reader may wish to calculate the 5-year cumulative incidence based on the baseline and midpoint denominators, and the person-years of observation. For advanced understanding of the concepts of incidence and prevalence, readers may wish to consult Rothman and Greenland (1998).

Table 7.7 Answers to questions in Box 7.11 on incidence and prevalence of myopia

Cumulative incidence of myopia	$\dfrac{100 \text{ new cases}}{10\,000}$	$= 0.01$	$= 1\%$
Cumulative incidence using midpoint estimate of population at risk	$\dfrac{100}{9950}$	$= 0.01005$	$= 1.005\%$
Incidence rate using person-time	$\dfrac{100 \text{ new cases}}{10\,000 \text{ years}-50 \text{ years} = 9950}$	$= 0.01005 = 1005$ cases per 100 000 years of observation	

Point prevalence rate:

– beginning	$= \dfrac{0}{10\,000}$	$= 0$
– middle	$= \dfrac{50}{10\,000}$	$= 0.5\%$
– end of year	$= \dfrac{100}{10,000}$	$= 1\%$
Period prevalence	$= \dfrac{0 + 100}{10\,000}$	$= 1\%$
Period prevalence over 5 years	$= \dfrac{0 + 100 \times 5}{10\,000}$	$= 5\%$
Point prevalence at midpoint (2.5 years)	$= \dfrac{\text{Cases at midpoint of interval}}{10\,000}$	$= \dfrac{250}{10\,000}$ $= 2.5\%$
Average duration of myopia	$= \dfrac{\text{Point prevalence at midpoint}}{\text{Annual incidence rate}}$	$= \dfrac{250}{10\,000} \div \dfrac{100}{10\,000} = 2.5$ years
Point prevalence over 5 years based on formula	$= \dfrac{\text{Annual incidence rate} \times \text{duration}}{10\,000}$	$= \dfrac{100 \times 2.5}{10\,000} = \dfrac{250}{10\,000} = 2.5\%$
Incidence rate based on formula	$= \dfrac{\text{Point prevalence rate}}{\text{Duration}}$	$= \dfrac{250}{2.5} = 100$

7.8 **Choice of incidence or prevalence measures**

As a general principle, for studies of the causes of disease, the incidence rate is preferred because it is not affected by variation in treatment and case-fatality, so differences between populations are easier to interpret. For studies of the burden of diseases of short duration (e.g. measles, influenza, diarrhoea, transient ischaemic attacks, ankle sprains, acute low backache), incidence is also preferred because point prevalence would underestimate the problem. The point prevalence figure would miss the recovered or dead cases. The period prevalence adds little to understanding here.

The prevalence rate is generally preferred as the measure of burden for long-lasting diseases even when these are rare (e.g. multiple sclerosis, renal failure). For health behaviours and other disease risk factors prevalence is the preferred measure (even in studies of disease causation). Prevalence is sometimes perceived in epidemiology as inferior to incidence. It is not. Both measures have inherent weaknesses and strengths, and different value in various circumstances. Both measures are prone to the numerator and denominator errors discussed in sections 7.4 and 7.5.

7.9 **Presenting rates: overall and specific**

Rates can be presented for the whole population under study or for subgroups of that population. For example, the population of Scotland in 1999 was 5.195 million, and there were 60 277 deaths, giving an overall mortality rate of 60 277/5 195 000 = 0.0116 = 11.6 per 1000. Such an overall rate is commonly referred to as the crude rate. As the word crude has negative connotations a better term is actual. The actual rate can be subdivided by any characteristic of the population of epidemiological interest (e.g. age, sex) and calculated for different places and times. Such subdivided rates are called specific rates (e.g. age- or sex-specific rates) and this is called stratified analysis.

Commonly used variables for subdivision of rates include age group, sex, ethnic group, race, social class, educational status, and marital status. Such variables are, of course, commonly referred to as epidemiological variables (discussed in Chapter 1). Obviously, to calculate specific rates we need to be able to subdivide the population counts by these variables. We need to know, for example, the number of people in each ethnic group in the underlying population before we can calculate ethnic group specific rates. Such information may not be available, especially in small geographical areas and at times other than the census year.

Specific rates permit rational and easy comparison of disease patterns in different places and times for they can be directly compared with each other, and questions asked about why differences occur. The answers are usually complex and elusive. Simple observations of difference in disease rates may lead to inspiration, as in the example of Semmelweiss's hypothesis of a transmissable cadaverous particle, arising from his reflection on mortality in two clinics (discussed in Chapter 5). More often the observations are merely noted or give rise to untested hypotheses. For example, long-standing observations of greater lifespan (and lower mortality rates) in women compared with men are largely unexplained in specific biological or social terms as are differences in chronic diseases at different ages. Explaining differences in disease rates is exceptionally difficult epidemiological science.

Although there are still intriguing and unexplained differences in disease by sex and age, these variables are usually treated as confounding variables. (It is good practice, however, to check for effect modification—interaction—before treating these variables as confounders.) Imagine that we observe that a seaside resort town such as Bournemouth has a higher actual overall (or crude) mortality rate from stroke than, say, a city such as Bristol. The likely explanation is one of low scientific interest; the seaside resort has more elderly people, for it is a place people move to after retirement. The overall higher rate, though true, is usually adjusted to take account of these differences in age structure of the population of the two cities using methods discussed in the next chapter. We would not usually investigate the role of age in causing differences in stroke between these cities because it is a basic explanation of little epidemiological interest nowadays. That is not to deny the continuing question of how ageing alters biology and disease. Just occasionally the pattern of disease by age group becomes of intense interest, e.g. we are witnessing the resurgence of CHD in younger age groups in countries such as the USA.

7.10 **Conclusion**

Epidemiology is a practical and pragmatic science that is focused on measuring and explaining risk of disease in populations. This requires three distinct types of data in context of time and place: on diseases, on the factors that potentially cause disease, and the size and characteristics of the populations under study. Obtaining these data with a high degree of accuracy is a serious obstacle to epidemiology, even in the most economically advanced populations.

The art of epidemiology lies in making judgements on the appropriate interpretation of, inevitably, inaccurate data. Epidemiological and other theories of health and disease, and frameworks for data analysis and interpretation, are vital to guide such judgements.

Theoretical considerations around measurement and presentation of risk, and mathematical and statistical ideas on measurement of disease occurrence, underpin the practice of data collection. These are the factors that have driven change and advancement in an aspect of epidemiology that is based on mathematics. The increasing use of the person-time denominator is one example of such change.

The rate of disease, where a measure of the quantity of disease or risk factor for disease (the numerator) is considered in relation to a measure of the quantity of population (the denominator), lies at the core of the epidemiological method. These rates are the hammers, screwdrivers and spanners of the epidemiological toolbox. Two types of rates are dominant in epidemiology, incidence and prevalence. The two are clearly distinguished by being concerned with either new events (incidence) or events old and new (prevalence). Epidemiologists should examine these building blocks of their data extremely carefully, questioning the veracity of the numerator and denominator. Numerous false starts and misleading turns would be avoided by careful scrutiny of the rates, both overall and specific. Only when these fundamentals are sound should data manipulation proceed. These two measures are manipulated in epidemiology to produce a multiplicity of perspectives on population patterns of health and disease—and that is the subject of the next chapter.

Summary

Risk is the possibility of harm. In epidemiology risk refers to the likelihood, or in statistical language probability, of an individual in a defined population developing a disease or other adverse health problem. In epidemiology the association between risk of disease and both individual and social characteristics (risk factors) is often the starting point for causal analysis. Epidemiological studies measure, present and interpret disease frequency, usually by comparing the patterns in one population relative to another. The prime measures of disease frequency that provide the basis for such comparisons are incidence and prevalence rates.

  The incidence rate is the number of new cases in relation to a population, time, and place. Two forms of incidence rates are in common use, usually distinguished by terms such as cumulative incidence and person-time incidence rate. In cumulative incidence the denominator is the population, in person-time incidence the denominator is the sum of the time periods for which the individuals in the population have been observed. Prevalence rate measures all disease in a population either at a particular time (point prevalence) or over a time period (period prevalence, lifetime prevalence). There is a mathematical relation between the two measures, such that in a fixed population prevalence rate is approximately equal to the incidence rate multiplied by the duration of the disease. As epidemiology concerns dynamic populations this relationship is seldom useable. Rates are most accurately presented by age and sex groups ('specific' rates), but for ease of interpretation they may be grouped as overall actual (so-called crude) rates, which can be adjusted for age and sex differences between compared populations. The collection of both disease and population data to achieve accurate figures of incidence and prevalence is problematic, and remains a major challenge.

Sample examination questions

Give yourself 10 minutes for every 25% of marks.
Many of the examination questions in Chapters 8 and 9 are relevant to this chapter.

Question 1 Why are (point) prevalence rates useful in epidemiology? List at least five factors which may lead to either an increase or decrease in the prevalence rate. (25%)
Answer Prevalence rates indicate the burden of health problems and their causes or risk factors. They point to priorities and help target priority groups for health and

medical services. Prevalence rates may also serve as baseline indices for subsequent evaluations of health services in the groups served.

The prevalence rate is increased by:

◆ Immigration of cases

◆ Emigration of healthy people

◆ Immigration of susceptible cases or those with potential of becoming cases, for example, the aged

◆ Prolongation of life of cases without cure (increase in duration of disease)

◆ Increase in new cases.

The prevalence rate is decreased by:

◆ Immigration of healthy people

◆ Emigration of cases

◆ Improved cure rate of cases

◆ Increased death rate of cases

◆ Decrease in occurrence of new cases

◆ Shorter duration of disease.

Question 2 900 residents in a retirement home (350 with low salt intake and 550 with high salt intake) who do not have hypertension participate in a study to assess the incidence of hypertension. Assume that the populations remain stable over one year of follow-up. Blood pressure is measured in everyone at the beginning of the year and again at the end. At the end 20 residents with low salt intake (low risk) and 70 with high salt intake (high risk) have hypertension. Assume the diagnostic methods are correct.

1 Place these data in an appropriate 2×2. (10%)

2 Calculate the incidence rate for high blood pressure using the person-time denominator (base your denominator on the estimated population at risk i.e. taking into account the time contribution of those with the outcome). (10 %)

3 Briefly state and discuss why the person-time denominator may be preferred over the population denominator. In this instance does it matter which denominator you use? Explain why. (30 %)

Answer 1

Risk factor	Hypertension		
	Yes	No	Total
High salt intake	70	480	550
Low salt intake	20	330	350
Total	90	810	900

Answer 2

Incidence of hypertension in high salt intake group:

$$\frac{70}{(70 \times 0.5) + (480 \times 1)} = \frac{70}{515} = 135.9 \text{ per 1000 person-years}$$

Incidence of hypertension in low salt intake group:

$$\frac{20}{(20 \times 0.5) + (330 \times 1)} = \frac{20}{340} = 58.8 \text{ per 1000 person-years}$$

Answer 3

Often people are followed for different lengths of time. Some drop out or come into the study at different times. In such cases, the denominator will not be the number of people but the accumulated periods of time each person is in the study. The person-years approach has been an effective method of utilizing information about each subject even if the period of follow-up is short. In other words, it uses all the data on participants in a follow-up study.

The incidence rates are not the same using the two different denominators. When using the population at risk denominator the following results are obtained: incidence rate in high salt intake group $(70/550) = 127.3$ per 1000; in the low salt intake group the incidence is $(20/350) = 57.1$ per 1000.

Question 3 The phrase 'risk factor' is often used in epidemiology. Explain the meaning of this phrase, and discuss how it differs from causal factor. (25%)

Answer Risk in epidemiology usually refers to the likelihood (probability) of dying or developing a disease, or its precursors. In epidemiology our prime interest is in the interaction between the probability of disease, or risk, and those environmental, individual and social characteristics which influence the risk. Where there is an association with an increased probability of disease in those with such characteristics, the characteristics are called risk factors.

The phrase 'risk factor' does not necessarily imply the characteristic has a causal effect (association is not causation). No causal relationship is presumed, though there is great interest in assessing whether one exists. When a causal relationship is agreed between disease and the risk factor the phrase causal factor, or simply cause, is used.

Question 4 Why is the count of the numerator in the rate of disease difficult to measure accurately? (25%)

Answer The numerator is difficult to measure because of the problems in accurately defining diseases; in making the measurement to see whether the definition applies; in applying these measurements in population settings; in collecting, analysing and interpreting the data; and in keeping track of changes over time.

An exercise on incidence and prevalence from the first edition

Incidence and prevalence of gunshot wounds

Imagine a population of 10 000 new army recruits. Your interest is in the incidence and prevalence of gunshot wounds on war duty. Assume all gunshot wounds lead to permanent visible damage. You follow the recruits for one year. All of the study population survive, all medical records are available, and all are available for interview and examination. Assume that the occurrence of gunshot wounds is spread evenly through the year, and that at recruitment none had such a wound. Over the year you find that 20 recruits had a gunshot wound.

♦ What is the cumulative incidence rate of gunshot wounds? What is the incidence rate based on the person-time denominator?

♦ What is the point prevalence rate of having had a gunshot wound at the beginning, middle, and end of the year?

♦ What is the period prevalence rate over the year?

♦ If the incidence rate remains the same over time, what is the prevalence rate of ever being scarred by the end of 5 years?

♦ What is the average duration of a gunshot wound, among those scarred, by the end of the first year?

♦ What is the estimate of the point prevalence over the 5-year period (effectively at the 2.5 year point)?

♦ What is the average duration of scarring over the 5 years?

Answer The incidence rate (cumulative) of first scarring wounds, based on the donominator at the beginning of the study, is 20/10 000 per year = 2/1000 or 0.2%. The alternative is to take the population at risk at the midpoint of the time interval, at 6 months. By then 10 people will have been scarred and hence are no longer at risk. The incidence rate then is 20/9990 = 0.2002%. The incidence rate estimated by the person-time denominator of first gunshot wounds is identical. The total person-years of observation is 9990 (9980 given by those unwounded, and 10 by those 20 people who were wounded for they give, on average, 0.5 years). The result is 20/9990 person years, that is, 0.002002 per person-year, or 2.002 per 1000 person-years, identical to the incidence rate based on mid-interval denominator.

The point prevalence at the beginning is zero, and at 6 months, on average, half of all cases will have occurred, so it is 10/10 000 and by the end of the year it is 20/10 000.

The period prevalence at one year is also 20/10 000. The actual duration of scarring among cases is, on average, half of the time of follow-up. The prevalence is low and the population is fixed so our simple formula on p. 224 will give a good estimate. The average duration of a scarring wound at one year is point prevalence at the midpoint of the interval ÷ 2 = 0.5 year. The predicted approximate point prevalence over the 5 years = annual incidence rate × average duration × years of observation.

> = 2 per thousand × 0.5 years × 5 = 5 per 1000 or 50 per 10000 (which is fairly meaningless in this context)

The approximate average duration of scarring over the 5 years is 5/1000 ÷ 2/1000 = 2.5 years.

The prevalence above slightly overestimates because there will be a decreasing number of cases in each successive year, as those who have already had a scarring wound cannot contribute twice to the prevalence of ever having had a gunshot wound, even though they can continue to contribute to the incidence of new scarring wounds (first and subsequent).

A better estimate of the period prevalence at 5 years is 99.6/10 000 (or 9.96/1000) as follows:

1st year incident cases = 20, leaving 9980 at risk

2nd year incident cases = 0.2 per cent of 9980 = 19.96, leaving 9960

3rd year incident cases = 0.2 per cent of 9960 = 19.92, leaving 9940

4th year incident cases = 0.2 per cent of 9940 = 19.88 leaving 9920

5th year incident cases = 0.2 per cent of 9920 = 19.84, a total of 99.6 cases

Appendix 7.1

A formula for instantaneous incidence rate.

$$\frac{\text{Probability that a person well at time } t \text{ will develop the disease in the interval from } t \text{ to } t \text{ plus change in } t \ (\Delta t)}{\text{Time from } t \text{ to } t \text{ plus change in } t \ (\Delta t).} \tag{A7.1}$$

Chapter 8

Presentation and interpretation of epidemiological data on risk

Objectives

On completion of the chapter you should understand:

- that the aim of manipulating epidemiological data is to summarize information and sharpen understanding of actual and relative risk of disease, but that distortions occur easily;
- that epidemiological studies measure, present and interpret risk, often comparing one population with another, using relative measures;
- the idea behind, definition of, strengths and limitations of, and means of calculation of: proportional mortality, proportional mortality ratio, directly and indirectly standardized rates (and the standardized mortality ratio), relative risk, odds ratio, attributable risk, population-attributable risk, years of life lost, population impact numbers, numbers needed to treat and prevent, the quality-adjusted life year, the disability-adjusted life year;
- that the principal relative measure is the relative risk while the odds ratio can approximate it in particular circumstances;
- that attributable risk and population-attributable risk are measures that help us to assess the proportion of the burden of disease that is caused by a particular risk factor;
- that the term avoidable mortality refers to the potential to avoid death or disability from the specified causes if the best possible health care actions were taken;
- that the number of years of avoidable life lost measures the impact of avoidable mortality and helps us to assess the effectiveness of health care;
- how epidemiological data contributes to assessing the health needs and health status of populations;
- the process of constructing summary measures of health status;
- that different ways of presenting the same data have a major impact on the perception of risk, so epidemiological studies should provide both relative and actual risk.

8.1 Introduction

Epidemiological data can be manipulated easily, with the purpose of summarizing information and/or extracting additional insights. Usually, but not always, the objective is to permit or sharpen up comparisons, whether over time or between places and population groups.

This chapter introduces the main ways in which data are manipulated, with a warning that the end results are often artificial measures that change (and sometimes distort) the perception and interpretation of risk, a matter of utmost concern to a science where communication between researchers, health professionals, and the public is critically important.

8.2 Proportional morbidity or mortality ratio

Sometimes the only reliable data we have are on cases. Comparisons are difficult without population denominators (to construct rates) but these may not be available or they may be inaccurate. For example, there are usually no accurate population denominators for comparing disease and mortality outcomes by workplace or hospital, because most workplaces and hospitals do not draw their workers and patients from a specific and defined population. Studies of ethnicity and health in the UK (and similarly in many countries) are thwarted by the fact that ethnic code has been collected only at two censuses (1991 and 2001) and that records providing information on disease do not record ethnicity accurately (e.g. the death certificate has country of birth but no ethnic code and in hospital admission records the ethnic code is often missing). Furthermore, some record systems and studies that do provide an ethnic code use a different classification from that in the census.

The proportional morbidity or mortality ratio (PMR) is commonly used to study disease patterns by cause where population denominators are not available, as illustrated here using mortality.

The total number of deaths (not the population) is used as the denominator, and the deaths from each specific cause as the numerator. The proportional mortality (PM) is the resulting fraction, usually expressed as a percentage. The formula is:

$$PM = \frac{\text{Number of deaths due to cause X}}{\text{Total number of deaths}}$$

(8.1)

Multiplying this fraction by 100 provides the PM as a percentage. The proportional mortality can be calculated by sex, age group or any other appropriate subdivision of the population. These figures can be compared between populations, places or time periods by calculating the PMR, which is simply the ratio of PMs in the two comparison populations, that is,

$$PMR = \frac{\text{PM in population A}}{\text{PM in population B}}$$

(8.2)

In this formula population A is called the study population, population B the standard or comparison population. The latter supplies the information on the expected proportion.

The PMR examines differences in the proportion of deaths attributable to disease X in one population compared with a second population. (Obviously, all-cause PM or PMR is always 100 per cent.) The PMR (formula above) can then be reconsidered as:

$$PMR = \frac{\text{Observed proportion of deaths from a specific cause (study population)}}{\substack{\text{Expected proportion of deaths from a specific cause} \\ \text{(from the standard population)}}}$$

(8.3)

Either the proportion in the overall standard population can be applied to obtain the expected proportion in all ages (the actual or crude PMR), or the age-specific proportions can be applied. If the latter is adopted the expected proportion is calculated for each specific age group, with the specific figures being summed (in effect standardizing for age, as explained in Section 8.3). The denominator may also be cause-specific. For example, we could look at deaths from coronary heart disease (CHD) as a proportion of deaths from stroke, or cancer, or accidents, rather than all causes.

Marmot and colleagues (1984), for example, were interested in whether people of Indian, Pakistani, Bangladeshi, and Sri Lankan ethnic origin (South Asians) living in England and Wales have a higher rate of mortality from coronary heart disease than the population as a whole. They studied mortality rates around the years of the 1971 census. The preliminary answer on the basis of mortality rates by country of birth was—possibly so. The problem was that some people born on the Indian subcontinent were of European ethnic origin. Further, some South Asians were born in England and Wales. Neither the 1971 census nor the death certificate recorded ethnic group, only country of birth. The solution Marmot *et al.* adopted was to calculate the age-adjusted PMR (see Table 8.1). They tested the hypothesis that the proportional mortality ratio in those with South Asian names (an indicator of ethnic group, not just birthplace), was different from that in those born in the Indian subcontinent without such names, from African New Commonwealth born, and from the whole population of England and Wales. The proportional mortality of the whole population of England and Wales provided the standard. A PMR of 100 per cent would, therefore, reflect no difference between the ethnic groups and the standard population. Before reading on do the exercise in Box 8.1.

The magnitude of the PM depends not only on the number of deaths from the cause under study but also the number of deaths from other causes. In comparing PM between populations, therefore, differences might arise from either differences in the disease under study, or differences in other diseases. In South Asians, for example, cancers are

Table 8.1 PMR for ischaemic heart disease in male immigrants born in the Indian subcontintent and the African New Commonwealth

	Observed deaths	PMR
Indian subcontinent-born		
Standard population		100
With Indian names, Indian ethnic origin	605	119
Without Indian names, 'British' ethnic origin	535	121
African New Commonwealth born		
With African names, African ethnic origin	28	56
With Indian names, Indian ethnic origin	23	120
With British names, British ethnic origin	39	84

Table developed from data in Marmot *et al.* (1984, p. 51—see Permissions).

Box 8.1 Assumption behind, and interpretation of, the PMR

Examine Table 8.1. How do the PMRs in the Indian ethnic group compare?

◆ What is the fundamental assumption that underpins valid comparisons between populations using PMRs?

◆ Were Marmot *et al.* correct in inferring that ischaemic heart disease was comparatively more common in the South Asian populations?

less common than in the population as a whole, so the high PMR could be due to either a higher level of CHD or a lower rate of cancer. While the data in Table 8.1 favour the view that ischaemic heart disease is comparatively common in South Asian-born the result is not conclusive (at least, on its own).

The PMR can be considered as a preliminary, or corroborative, analysis tool. This is because its fundamental assumption, that the distribution of deaths from causes other than the one under study is the same in the two populations, is often unlikely to hold. When it does, the standardized mortality ratio (SMR—see section 8.3) and the PMR are related, according to the formula given by Roman *et al.* (1984):

$$\text{SMR (for a specific cause)} = \frac{\text{All cause SMR} \times \text{PMR (for a specific cause)}}{100} \qquad (8.4)$$

When SMR can be calculated but only for all causes this formula might be useful. It is, however, rarely used.

Clearly, proportional mortality is a simple and potentially useful way of portraying the burden of a specific disease within a population, and the PMR provides a way to compare populations. PMRs can be used to examine the association between an exposure and a cause of death. In our example of Marmot *et al.*'s study (Table 8.1), the exposure is South Asian ethnicity and cause of death CHD. The PMR then is one measure of the strength of the association, but for reasons already discussed in relation to the exercise in Box 8.1, a potentially flawed one. It is most popular in occupational epidemiology.

8.3 Adjusted overall rates: standardization and the calculation of the SMR

When numerator and population denominator data are available, age- and sex-specific rates can be calculated and compared between times, places, and subpopulations (Chapter 7). These rates provide an undistorted view of the disease patterns in a population. Wherever possible, these rates should be presented.

Sometimes the numbers of study participants or study outcomes is small and age- and sex-specific rates are imprecise. The resulting data set may pose difficulties in interpretation. Age- and sex-specific tables are usually large and difficult to assimilate (e.g. Table 8.17). Nonetheless, for reasons given in Chapter 7 epidemiologists need to examine such data carefully before summarizing them. The obvious answer is to calculate a summary figure such as the overall actual (crude) rate. The result is truly reflecting the burden of disease X in that population.

For comparative research, however, overall actual (crude) rates may mislead. The usual problem is that the age and sex structure of the compared populations differs, in other words age and sex are confounding variables (see section 4.2.4). The simplest way to take this into account is to adjust (or standardize) the rates for age, sex or both, as discussed below. This is usual and good epidemiological practice. There are exceptions to this principle. Where the comparison populations are virtually identical in age and sex structure, age and sex adjustment will not alter the results. When age and sex differences in populations are potentially interesting or important explanatory factors for population disease patterns, rates should not be adjusted and age-specific and sex-specific data should be shown.

Adjusted rates have become the norm, but a warning is appropriate. The disadvantages of adjusted rates are substantial. As they are not true population-based rates, they do not accurately measure the health status of a population, and resulting estimates of health-care needs are wrong. For example, the age-adjusted rate for stroke in seaside resorts which attract the healthy but relatively old people who have retired, may be lower than in major commercial cities such as London but this is quite misleading. London's need for stroke services per unit of population is actually less than a place like a seaside resort.

Summarizing a set of age-specific rates into one age-adjusted figure loses information, which is particularly important when differences are not consistent across age group or sex. For example, Table 8.2 shows that the overall SMR for lung cancer for women living near industry (zones ABC) was higher than in the control area (S). (Study details are in Box 4.6.) The summary figure (SMR all ages) disguises the fact that mortality rates in the under-65-year-olds were much higher in zones ABC while rates in over-75-year-olds were actually lower in zones ABC than in zone S.

Where there are major differences in age and sex structure between populations, when adjustment is most needed, the method leads to the most distortion. These limitations

Table 8.2 Standardized mortality ratios for lung cancer in women at all ages and by age group in larger zones[1] (ABC) compared with an area in Sunderland (S)

Population women (census 1991)	ABC (N = 40332)		S (N = 22321)	
	SMR	N	SMR	N
All ages	217	288	173	152
0–64	287	136	170	55
65–74	190	98	165	56
75 +	161	54	192	41

[1]Standardized to England Wales population with 5-year age groupings. N, observed number of population or deaths; SMR, standardized mortality ratios. Adapted from Pless-Mulloli *et al.* (1998), Environmental Health Perspectives **106**, 189–96—see Permissions.

also apply to the same population being compared at different time periods; for example, CHD in the USA in 1994 compared with 1940. Until recently USA CHD mortality data were adjusted using the 1940 age structure, but for the 1996 analysis the population structure of the year 2000 was used. The calculation based on the 1940 structure gave a rate of 86.7/100 000, compared with 187.1/100 000 using the 2000 structure (the explanation for this extraordinary result is given below).

8.3.1 Direct standardization

Before reading on do, with much care, the exercise in Box 8.2, based on Table 8.3. Then, compare your results with Appendix Table A8.3. Remember the fundamental measures are the age and sex specific rates.

Table 8.3 shows three populations with radically different age structures. Population A is not untypical of industrialized countries, with similar numbers of people in the three decades. Population B is clearly an unnatural age structure. This could be the age structure of hospital specialist doctors, or university academic staff. This could also be the age structure in the aftermath of war, decimation by a disease such as AIDS or the result of the major industry closing down, for example, in a mining town, leading to emigration of the young. Population C is also unnatural in structure. It could be the population of soldiers, university students, doctors in the training grades, or the population in a new suburb with low-cost homes for families. These three populations will be used for several exercises below.

The age-specific rates (Appendix table A8.3) show that the disease rates are identical in the three populations and that they rise with age. The actual overall (crude) rates differ markedly. Why? Population B has high overall rates because it has a comparatively older population. The larger number of older people is weighting (exerting influence upon) the summary rate. In effect, the size of the population in each age group provides a set of weights that are reflected in the overall rates. While the actual overall rates are accurately describing the disease experience in each of the three populations, the comparison of the overall rates is misleading us into thinking there are differences between them, because the weights exerted by the population structure differ. These differential weights cause confounding. Age is the confounding factor.

There are two main techniques for standardizing the rates to nullify the effects of the differing age structures and make overall comparisons possible—direct and indirect.

Box 8.2 Interpreting age-specific and actual overall (crude) rates

What kind of populations might have these age structures shown in Table 8.3? Calculate the age-specific and actual (crude rates) yourself, based on the data in Table 8.3 (the results are in the appendix table A8.3). Consider the age-specific and actual overall rates in Table 8.3. Comment on the age structure, and the effect this has on the overall rate, which varies in populations A, B and C. Why does this effect occur? Do these three populations have the same disease rates or not?

Table 8.3 Population size, and cases: calculation of age-specific and actual overall (crude) rates in three populations of varying size

Age group	Population size	Cases	Rate (as %)
Population A			
21–30	1000	50	
31–40	1000	100	
41–50	1000	150	
Actual overall (crude) population, cases and rate	3000	300	
Population B			
21–30	500	25	
31–40	1500	150	
41–50	3000	450	
Actual overall (crude) population, cases and rate	5000	625	
Population C			
21–30	5000	250	
31–40	1000	100	
41–50	200	30	
Actual overall (crude) population, cases and rate	6200	380	

In the direct method the age-specific rates from the study population are applied to a standard population structure. Table 8.4 (a) shows the results of doing this with a relatively young population as the standard. Before reading on, reflect on the exercise in Box 8.3, including completing table 8.4 (b) yourself. Then compare your results with Appendix Table A8.4.

Whichever standard population is used, young (a) or old (b), the identical age-specific rates in populations A, B and C obtained from Table 8.3 lead to the same number of cases expected in each of Table 8.4 (a) and Table 8.4 (b) and, therefore, an identical overall (standardized) rate. Here the standard population structure supplies the weights and these are, therefore, the same in all comparison groups. The overall rates in Table 8.4(a), however, differ from those in Table 8.4(b).

The use of a young standard population leads to a low standardized rate (7.5 per cent), and an old standard to a high rate (13.9 per cent). This explains why the standardized rate of CHD in the USA rose greatly (see above) when a modern, older age structure replaced the younger, 1940 age structure. The problem is that the overall standardized results of 7.5 per cent in Table 8.4 (a) and of 13.9 per cent in 8.4 (b) are not real, and differ from the actual (and true) overall rates in Table 8.3. These are subtle but fundamental issues that you need to reflect on carefully.

Table 8.4 Standardization with the direct method: effect of young and old standard populations

Standard population	Population size	Applying age-specific rates from Table 8.3 to standard population: cases expected		
		Population A	Population B	Population C
(a) A young population (age group)				
21–30	3000	150*	150	150
31–40	1500	150	150	150
41–50	500	75	75	75
Overall	5000	375	375	375
Overall standard rate = 375/5000 = 7.5%				
(b) An older population (age group)				
21–30	200			
31–40	1000			
41–50	5000			
Overall	6200			

*Example: from Table 8.3 we see that the rate in the age group 21–30 in populations A, B, and C is 5%. In the young standard population (a) there are 3000 people. We expect, therefore, that 5% of them will develop the disease, i.e. 150 people.

8.3.2 Indirect standardization

The second approach is called indirect standardization. Here, the standard population supplies disease rates, not population structure. These rates are applied to our own study population structure to answer the question: how many cases would have occurred if the study population had the same disease rates as the standard population? The observed number of cases is divided by the expected number of cases. This resulting figure is the standardized morbidity (or mortality) ratio and is usually expressed as a percentage.

Table 8.5(a) shows a set of rates in the standard population, and these are high, while those in 8.5(b) are low. The original (crude) overall rates (Table 8.3) and, likewise, standardized rates in the three populations A, B and C differ. Why? Before reading on do the exercise in Box 8.4. Then, compare your results with Appendix Table A8.5.

Box 8.3 Effect of directly standardizing on overall rates

First calculate the cases expected when you apply the age-specific rates in Table 8.3 to the older population (b) in Table 8.4. Follow the same approach as for Table 8.4(a). Consider the age structure of the standard populations, and the age-specific and overall rates in Table 8.4. What is the relationship between the overall standardized rates in Table 8.4 and those in Table 8.3? Why are the overall rates now the same in populations A, B and C? What is the influence of a relatively young and a relatively old standard population?

Table 8.5(a) Standardization with the indirect method

Standard population (high rates)

Age group	Population	Cases	Rate (%)
21–30	40 000	4000	10
31–40	50 000	7500	15
41–50	60 000	12 000	20
Total	150 000	23 500	15.7

	Population A		Population B		Population C	
	Population	Cases expected	Population	Cases expected	Population	Cases expected
21–30	1000	100	500	50	5000	500
31–40	1000	150	1500	225	1000	150
41–50	1000	200	3000	600	200	40
Total	3000	450	5000	875	6200	690
Observed[*]/expected (standardized morbidity/ mortality ratio, SMR)	$\dfrac{300}{450} = 66\%$		$\dfrac{625}{875} = 71\%$		$\dfrac{380}{690} = 55.1\%$	

[*]Observed from Table 8.3—no. of cases in total.

Table 8.5(b) Standardization with the indirect method

Standard population (low rates)

Age group	Population	Cases	Rate (%)
21–30	40 000	2000	
31–40	50 000	3750	
41–50	60 000	6000	
Total	150 000	11 500	

	Population A		Population B		Population C	
	Population	Cases expected	Population	Cases expected	Population	Cases expected
21–30	1000		500		5000	
31–40	1000		1500		1000	
41–50	1000		3000		200	
Total	3000		5000		6200	
Observed[*]/expected (standardized morbidity/mortality ratio, SMR)						

[*]Observed from Table 8.3—no. of cases in total which is the same as the observed in Table 8.5 (a)

Box 8.4 Calculating and interpreting indirectly standardized rates

Reflect carefully on Table 8.5(a) and the calculation of cases expected and the resulting SMR.

Follow the same approach to do the calculations on Table 8.5 (b), before comparing your results with appendix Table A8.5(b).

Why are the SMRs for populations A, B and C different when the same standard rates in 8.5(a) are applied? Why are the standardized mortality ratios higher in Table 8.5(b) compared to 8.5(a)?

The standardized mortality ratios differ because the standard rates are weighted differentially by the different population structures. Here the population structures from populations A, B and C are weighting the standard rates once again. This is entirely analogous with the weighting effects in Table 8.3.

Rates adjusted by the indirect method are, to re-emphasize, weighted (or biased) in relation to the age and sex structure of the population under study. The summary output from such adjustment is the SMR. This means that SMRs from several study populations cannot be compared with each other. Only SMR comparisons between the study population and the chosen standard population are, strictly speaking, valid. This principle is often breached, sometimes knowingly. Where comparisons are to be made between several populations, strictly, either specific rates, or those adjusted by the direct method should be examined. Reconsider Table 8.2, bearing in mind that the SMRs were calculated using the age-specific mortality rates of England and Wales applied to the population structures of the geographical areas ABC and S. Now do the exercise in Box 8.5 before reading on.

The SMR of 217 shows that the number of cases observed in area ABC was 2.17 greater than the number expected if this area had the same age-specific death rates as England and Wales. Area S had 1.73 times the expected number. As we do not know the population structure of areas ABC and S, strictly speaking we cannot directly compare ABC with S. If the population structures were the same then there is no purpose in

Box 8.5 Interpreting SMRs in Table 8.2

◆ What is the correct interpretation of the all-ages SMR in area ABC and area S?

◆ Is it correct, strictly speaking, for the two SMRs (217 and 173) to be compared directly?

◆ In practice, why might the comparison above be acceptable?

◆ What about the age specific comparison (0–64, 65–74 and 75+ years)? Answer the questions above for these more specific comparisons.

indirect standardization. The all-cause, all-age actual (crude) rates could be compared without any confounding. As areas ABC and S are only 20 miles apart in the north-east of England, we would expect (and can demonstrate) only small differences in age structure. In practice, therefore, direct comparisons, inferring that area ABC has a higher SMR than area S, is reasonably safe. Readers will learn that such direct comparisons of SMRs are commonplace, even though on occasion they are seriously misleading (usually they are not).

The authors also calculated SMRs within age groups. At first glance, that is odd. This is to exclude residual confounding caused by age differences within age groups. It is conceivable that in the age group 65–74 in area ABC people in area ABC have an average age of 71 while those in area shave an average age of 69. This could make a big difference for an age-sensitive outcome such as cancer. The reasoning above applies here. We are on sounder ground in making direct comparison of the age-specific SMRs, especially if these can be in tight age ranges, e.g. 60–65 yrs or even 60–61 yrs.

The procedure of standardization can be extended to include sex and further variables, but the principles are the same as for age.

8.4 Relative measure: relative risk

The incidence rate (cumulative) is the prime measure of the probability of the outcome, i.e. risk, in epidemiology. To see how the risk varies between populations (say, those with and without a particular risk factor) the incidence rates (age-specific, overall, or directly standardized) can simply be compared. Alternatively, we can calculate the relative risk (Table 8.6) which is the ratio of two incidence rates: that in the population of interest divided by the rate in a comparison (or control or reference) population. (When the incidence rates are based on the person-time denominator the ratio is sometimes named the rate ratio, but mostly it is also called the relative risk.)

The phrase is derived from the fact that we are relating the risk of disease in those with the risk factor to those without. Relative risk, as with the phrase risk factor, is often used

Table 8.6 Incidence rate, relative risk (RR), odds ratio (OR), and 2 × 2 tables

Risk factor/exposure	Clinical outcome		Total
	Diseased	Not diseased	
Present (exposed)	a	b	$a + b$
Absent (not exposed)	c	d	$c + d$
Total	$a + c$	$B + d$	$a + b + c + d$

(a) Incidence rate in those with the risk factor = $a/a + b$. (With the baseline population as the denominator.)

Incidence rate in those without the risk factor = $c/c + d$.

(b) $RR = \dfrac{\text{incidence rate in those with risk factor}}{\text{Incidence rate in those without risk factor}} = (a/a + b) \div (c/c + d)$.

(c) OR = cross product ratio = $\dfrac{a \times d}{c \times b}$.

loosely where rates of any kind are compared. The relative risk is the most important summary measure of the size of the effect of the risk factor on disease rates and, hence, the strength of the association (see Chapter 5) in epidemiology. Correlation is another method of measuring association that has lesser utility in epidemiology (see section 9.11.5). The formula for relative risk based on cumulative incidence rates is simple (see Table 8.6), but the interpretation is not.

The relative risk (RR) can be calculated from all studies providing incidence data: cohort studies, disease register studies with valid estimates of the denominator, trials and (most exceptionally) cross-sectional surveys (see Chapter 9). The RR can never be calculated from case–control studies (see Chapter 9) which do not give incidence data. As discussed in Section 8.5, in some circumstances the odds ratio provides an acceptable estimate of the relative risk and in others an exact equivalent. Before interpreting any relative risk always critically review the underlying data to judge the likelihood and extent of error and bias in the incidence rates. Before reading on do the exercise in Box 8.6.

The problems lie in the measurement of disease incidence (Chapter 7). Differences between populations may reflect differences in the accuracy with which the diagnosis is made (numerator inaccuracy) or the population counted (denominator inaccuracy). For example, young people are less likely to consult for medical care, are more likely to be undercounted at census, and most likely to be lost to follow-up or be a non-responder in surveys. A different incidence of a disease in 15–24 year olds, compared to 25–34 year olds, may reflect such factors, rather than, say, effect of age. The time periods for the measurements of incidence need to be comparable to avoid spurious differences arising from time trends. Data are often collected for large areas and presented for small areas. This process may create errors by incorrectly attributing cases and population at risk to the smaller areas. These and other factors need to be checked before calculating and interpreting relative risk. Now do the exercise in Box 8.7 before reading on.

The relative risk of lung cancer in the polluted city is:

$$\frac{\text{Incidence rate in A}}{\text{Incidence rate in B}} = \frac{20/100\,000}{10/100\,000} = \frac{20}{10} = 2 \qquad (8.5)$$

The relative risk of lung cancer in city B compared with A is:

$$\frac{\text{Incidence rate in B}}{\text{Incidence rate in A}} = \frac{10/100\,000}{20/100\,000} = \frac{10}{20} = 0.50 \qquad (8.6)$$

Box 8.6 False estimates of relative risk

Consider why the relative risk might provide a false picture of the effect of the risk factor on disease and hence the strength of the association.

Box 8.7 Calculating and interpreting relative risk

Imagine that the incidence of lung cancer is compared in two cities, one with polluted air (A), the other not (B). In the polluted city there were 20 cases in a population of 100 000; in the other city 10 cases in a population of 100 000. Assume accuracy in the numerators and denominators.

- What is the relative risk of lung cancer in the polluted city (A)?
- What is the relative risk of lung cancer in the less polluted city (B)?
- Do we know the precision of this estimate of relative risk?
- What explanations are there for the higher relative risk in the polluted city?
- What alternative explanations (and technical approaches to testing them) will you consider before concluding that there is a real association between pollution and lung cancer?

The precision of the estimate can be assessed by calculating confidence intervals around the point estimate (the reader should consult a statistics textbook on how to do this).

The obvious explanation is that the pollution in town A causes lung cancer, and doubles the risk. Before reaching this conclusion, however, the investigator needs to ask questions such as these:

- Is the age distribution of the populations being compared similar? As lung cancer is more common in older people it may be that town A has more older people. The solutions to this potential problem are to base relative risk calculations on age-specific rates or use age standardized rates (Section 8.3).

- Are the prevalences of the known causal and protective factors for lung cancer different in town A from those in town B? If town A has a higher prevalence of smoking or other causal factors (or less exposure to protective factors such as a high fruit and vegetable consumption) then the increased relative risk may not be attributable to pollution. The solution is to do prevalence studies in cities A and B on the major causal and protective factors.

- Were the risk exposure patterns several decades ago, when the disease was induced, similar to those in the present? (Data on exposure patterns in the distant past may not be available.)

- Were there differences in health care in the two cities?

Health care differences between towns A and B are unlikely to explain the differences in lung cancer incidence unless they prevent disease, i.e. tobacco and pollution control campaigns delivered or influenced by health care systems in town B may have been more effective than in town A. If the study had been of lung cancer mortality, rather than incidence, however, differences in diagnostic acumen leading to earlier detection of disease in town B, or better and more effective treatment in town B, are potential explanations. Equally, if the cancer under study were breast cancer or cervical cancer, then a higher quality of the screening programme in town B would be a potential explanation for differences in both incidence and mortality.

Once these explanations are considered and due adjustments to the RR made, the investigator can consider the relative risk as a fair measure of the strength of the association and can apply frameworks for causal thinking to judge whether pollution is the probable cause of the higher relative risk in town A (see Chapter 5). The methods by which adjustments to the RR are made, except by standardization of the incidence rates as already discussed, are beyond the scope of this book. The commonest approach is to use regression methods, that can include a number of interacting and confounding factors in a mathematical model (see also section 9.11 on correlation and regression).

8.5 The odds ratio

The odds ratio (OR) is a popular measure of association in current epidemiological practice, and is invaluable in case–control studies (Chapter 9.5). The term odds ratio is an apt description, for it is simply one set of odds divided by another. The odds are the chances in favour of one side in relation to the second side.

In the epidemiological context, the odds are the chances of being exposed (or diseased) as opposed to not being exposed (or diseased). In a standard 2×2 table (Table 8.6) the odds of exposure to the risk factor for the group with the disease are then $a \div c$ and for the group without disease, $b \div d$. The odds ratio for exposure in those with and without disease is simply the odds $a \div c$ divided by the odds $b \div d$. Similarly, the odds of disease in those exposed to the risk factor are $a \div b$, and for those not exposed, $c \div d$. The odds ratio here is a $\div$ b divided by c $\div$ d.

These formulae can be expressed as:

$$\text{Exposure odds ratio} = \frac{a}{c} \div \frac{b}{d} \quad \text{and, disease odds ratio} = \frac{a}{b} \div \frac{c}{d} \quad (8.7)$$

Arithmetically, it is usually easier to multiply than divide two fractions, so to simplify this formula we use the arithmetical rule that division by a fraction is equivalent to multiplication by the inverse of the fraction; for example, division by 1/3 equals multiplication by 3/1. So, the odds ratio can be expressed as:

$$\text{Exposure odds ratio} = \frac{a}{c} \times \frac{d}{b} \quad \text{and, disease odds ratio} = \frac{a}{b} \times \frac{d}{c} \quad (8.8)$$

This equation (8.8), usually expressed as $\frac{`a \times d`}{b \times c}$ which is arithmetically the same, is known as the cross-product ratio. It is exactly the same for exposure odds ratio and disease odds ratio. As it is so easy it has become the standard way of calculating the odds ratio. Product is another word for multiplication, so the phrase cross-product ratio is descriptive of the criss-cross multiplication in a 2×2 table (Table 8.6).

The drawback of the cross-product ratio is that the epidemiological idea behind the the odds ratio is lost. The epidemiological idea is a simple one: if a disease is associated with an exposure, then the odds of exposure in the diseased group will be higher than the corresponding odds in the non-diseased group and the odds ratio will exceed 1. If there is no association, the odds will be the same and the odds ratio will be one. If the exposure is protective against disease, the odds ratio will be less than one. This idea fits in with the basic question behind a case–control study (Chapter 9). For a cohort study (see Chapter 9) the corresponding idea is that if an exposure is associated with a disease then the odds of disease in the exposed group will be higher than in the non-exposed group, so the disease odds ratio will exceed 1.

The odds ratio is a means of summarizing and quantifying these differences, just as a relative risk provided a way of summarizing differences in incidence rates. Before reading on, do the exercise in Box 8.8.

If a disease is caused by an exposure the cases of the disease will have more exposure than controls, so in the first study in Box 8.6 (a case–control study) the odds of exposure, lack of exercise, will be higher in cases and the odds ratio will exceed 1. In the first study the relative risk cannot be calculated because we have no incidence data. In the second study, which is a cohort study, the exercise group will have the lower odds of disease. This study will provide incidence data, so relative risk and the odds ratio can be calculated.

In the second study, for both the odds ratio and the relative risk, the numerators (a, and c, as in Table 8.6) are identical. The denominators are different, that is, b and d, respectively, in the odds ratio, and $a + b$ and $c + d$, respectively, in the relative risk. When b is similar to $a + b$, and d is similar to $c + d$, the odds ratio and relative risk will be similar. This happens when the disease is rare, that is, when a and c are small in relation to b and d. Before reading on do the exercise in Box 8.9.

Table 8.7 shows the data and the results for the calculation of odds ratios for the exercise in Box 8.9. The first calculation (exposure odds) follows the epidemiological logic, but it gives the same answer as the alternative formula which is easier to calculate.

Box 8.8 Disease, relative risk, and odds ratios

Imagine that a disease is caused by lack of exercise (exposure).

You compare the exercise habits of 1000 cases of this disease with 1000 similar people who are disease free. You set out your data as in Table 8.6. Which group will have the higher odds of not taking exercise? Will the odds ratio be more or less than one? Can you calculate the relative risk in this example?

Now, imagine you follow up 1000 people over time who do take exercise and 1000 who do not and count the number of cases over time. Which group will have the higher odds of becoming diseased? Can you calculate the relative risk in this example?

In these two examples in what circumstances will the OR approximate the RR? Why? Based on Table 8.6, try to figure this out for yourself before reading on.

(You may find this exercise easier if you put some figures into a table laid out as in Table 8.6. For example, you may wish to vary the number in a, b, c and d to see what happens.)

Box 8.9 Calculating odds ratios

A study of a disease compared cases with non-cases, and found that 25/100 cases took no exercise compared with 10/100 of the non-cases.

- ◆ Develop a 2 × 2 table to display the data.
- ◆ Calculate the odds of exposure in cases and non-cases.
- ◆ Calculate the odds ratio using equations (8.7) and (8.8) given earlier.
- ◆ How does the difference between the two prevalences of exercise (25 per cent vs 10 per cent) compare with the odds ratio?
- ◆ Which is the more accurate way of assessing the differences between the two groups, the odds ratio or the comparison of prevalences?
- ◆ Which gives the better feel for the degree of association between the disease and exposure, prevalence rate ratio or odds ratio?

In epidemiology one of the key goals is to compare the health experience of one group with another, so our measures should give a feel for the degree of difference between groups. Here we see a 2.5-fold difference in the prevalence rate (25 per cent vs 10 per cent) change to a threefold difference in odds ratio. Clearly, the two approaches are giving different results. Before reading on, try the exercise in Box 8.10.

The odds ratio approximates the prevalence rate ratio when the exposure is infrequent, but not when it is common, as shown in Table 8.8. When $a{:}c$ (odds) is similar to $a/a + c$ (prevalence rate) and $b{:}d$ (odds) is similar to $b/b + d$ (prevalence rate) the odds ratio and

Table 8.7 Odds ratio relating to Box 8.9

Risk factor/exposure	Disease group	
	Case	Control
No exercise	25(a)	10(b)
Exercise	75(c)	90(d)

The odds of exposure in:
case group: $a \div c = 25 \div 75 = 1/3$;
control group: $b \div d = 10 \div 90 = 1/9$.

The odds ratio:

$$OR = \frac{a \div c}{b \div d} = \frac{25 \div 75}{10 \div 90} = \frac{1/3}{1/9} = 3.0 \; (= \text{ exposure odds})$$

$$OR = \frac{a \div c}{b \div d} = (a \div b) \times (d \div c) = \frac{a \times d}{b \times c} = \frac{25 \times 90}{10 \times 75} = \frac{2250}{750} = 3.0$$

(= cross-product ratio)

> # Box 8.10 Varying prevalence of exposure: impact on odds ratio and its validity as an indicator of differences between populations
>
> ◆ What happens to the difference between the picture provided by the prevalence rate ratio and the odds ratio if the percentages exposed in the disease group were 15 per cent and in the control group 6 per cent (scenario 1)?
> ◆ What happens if the percentages were 50 per cent in the diseased group and 20 per cent in the control group (scenario 2)?
>
> In both these scenarios, as in Box 8.9, the prevalence in the disease group is 2.5 times that in the control group.

prevalence rate ratio approximate each other. This happens when the prevalence is low. Before reading on do the exercise in Box 8.11, which concerns incidence.

The results are given in Table 8.9. The odds ratio is higher than the relative risk in both instances, and is greater when the disease incidence is higher (in people with diabetes). In cohort studies, the odds ratio best corresponds to relative risk when the disease incidence is low (which is often the case over short-term follow-up).

The odds ratio is an extremely popular summary measure in epidemiology, despite its disadvantages, for three main reasons. First, in some circumstances it approximates well to the relative measures of prevalence rate ratio and relative risk so provides an alternative measure of association. Second, in case–control studies where relative risk cannot be calculated, it provides an estimate of this. Third, the odds have desirable mathematical properties permitting easy manipulation in mathematical models and statistical computations, as,

Table 8.8 Odds ratios in relation to exercise in Box 8.10: effect of changing prevalence

	Case	Control
Scenario 1		
No exercise	15	6
Exercise	85	94

$$OR = \frac{15 \times 94}{85 \times 6} = \frac{1410}{510} = 2.76$$

	Case	Control
Scenario 2		
No exercise	50	20
Exercise	50	80

$$OR = \frac{50 \times 80}{50 \times 20} = \frac{4000}{1000} = 4.0$$

Box 8.11 Effect of changing incidence on OR

Imagine that an exposure to a causal factor triples the incidence of a disease, that is, the relative risk is three. This disease has a baseline incidence of 1 per cent per year (in the non-exposed group). Imagine also that the baseline incidence is double in people with diabetes, that is, 2 per cent, and that the relative risk associated with exposure is the same, 3. You follow up 100 non-diabetic and 100 diabetic subjects with the exposure, and an equivalent number without the exposure. The study lasts 5 years. Work with 5-year cumulative incidence and a denominator of 100.

Create two 2 × 2 tables to show the data for people with and without diabetes and calculate the OR of disease in the exposed group in relation to those not exposed. Compare the odds ratio with the RR of 3.

---

for example, in multiple logistic regression. For example, in epidemiology we are usually focused on the disease or other adverse outcome. If, however, non-occurrence of disease is of equal interest the OR provides a symmetrical result while the RR does not as shown below.

From the preceding data on people without diabetes in Table 8.9 the RR for being diseased is:

$$\frac{a}{a+b} \div \frac{c}{c+d} = 3.00 \tag{8.9}$$

The RR for not being diseased is:

$$\frac{b}{a+b} \div \frac{d}{c+d} = \frac{85/100}{95/100} = 0.89 \tag{8.10}$$

Table 8.9 Relative risk and odds ratios associated with an exposure in people with and without diabetes: annual disease incidence at baseline = 1% and RR = 3 (5-year follow-up)

	Not diabetic		People with diabetes	
	Diseased	Not diseased	Diseased	Not diseased
Exposed	15	85	30	70
Not exposed	5	95	10	90

$$RR = \frac{15/100}{5/100} = 3.00 \qquad\qquad RR = \frac{30/100}{10/100} = 3.00$$

$$OR = \frac{15/85}{5/95} = \frac{15 \times 95}{5 \times 85} = 3.35 \qquad\qquad OR = \frac{30/70}{10/90} = \frac{30 \times 90}{10 \times 70} = 3.86$$

The relative risk of not being diseased (0.89) is not the reciprocal of 3, which is 1/3.

The OR for being diseased is 3.35 and the OR for not being diseased is:

$$\frac{85 \times 5}{95 \times 15} = \frac{425}{1425} = 0.298 \qquad (8.11)$$

This odds ratio (0.298) is the reciprocal of 3.35. The OR has this arithmetical advantage.

There is a vigorous debate on the merits and problems with odds ratios. Epidemiologists need to be aware that misinterpretation of the odds ratio is common, so care is needed when reading papers reporting it. Many writers, wrongly, treat the odds ratio as if it always were a true measure of relative risk. Statistical packages may label the output of odds ratio analysis as relative risk, creating a trap for the unwary investigator and reader. Some researchers, wrongly, use relative risk as a general term for any summary measure of comparison between groups.

Odds ratios give a fair estimate of the following:

- The prevalence rate ratio when the prevalence of exposure is low.

- Relative risk in a cohort study when the disease incidence is low in the control group, usually taken as less than 10–20 per cent, which is usually true for specific causes, except in very long-term studies.

- The relative risk in a case–control study when the exposure in the control group represents the population from which cases derive (and, in some designs, when the disease is care). (See also section 9.5).

As with relative risk, the OR only makes sense if the study is well executed and can be related to a population. These conditions are sometimes not met. The odds ratio must be interpreted with care.

Odds ratios are not comparable across times, populations and between places if the exposure levels and incidence rates differ substantially. If we are interested, for example, in the size of the association between smoking and lung cancer in men and women, the odds ratios are not comparable across sexes if the underlying smoking prevalence differs in men and women. The odds ratio from a study done in London is likely to differ from one in Tokyo simply because the exposure status in the control group differs even when the relative risk is identical (the point is illustrated in Table 8.9).

Prevalence rate ratio and RR are stable and independent of exposure or incidence levels, respectively, but the odds are not. While it is true that the incidence of most diseases is rare, it does not apply to long-term cohort studies, especially in people with concomitant disease that increases the risk. The implications of this are often ignored. While the relative risk is virtually never calculated in cross-sectional studies for incidence data are rarely available from cross-sectional studies, the odds ratio often is (in preference to the prevalence rate ratio). In these circumstances its interpretation as an estimate of relative risk is erroneous. It estimates the prevalence rate ratio. As a measure of association, and an alternative to the prevalence rate ratio, it has the disadvantages demonstrated above. In cross-sectional studies the prevalence of exposures is usually high (and the prevalence of disease is sometimes so) and the odds ratio may be a poor estimator of prevalence rate ratio. The error in interpretation is often important. Ease of calculation of the odds ratio should not override its limitations. Statistical methods for adjusting the OR so it more closely approximates the RR are available (see references), but are too rarely used. Whenever possible in cross-sectional studies the prevalence rate ratio should be modelled and in cohort studies relative risk should be modelled.

8.6 Measurements to assess the impact of a risk factor in groups and populations: attributable risk and related measures

As discussed in Chapter 5, knowledge of the causes of diseases is the surest route to their prevention and control. In a few diseases there is a unique, known causal factor, for example, nutritional disorders such as scurvy, infections such as measles, and environmental diseases such as asbestosis. All cases of such diseases are attributable, by definition, to one cause. By removing asbestos from the environment we can eliminate asbestosis, and by removing the measles virus we eliminate measles. Cases of diseases that clinically mimic scurvy, asbestosis, and measles will, by definition, be a result of different causes and be different diseases. Often, however, removal of the causes is impossible because we do not know what they are, or removing them is too difficult or costly, or the causes are multiple and complex.

Indirect methods to estimate the effect of reducing the causal factor may therefore be needed. For example, for some chronic diseases there are several risk factors. Stroke, ischaemic heart disease, and cancers such as those of the breast and the colorectal tract are such diseases. The problem that now arises is choosing between alternative actions for there is limited time, money, energy, and expertise. We need ways of helping to make choices by predicting the possible consequences.

Attributable risk provides a way of developing the epidemiological basis for such decisions. An extension of the concept—population-attributable risk—is discussed in section 8.6.2. Attributable fraction/proportion and population-attributable fraction/proportion are among several synonyms for this concept.

Before reading on reflect on the exercise in Box 8.12.

Some of our information needs are as follows:

• Solid evidence that each of these risk factors is a component of the causal pathway and not merely artefactually or statistically associated with the disease. Actions directed at non-causal associations will not achieve the goal set in box 8.10. Such data usually comes from case–control studies, cohort studies, and trials (Chapter 9), together with supporting information from the laboratory and clinical sciences, to provide understanding of the biological basis of the disease. We need to specify the causal model we are using to judge the evidence (Chapter 5).

• Knowledge of the frequency of each risk factor in the population (Chapter 7). If a risk factor is rare then action to reduce it will have little effect on the incidence of the disease in the population. For controlling coronary heart disease, for example, diabetes will be a more important risk factor in South Asian and African and African Caribbean

Box 8.12 Epidemiological information to choose between priorities

Several hundred factors have been associated with coronary heart disease. That said, the following modifiable risk factors have been established as important:

- high levels of some lipids in the blood, particularly low-density lipoprotein (LDL) cholesterol;

- high blood pressure;

- smoking;

- low levels of physical activity;

- obesity;

- diabetes.

Imagine that there are insufficient resources to tackle all six of these risk factors. What epidemiological information would help us to choose between them to reduce coronary heart disease in a population?

---

origin populations than in European origin populations, simply because diabetes is about three to four times more common in these populations.

- A precise estimate of the additional risk that each risk factor imposes on our population. If the relative risk of CHD among those with diabetes was 1.1 (a 10 per cent increase) the impact of controlling diabetes would be much smaller than if the RR was 3 (a 200 per cent increase).

- An understanding of the actions that are (or might be) effective in reducing the prevalence of the risk factor and their costs (this latter subject, health economics, is beyond the scope of this book but see section 8.10).

- Assuming success in reducing the prevalence of the risk factor, the expected reduction in disease outcome (attributable risk). The formulae to calculate attributable risks are shown in Tables 8.10 and 8.11 and are discussed in Sections 8.6.1 and 8.6.2.

8.6.1 Attributable risk/exposed group: estimating benefits of changing exposure in the at-risk group

The question being answered by attributable risk is—how many cases would not have occurred if a particular risk factor had not been present? Another way of framing the same question is, what proportion of disease incidence in those exposed to the risk factor is attributable to that particular risk factor? Finally, in shorthand, what is the attributable risk associated with a risk factor?

The answer is conceptually simple. From the total number of cases, subtract the number that would have occurred anyway, even if the cases had not had the risk factor. This number

Table 8.10 Formulae for attributable risk (synonym: attributable fraction)

Attributable risk (AR) answers the question: What proportion of the risk in those *exposed* is attributable to risk factor X?

$$AR = \frac{Risk\ in\ exposed - background\ risk}{Risk\ in\ exposed} \qquad \text{(equation 1)}$$

$$= \frac{Incidence\ in\ exposed\ (I_e) - Incidence\ in\ unexposed\ (I_u)}{Incidence\ in\ exposed\ (I_e)} = \frac{I_e - I_u}{I_e} \qquad \text{(equation 2)}$$

$$= \frac{RR_e - RR_u}{RR_e} \qquad \text{(equation 3)}$$

$$= \frac{RR - 1}{RR} \qquad \text{(equation 4)}$$

When RR can be estimated by OR $= \qquad \dfrac{OR - 1}{OR} \qquad$ (equation 5)

To express AR as a percentage we multiple by 100

AR, attributable risk; RR, relative risk; I, incidence; e, exposed; u, unexposed; OR, odds ratio.

can never be known as a fact, but it can be estimated from the control, or unexposed, group. These 'excess' cases represent those attributable to the risk factor. It is more elegant to express this excess risk as a percentage. Table 8.10 shows five formulae (these are easy to understand when applied to a practical example, as will be done below). In equation 1 the background risk (estimated from the control group) is subtracted from the risk in the exposed (study) group and expressed as a fraction of the risk in the exposed group. The difference in the two risks is the excess risk. Equation 2 simply substitutes incidence rates for risk.

Table 8.11 Formulae for population-attributable risk (PAR) (synonym: population-attributable fraction) PAR answers the question: What proportion of the incidence in the population as a whole is attributable to risk factor X?

$$PAR = \frac{Risk\ in\ total\ population - Risk\ in\ unexposed\ population}{Risk\ in\ total\ population} \qquad \text{(eqn 1)}$$

$$= \frac{Incidence\ in\ total\ population\ incidence\ in\ unexposed\ population}{Incidence\ in\ total\ population} = \frac{I_p - I_u}{I_p} \qquad \text{(eqn 2)}$$

or an alternative formula based on relative risk and prevalence data

$$PAR = \frac{P_e(RR - 1)}{1 + P_e(RR - 1)} \qquad \text{(eqn 3)}$$

or an alternative formula based on odds ratio and prevalance data $= \dfrac{P_e(OR - 1)}{1 + P_e(OR - 1)} \qquad$ (eqn 4)

I, incidence; p, population; u, unexposed population; e, exposed population; P, prevalence of risk factor (P_e = proportion of population exposed); RR, relative risk; OR, odds ratio.

Box 8.13 Calculating attributable risk

From Table 8.12, calculate the attributable risk associated with smoking based on equation (2) and (4) given in Table 8.10 and the data in Table 8.12. Now do the same for smoking and coronary heart disease.

Attributable risk (AR) is, therefore, the excess risk expressed as a fraction of total risk in the exposed group. The excess risk can also be derived as the relative risk in the exposed group minus the relative risk in the unexposed group which is, by definition, 1 (equation 3 and 4). The total risk in this exposed group is simply the relative risk. The benefit of this formula is that when the odds ratio is an accurate estimate of RR, it can be used to provide AR even without incidence data (equation 5).

Before reading on do the exercise in Box 8.13.

So, from the cohort study data in Table 8.12, among heavy smokers the excess risk of lung cancer associated with smoking is 166–7 = 159 cases = 159/100 000 persons annually. We can express this as attributable risk by using equation 2 in Table 8.10 with the total rate as the denominator, and the excess risk in the exposed group as the numerator, as shown in the table (159/166 × 100 = 95.8%). This percentage is identical to that obtained using relative risk (equation 4 in Table 8.10).

We are claiming, therefore, that among heavy smokers 95.8 per cent of the lung cancer cases were attributable to smoking. By implication, if the cause could be removed, in heavy smokers the disease would be reduced by up to 95.8 per cent and 159 lives would be saved per 100 000 of the population of heavy smokers. The attributable risk for CHD was 29.5 per cent.

It is worth noting that the excess risk is dependent on the actual incidence rate. Table 8.12 shows that even though the relative risk of coronary heart disease in heavy smokers was 1.4, the excess risk of deaths (177) was greater than that for lung cancer (159), where the relative risk was 23.7. The public health impact of stopping smoking, at least in this population, is potentially even greater via CHD prevention than with lung cancer prevention.

Since the removal of the cause may arise from preventive health programmes, attributable risk estimates their potential benefits. The concept of attributable risk is a powerful tool in public health practice but we should critically appraise the underlying assumptions. Before reading on, you may wish to reflect on these.

The foremost assumption is that the risk factor is a causal one. If not, the calculation of attributable risk is merely an arithmetical exercise, which makes false promises. (At best, it answers the question: if the association turn out to be causal, what will be the attributable risk?) The second assumption is that the incidence data apply elsewhere to other populations. It may be that in other populations the relative risk is the same, but the incidence of lung cancer in the unexposed population is lower, say 3.5 per 100 000.

Table 8.12 Relative, excess, and attributable risk: study of lung cancer and coronary heart disease in heavy smokers and non-smokers. See base of page for calculation

	Annual death rates per 100 000	
	Lung cancer	**Coronary heart disease**
Heavy smokers	166	599
Non-smokers	7	422
Relative risk (RR)	23.7	1.4
Excess no. of cases caused by smoking based on incidence formula	166–7 = 159	599–422 = 177
Excess risk	159/100 000	177/100 000
Attributable risk given as a percentage of all risk; based on incidence	$\dfrac{159}{166} = 95.8\%$	$\dfrac{177}{599} = 29.5\%$
Attributable risk based on relative risk formula given as a percentage; based on RR	$\dfrac{23.7-1}{23.7} = 95.8\%$	$\dfrac{1.42-1}{1.42} = 29.5\%$

Adapted from Mausner and Kramer (p. 170); original data from Doll and Bradford Hill, *British Medical Journal* (1956), pp. 1071–1081, with permission from the BMJ Publishing Group.

Then, the incidence in the exposed populations would be 83 per 100 000 (3.5 × 23. 7, i.e. baseline incidence times relative risk), and the excess risk 79.5 per 100 000. When expressed as a percentage, the attributable risk would remain at 95.8 per cent, but the potential for lives saved by the intervention is substantially less at 79.5 lives per 100 000 of the population. This will have a big impact on the cost per life saved.

The third assumption is that the study is valid and accurate. The true incidence rates and relative risk may not be the same as the point estimates, so allowance needs to be made in calculating attributable risk. The precision of these estimates can be reflected in confidence intervals though these only reflect sampling imprecision. So it may behove planners to use various incidence rates and relative risks and estimate costs and impacts within the range given by the confidence intervals.

There is also a need to understand the underlying natural history of disease and causal model to achieve the predicted benefit. How does smoking operate as a carcinogen? What are the causal mechanisms? Is there a threshold effect? Will smokers personally benefit from stopping or has the carcinogenic damage been done already? Without this understanding we cannot properly interpret the attributable risk or offer rational advice to smokers. If the damage is irreversible, the potential lives saved according to the attributable risk may not be achievable and public health efforts might concentrate on preventing children taking up smoking. If the damaging effects are reversible then smoking cessation is a higher priority. (The latter is the case.)

Another important consideration is whether smoking interacts with other factors to cause lung cancer or whether it acts alone. If it acts alone then an intervention to reduce smoking will achieve the promise indicated by the attributable risk. If, however, there are other interacting factors the effect may be greater or less than predicted. To take a well-known example, smoking and asbestos interact in the causation of lung cancer and increase the incidence rate greatly. Stopping smoking in a community of shipbuilders previously exposed to asbestos may yield benefits far greater than predicted from a study based on British doctors.

8.6.2 **Population-attributable risk and population impact number: estimating the benefits of reducing exposure in the population as a whole**

From a public health perspective we are interested in the benefits of an intervention to the whole community. The question of interest to the whole community is, what proportion of the disease experience in the population (not just the exposed population) is attributable to a particular exposure? This clearly depends on how common the exposure is. If a community had no or very little exposure to smoking, as in Sikh women living in the Punjab, India (and in many parts of the world), then cases of lung cancer in that population must be caused mainly, if not wholly, by other factors.

The measure that answers this question is known as the population-attributable risk (or fraction or proportion). The formulae are in Table 8.11. Essentially, equations (1) and (2) are similar to that for attributable risk except that the risk or incidence is not in the exposed group but in the entire population (or a random sample of the population). As such studies are rare, population-attributable risk is often calculated by combining data from representative cross-sectional studies providing prevalence of exposures, and relative risks from cohort studies usually from selected populations as in equation (3) and its equivalent for odds ratios when the OR approximates the RR (equation (4)). The attributable risk is, effectively, being weighted by the prevalence of the exposure in equations (3) and (4).

Population-attributable risk can overturn perceptions and conclusions derived from studying relative risks. The population-attributable risk rises as the excess risk, the relative risk, and the prevalence of exposure rise. In contrast, relative risk is unaffected by change in prevalence of exposure.

The population-attributable risk can help to answer questions such as: if a choice needs to be made on which exposure to reduce, which will have the bigger impact on disease incidence? Try the exercise in Box 8.14.

Table 8.13 shows the result. Given the assumptions, the population-attributable risk calculation supports a programme to increase exercise uptake. Clearly, this is a simplistic example. Nonetheless, the calculation makes the expectation of risk reduction explicit.

Both population-attributable risk and attributable risk are theoretical exercises which provide estimates to help pose and debate options. To assess the benefits in practice, trials need to be done (Chapter 9). In the absence of such trials the validity of population-attributable risk/attributable risk estimates remains questionable. This kind of reasoning is under continuing development, with formulae now available for population impact numbers, and disease impact numbers (Gemmell, 2005, 2006).

Box 8.14 Choosing between options for public health campaigns

Let us say that a sum of £100 000 is available for a health promotion programme to reduce coronary heart disease mortality. We can spend it on either reducing smoking *or* increasing the level of exercise. Assuming that the relative risk associated with both risk factors is 2, that changes of prevalence are equally permanent, and that the cardio-protective effect occurs quickly, which choice will give a better return in lives saved?

First make a judgement on which of the two preventive programmes you prefer.

Now consider which is more common, smoking or lack of exercise? Does this change your opinion?

Calculate population-attributable risk with prevalence of smoking of 20, 30, 40 and 50 per cent and prevalence of lack of exercise 60, 70 and 80 per cent. (These are realistic prevalences in the context of industrialized countries.) Has the result altered or substantiated your earlier judgement?

To describe the impact of a risk factor on causing ill health and disease the Population Impact Number of Eliminating a Risk factor (over a time period) (PIN-ER-t) is defined as 'the potential number of disease events prevented in a population over the next t years by eliminating a risk factor'. The PIN-ER-t extends the well-known population-attributable risk (PAR) to a particular population and relates it to disease incidence

Table 8.13 PAR* for smoking and not taking exercise

	PAR (%)
Prevalence of smoking (%)	
20	16.7
30	23.1
40	28.6
50	33.3
Prevalence of not taking exercise (%)	
60	37.5
70	41.2
80	44.4

*Formula: $\dfrac{P_e \times (RR-1)}{1+P_e \times (RR-1)} \times 100$

e.g. for first row

$$PAR = \frac{0.20 \times (2-1)}{1+0.20 \times (2-1)} \times 100 = \frac{0.2}{1.2} \times 100 = 16.7\%$$

Gemmell et al. used population impact measures to help prioritize strategies for reducing the population burden of coronary heart disease (CHD) in England.). They calculated that if lifestyle targets for primary prevention were met, 73 522 (95% CI 54 117 to 95 826) CHD events would be prevented per year, with the greatest gain coming from reduced cholesterol and blood pressure levels. In those at high risk of developing CHD, achieving target levels for lifestyle interventions would prevent 4410 (95% CI 1993 to 8014) CHD events and for pharmacological treatments 2008 (95% CI 790 to 3627) CHD events.

The formula is:

$$\text{PIN-ER}-t = N*Ip*PAR$$

where: N is the number of people in the population; Ip the baseline risk of the outcome of interest in the population as a whole during the time period of interest; t is the time period over which the outcome is measured

8.7 Presentation and interpretation of epidemiological data in applied settings

The interpretation of epidemiological findings, and of the picture or pattern that arises, is greatly influenced by the mode of presentation of data. If practical decisions are to be made, then providing data in several formats is essential. Two principles nearly always hold: (1) give the actual figures in addition to the summaries arising from statistical manipulation and (2) present absolute and relative rates. Pressures of space and time acting against following these principles should be resisted. Table 8.14 summarizes some of the requirements in presenting disease data. Before reading on do the exercise in Box 8.15.

The first column gives the disease or condition. The value of this is self-evident. What is not self-evident is that a label for a disease may differ across times and places and even between diagnosticians working in the same health service. As discussed earlier (Chapters 1 and 7), standardized definitions applied by trained observers are necessary. The simplest way to provide a definition is to give the standard name of the disease or condition and give its ICD code (or use other standardized coding systems). Without definitions, the data have little lasting value, especially in terms of comparison. Worse, the data may be misinterpreted. For example, the label heart disease is not enough, and is open to erroneous interpretation, particularly in places where ischaemic heart disease arising from atherosclerosis is not dominant (e.g. where rheumatic heart disease is common).

Table 8.14 A standard table for organizing information for the assessment of the pattern of disease in applied settings

		Absolute measures		**Relative measures**	
Disease or condition	Number of cases	Rate (incidence or prevalence)	Rank position on number of cases or rate	PMR/SMR/relative risk/odds ratio	Rank on SMR

Box 8.15 Need for data as in Table 8.14

◆ What unique information or interpretation does each column supply?

◆ What difficulty would the absence of the information cause to the user of the information?

◆ What harm could arise from the misinterpretation arising from such omissions?

The second column states the number of cases for each specific cause. (The less satisfactory alternative is to give the total number of cases for all causes as the denominator and the percentage relating to each disease/condition.) This information has unique value to health service planners and professionals delivering care, in deciding the staffing, accommodation, and supplies needed or used. The numbers also give the best idea of the scale of the health problem and hence help to develop a sense of priority. The diseases may be ranked as numbers to help assess priority. The numbers are also needed to assess whether the sample size is adequate, to permit alternative presentations and analyses of data and to check for errors, which are hidden by all summaries.

The rate is the primary epidemiological tool to permit comparisons over time and between places and populations, but it does not have the immediacy of case numbers. That there were 5000 deaths from a particular disease in a community of 500 000 people last year gives a different impression from knowing the death rate was 10 per 1000 per year, though one can be calculated from the other.

Age-specific and actual overall (crude) rates have the advantage that they can be easily understood and applied to different populations. When the rates are adjusted for confounding factors the resulting rates have no reality and cannot be used directly for health care planning. This is the penalty paid for increased comparability. Depending on the context, there may be a need for both actual overall (crude) and adjusted rates. The source of the population denominators used to construct rates needs to be recorded, preferably as a footnote to the table, or space permitting, somewhere in the paper or report. Unlike case numbers, population denominators are usually easily accessible.

The directly adjusted rate is, to some extent, a relative measure of disease frequency and not, as at first sight, an absolute one. It is the disease experience in relation to the standard population. (The standard population used in adjustment needs to be described.) This and other relative measures, such as the SMR (indirectly adjusted rates), RR, and OR, can be used to refine the picture using the power of analysis of similarities and differences. Finally, the diseases/conditions can be ranked on these relative measures. Such rankings aid interpretation and evaluation of the importance of different diseases/conditions, particularly for future aetiological work.

Relative measures unleash the potential to generate hypotheses to explain differences. The problem is that attention tends to be focused on differences at the expense of similarities, and more attention is given to diseases that are relatively common, even though they may be less important as a cause of illness and death than those which are relatively less common. These points are illustrated in Table 8.15. The list of diseases/conditions highlighted by an analysis focused on absolute (actual) frequency is quite different from that highlighted by the relative approach. Table 8.16 lists the main epidemiological measures of disease frequency as absolute, adjusted, or relative. Life-years lost are discussed in the next section and numbers needed to treat thereafter.

8.8 Avoidable morbidity and mortality and life-years lost

Death and much sickness, disability, and disease is unavoidable, so the idea of avoidable mortality or morbidity can be confusing. Avoidable mortality (or morbidity) is the idea that there is potential to avoid death (or morbidity) from specified causes if the best possible public health and health care actions are taken. For example, death from appendicitis is avoidable given early diagnosis and treatment and some morbidity from that ought to be (e.g. rupturing of the appendix). The causes of avoidable mortality and morbidity are chosen on the potential for prevention or cure so they change with advances in knowledge.

Table 8.15 Deaths and SMRs* in male immigrants from the Indian subcontinent (aged 20 and over; total deaths = 4352)

Cause	Number of deaths	% of total	SMR
By rank order of number of deaths—actual/absolute approach			
Ischaemic heart disease	1533	35.2	115
Cerebrovascular disease	438	10.1	108
Bronchitis, emphysema and asthma	223	5.1	77
Neoplasm of the trachea, bronchus and lung	218	5.0	53
Other non-viral pneumonia	214	4.9	100
Total	**2626**	**60.3**	–
By rank order of SMR—relative approach			
Homicide	21	0.5	341
Liver and intrahepatic bile duct neoplasm	19	0.4	338
Tuberculosis	64	1.5	315
Diabetes mellitus	55	1.3	188
Neoplasm of buccal cavity and pharynx	28	0.6	178
Total	**187**	**4.3**	–

*Standardized mortality ratios, compared with the male population of England and Wales, which was by definition 100.

Source of original data for the construction of this table: Marmot *et al.* (1984).

This table is adapted from that published by Senior and Bhopal, *BMJ* 1994; **309**, 327–30. Published with permission of the BMJ Publishing Group.

Table 8.16 Actual, adjusted, and relative measures

Actual/absolute measures	Adjusted measures, relative but not explicitly so	Relative measures
Numbers	Weighted/adjusted numbers	Proportional mortality ratio
– Overall		Standardized morbidity or mortality ratio
– Specific to age, sex, class, etc.		
Percentages	Weighted/adjusted percentages	Prevalence rate ratio
Proportional mortality		Relative risk
Age specific and actual overall rates (crude)	Weighted/adjusted rates	Odds ratio
Attributable and population-attributable risks		
Life-years lost		
Numbers needed to treat		

The avoidable causes of death tend to be those where a preventive and therapeutic intervention has been developed, and the causal chain understood sufficiently to break the link through intervention. The research challenge for these conditions is to implement (and evaluate) effective services. For non-avoidable conditions the challenge is to develop new interventions and, usually, this will need causal understanding.

Calculating how many years of life would potentially be saved if all avoidable deaths were averted (years of life lost) measures the impact of avoidable mortality in a population, assesses the potential benefits of actions to reduce avoidable mortality, and is a test of the health care system. The age at which death would have occurred naturally if the avoidable cause of death had not occurred, the key data item, is of course unknown so it is estimated. Usually, the expected age at death is set at the average life expectancy in the population. For example, assuming the life expectancy was 75 years, a 74-year-old woman dying of lung cancer would have lost one year of life. In fact, life expectancy for a person who has reached the age of 74 is about 10 years, so in truth about 10 years of life were potentially lost. It would be more accurate, though not so simple, to calculate the anticipated life expectancy of the dead individual based on the population average at that age.

Sometimes a lower age cut-off (65 years usually) is taken as a measure of premature mortality. Clearly, the idea of premature death is arbitrary and refers simply to chronological age. Deaths over this age, however, may be premature if the health status of the deceased was good, while some persons below 65 years may be riddled with disease and their deaths may be timely.

The years of lost life approach gives emphasis to deaths in the relatively young. Given an expectation of life of 75, a death at the age of 10 would yield a years of life lost figure of 65 years, the same as 13 deaths at the age of 70. Clearly, there is no moral, social, legal, or religious set of values to justify equivalence of these yields. Yet here is a rationale for, and echo of, the fact that societies usually hold the prevention and treatment of death in childhood as a higher priority than death in older ages.

Years of life lost can change the perceived importance of problems, which seem relatively unimportant in the light of disease rates. For example, injury has emerged from the shadows partly because of the powerful impact of years of life lost analysis (see Chapter 10, Section 2, on priority setting).

The years of life lost approach provides a common denominator for judging the priority to be given to each cause of mortality. The concept provides a means of comparing the performance of the health care system with the best possible and can be used to set targets. For example, it would be reasonable to say that the organization of the health care system as a whole should mean that patients with appendicitis are sufficiently well-informed that they seek advice early, and that doctors are able to make the diagnosis and operate to prevent deaths. The setting of targets relating to avoidable mortality and evaluation of their achievement provides a powerful means of health care audit.

The years of life lost approach can be refined further by incorporating disability and quality of life as discussed below. Before doing so let us look at Lee's analysis of 10 health status measures.

8.9 **Comparison of summary measures of health status**

Lee explored age-specific mortality rates for pneumonia and suicide in Taiwan, 1995, using 10 summary measures, including years of life lost. Table 8.17 shows age-specific population size, number of deaths, and rates. Before reading on, readers may wish to summarize the results of the table, in terms of the pattern of deaths.

There were more deaths from pneumonia (3070) than from suicide (1618). Pneumonia deaths occurred mainly in the age groups over 55 years and the number of deaths rose with age, except in the 85-years-plus group. By contrast most deaths from suicide were in the 20–74 age groups with the peak number in the 25–44 age groups. The age-specific rates generally confirm the picture derived from case numbers for pneumonia but show that the highest rates were in the 85-years-plus group. For suicide age-specific rates indicate an increasing problem with age, the greater number of deaths in the 25–44 age group simply being a function of larger population size. The differentials in the rates for pneumonia are huge; for example, the 80–84-year-olds have a relative risk of pneumonia mortality about 1255 times that in the 20–24 age group. By contrast, the equivalent relative risk for suicide is 6.7.

What happens to this picture when summary measures are used? Lee used ten summary measures, but for simplicity the number has been reduced to six here. Table 8.18 shows that both the crude rate and the age-standardized rate show pneumonia deaths to be about twice as common as suicide mortality. The cumulative rate and life-table risk are much greater for pneumonia. The measures of years of life lost (YPLL and CRPLL), however, show these to be much lower for pneumonia than for suicide. The point is that the perception of the relative burden of disease depends on the choice and mode of

Table 8.17 Population size and mortality due to pneumonia and suicide in Taiwan, 1995

Age	Population	Pneumonia death	Mortality[a]	Suicide death	Mortality[a]
0–4	1 596 058	59	3.70	0	0.00
5–9	1 608 446	14	0.87	0	0.00
10–14	1 918 327	11	0.57	12	0.63
15–19	1 988 479	11	0.55	44	2.21
20–24	1 790 146	6	0.34	105	5.87
25–29	1 886 651	18	0.95	163	8.64
30–34	1 959 013	31	1.58	165	8.42
35–39	1 846 480	27	1.46	145	7.85
40–44	1 632 355	36	2.21	154	9.43
45–49	1 060 675	29	2.73	92	8.67
50–54	866 026	65	7.51	102	11.78
55–59	799 674	90	11.25	114	15.86
60–64	718 617	167	23.24	114	15.86
65–69	655 406	266	40.59	125	19.07
70–74	457 317	431	94.25	131	28.65
75–79	263 482	583	221.27	66	25.05
80–84	149 406	638	427.02	59	39.49
85+	71 094	588	827.07	27	37.98
Total*		3070		1618	

[a]Per 100 000 population.*Added by the author.

Adapted from Lee, *Int J Epidemiol* 1998; **27**, 1053–6—see Permissions.

Table 8.18 Comparison of various health-status measures in quantifying the impacts of pneumonia death and suicide in Taiwan, 1995

Measure[a]	Pneumonia	Suicide	*Ratio of pneumonia/suicide
Crude rate	14.44[b]	7.61[b]	1.9
ASR	14.55[b]	7.06[b]	2.1
CR	0.0834	0.0122	6.8
Life-table risk	0.0353	0.0080	4.4
YPLL	20 208	43 500	0.5
CRPLL	35.1[c]	55.0[c]	0.6

[a]ASR, age-standardized rate; CR, cumulative rate; YPLL, years of potential life lost; CRPLL, cumulative rate of potential life lost.

[b]Per 100 000 population. [c]In days. *Column added by the author.

Adapted from Lee, *Int J Epidemiol* 1998; **27**, 1053–6—see Permissions.

data presentation. Table 8.19 summarizes the qualities of these measures, as a stepping stone to more advanced studies for readers interested in this kind of applied epidemiology.

8.10 Disability-adjusted life years and quality-adjusted life years

The underlying idea behind disability-adjusted life years (DALY) and quality-adjusted life years (QALY) is that life expectancy free of disability or impairment is of greater value than the same life expectancy with such problems. A year of life with a disability or illness such as stroke, diabetes, or multiple sclerosis is said to be worth less to an individual than a year of life without. This is an idea that is controversial. The logical, but morally and ethically dubious, extension of this idea is that a year of life of a disabled or sick person is worth less than that of another person free of such disability or sickness. At the individual level, many contemporary societies have human rights laws and policies that prevent the application of this idea.

In population settings these measures provide a means of gauging the burden of disease. In contemporary times, unlike other eras, the equal worth of different populations is rarely questioned. In making choices between health-care interventions, and by implication populations to be served, these concepts have provided a way of presenting information and spurring debate and, fortunately, not for discriminating between individuals as to who gets services.

The key question is this: how much less is a year of life with a particular disability worth than a year free of that disability? In the quality-adjusted life year approach the answer is derived by asking people, usually those with the disability and their relatives, and others without a disability. This type of questioning yields a so-called utility value for particular health states, usually expressed on a scale of 0 to 1. Such surveys show that some states, like irreversible coma, may be judged to be worse than death. A year of

Table 8.19 The properties of some health-status measures as summarized by Lee

Measures[a]	Between-group comparison	Need for an external standard	Value judgement on death	Lifetime projected risk	Individual-level interpretation
Crude rate	No	No	No	No	No
ASR	Yes	Yes	No	No	No
CR	Yes	No	No	Yes	Yes
Life-table risk	Yes	No	No	Yes	Yes
YPLL	No	No	Yes	No	No
CRPLL	Yes	No	Yes	Yes	Yes

[a]ASR, age-standardized rate; CR, cumulative rate; YPLL, years of potential life lost; CRPLL, cumulative rate of potential life lost.

Adapted from Lee, *Int J Epidemiol* 1998; **27**, 1053–6—see Permissions.

life in coma, for example, may have no value (or even a negative one). In contrast, a year of life with a minor disability, say correctable short-sightedness, may have little or no negative impact on perceived quality of life and hence the QALY. The QALY provides a means of adjusting the value of life expectancy, and hence years of life lost, taking into account the disability. Clearly, however, the adjustments are based on subjective judgements which depend on who is asked, by whom, when, and how. The judgements are unlikely to be lasting, as social values change and advances in management of disease occur. The QALY has proved to be particularly useful in health economics, where it has provided an outcome against which costs can be considered (cost–utility studies).

Disability-adjusted life years are similar in concept to quality adjusted life years. The main difference is that disability is used directly to value the life year lost or gained, and not the perceived effect on value of life as in the QALY. The life years lost for each individual are, as usual, based on potential life expectancy minus years actually lived. To this value is added the loss caused by disability, after weighting. The weights vary for each diagnosis, for example, for angina the weight used in the Global Burden of Disease Project (see Murray *et al.* 1997) was 0.095, for congestive heart failure it was 0.171 and for acute myocardial infarction it was 0.395. Assuming that cases of acute myocardial infarction are disabled for 3 months (0.25 of a year), on average, then 100 cases would contribute 9.8 years of DALY (100 cases × 0.25 years × 0.395 (weight) = 9.8). Some will go on to develop angina (9.5 DALY per 100 cases of angina per year) and heart failure (17.1 DALY per 100 cases per year). The value of these morbidity weights is critical. The weights were changed in the Global Burden of Disease (GBD) Project between 1994 and 1996. Mental disorders moved from third to first ranking cause of DALY after the change.

The DALY calculations can be refined by including a discount rate, age weighting, sensitivity testing using different disability weightings, and restriction of analysis to avoidable causes of death and disease. The discounting argument hinges on the view that a health benefit now is worth more than a health benefit in the future. Not surprisingly discounting features heavily in health economics. The argument is as for money, for a pound (or dollar) now is worth more than a pound made available in 5 years time. So, a disability-adjusted life year lost or gained is weighted in accord with the discount rate (3 per cent in the Global Burden of Disease Project). Saving one life at age 0 would result in 80 life years saved using the World Bank standard life table (which uses a life expectancy of 80 at birth, and about 85.17 once 75 years are achieved), and saving the life of a 75-year-old saves 10.17 years. Without discounting, however, the infant life is worth about 8 lives at 75 years. With discounting this is not the case, because the short-term benefits gained by 10 people aged 75 years exceed the very long-term benefits to be gained by the one infant.

In the Global Burden of Disease Project DALYs at age 25 were valued highest and those in infancy and old age lowest. Age weighting is a controversial matter that openly accepts a stance that is ageist.

The quality-adjusted life years and disability-adjusted life years are summary measures suitable for policy analysis. Others are being or have been developed that follow similar principles e.g. the health adjusted life year (HALY). A summary measure useful for clinicians and patients is the number needed to treat or prevent.

8.11 **Number needed to treat or to prevent, and the number of events prevented in your population**

The accurate perception of risk is vital to making decisions, particularly where the patient must give informed consent and understand the risks and potential benefits. The number needed to treat (NNT) is a measure that combines directness with simplicity. It simply states the number of people who need to be treated for one patient to benefit. Conceptually, the same measure could be applied to preventive measures (numbers needed to prevent, or NNP) but this is done less often.

The calculation of an accurate NNT needs incidence rates for outcomes, from a well-conducted trial (Chapter 9). So if in a reliable trial we found:

- incidence of outcome per year in the untreated group = 30/1000 and
- incidence of outcome per year in the treated group = 25/1000 then
- the reduction in risk $= \dfrac{30-25}{1000} = 5/1000$ per year and
- NNT = 1000/5 = 200

In this trial five people in every thousand benefit, 0.5 per cent. In other words 1 in 200 benefit, or alternatively, 200 need to be treated for one to benefit. The reduction in risk is known as the absolute risk reduction (and it is similar in concept to excess risk). The NNT is the reciprocal of the absolute risk reduction. Before reading on, reflect on the exercise in Box 8.14.

The physician can explain to the patient that the annual risk (incidence) of disease will decline from 30/1000, or 3 per cent, to 25/1000, or 2.5 per cent. While the rates may not be easily understood, the percentages will be. The absolute risk reduction can simply be stated as 5/1000 or 0.5 per cent per year (the excess risk is 5/1000). These all suggest modest benefits. These are all measures of absolute risk.

The relative risk here (the treated group is exposed) is

$$\frac{25/1000}{30/1000} = 0.83$$

The odds ratio is essentially the same here.

The relative risk (and OR) imply a 17 per cent reduction in risk, a seemingly large benefit. Essentially, there is a substantial benefit on a very low baseline, for the risk of the

---

Box 8.16 NNT in relation to other summary measures

Compare the directness and value of this information with alternatives, e.g. stating the two incidences possibly as percentages, the excess risk, the attributable risk, the relative risk, or the odds ratio.

adverse outcome is very low even in the absence of treatment. This is another example of relative and absolute measures leading to very different perceptions.

The NNT tells the patient that for every 200 people treated one will benefit. By comparison with the other measures, this one requires no technical knowledge or sophistication in mathematics.

The NNT based on results in a trial, of course, may not apply to real health care settings, simply because trials enrol highly selected patients. The NNT, nonetheless, usually provides a more sobering assessment of benefits than the relative risk or the odds ratio. Policy-makers and clinicians have been quick to apply NNTs to therapies but not to preventive actions. This may reflect a fear that public support may be lost by this approach, for the NNP tends to be large. The NNP and NNT can be calculated from cohort and case register studies providing incidence data, but such figures might not be as reliable as those from a good trial (Chapter 9).

Gemmell and colleagues (2005) have been working on a new set of population impact measures to help public health policy decisions. One of these extends the NNT idea to the population. The number of events prevented in a population (NEPP) is defined as 'the number of events prevented by the intervention in your population over a defined time period'.

Using this measure they reported that in moving from current to best practice for beta-blockers and smoking cessation among those who have had a myocardial infarction in a population of 100 000 people in England and Wales will prevent 11 deaths in the next year (or gain 127 life-years), and 4 deaths (or 42 life-years) respectively for beta blockers and smoking cessation; and the cost per event prevented in the next year, or life year gained, is less for beta-blockers than for smoking cessation.

The formula for NEPP is

$$NEPP = n \times P_d \times P_e \times r_u \times RRR$$

where

n = population size

P_d = prevalence of the disease

P_e = proportion eligible for treatment

r_u = risk of the event of interest in the untreated group or baseline risk over appropriate time period (can be multiplied by life expectancy to produce life-years)

RRR = relative risk reduction associated with treatment.

8.12 Describing the health status of a population

One of the vital contributions of epidemiology is the measurement of the health status of a population. The first challenge is to define health. Based on the WHO definition, health is not merely the absence of disease or infirmity but a state of physical, mental, and social well-being. To be healthy it is necessary to be alive, functioning, and to have a sense of well-being. Before reading on do the exercise in Box 8.15.

Box 8.17 Describing health status: choice of measures

Imagine you are asked to describe, as comprehensively as possible, the health status of your population to a new minister of health. The minister has no previous background in the health field. What kinds of measures would you choose to portray the health of your community?

Consider not only the specific types of data, but also the qualities of the data you would seek out.

Obviously, your data presentation to the Minister of Health will comprise a mix of health and disease measures, but less obviously, it ought to include both qualitative and quantitive information. Qualitative information may include the public's and professionals' values, beliefs, and attitudes in relation to health and disease. Quantitative measures will be both self-reported such as on smoking, alcohol, and exercise habits, and directly measured such as height, weight, visual acuity, blood pressure, and cholesterol. There may be information on actual health-related events, such as recent mortality and morbidity rates and life expectancy, and future anticipated trends. The portrait of health would be incomplete without an indication of the health care facilities and services and the effects of such services. These might be described as structures (number of doctors, nurses, hospitals, etc.), processes (consultation and hospitalization rates, etc.), and outcomes (effect on morbidity, mortality, and well-being). These points are captured in Tables 8.20, 8.21 and 8.22.

The next step, beyond description, lies in explanation. This requires relating the determinants of health status such as age, sex, social and economic status, ethnicity, and health-related behaviours, to the measures of health status, and through study of the relationships, deriving conclusions about cause and effect. To complete the description of health status, therefore, the minister should be informed on these matters too.

Population-based data tend to be rich in information on death rates, and poor on function and well-being. As comparing health status between time periods and between populations and places is likely to be important in developing and interpreting the profile, the minister will need to be reassured that the validity and quality of measurement is high.

Table 8.20 Creating a health portrait: some qualities of required health status data

Health and disease
Qualitative and quantitative
Self-reported and measured (e.g. weight)
Actual death rates and anticipated disease trends
Health service structure, number of doctors, processes (e.g. consultation), and outcomes (e.g. death)

Table 8.21 General classification of some indices of health status

Socio-economic
Demographic
Behavioural
Physiological/biochemical/anatomical/pathological/microbiological
Genetic
Psychological
Morbidity
Mortality
Health care

In summary, the health minister might reasonably expect your presentation to include specific information on:

- the population and its demographic and socio-economic characteristics, generally;
- life expectancy, disease states, and causes of disability and infirmity;
- measures of physical well-being;

Table 8.22 Specific examples of some health status measurements

Biological function	Social function	Well-being	Disease and death	Health service utilization
Physical measures such as height weight body shape and obesity	Reproductive status of the population, e.g. fertility rates	Mental well-being, e.g. General Health Questionnaire	Mortality and morbidity rates overall and by cause	Consultation activity
Physiological function, e.g. blood pressure, heart rate	Activities of daily living	Well-being, e.g. as self-reported	Life expectancy, as measured from current mortality rates	Effectiveness of services
Biochemical status, e.g cholesterol level, plasma glucose, antioxidant levels	Social networks	Attitudes to health and health-related behaviours	Predicted disease and life expectancy patterns	Equity of health service use
Genetic profiles, e.g. prevalence of sickle cell trait or cystic fibrosis gene	Health-related behaviours		Disability: prevalence and severity	

- measures of mental and social well-being;
- measures of functioning;
- measures relating to health services;
- explanation of variations.

The next section discusses how these measures can be expressed in a consistent and easily understood way.

8.13 The construction and development of health status indicators

Having chosen an aspect of health—whether life expectancy, death rates, or fertility—we need to define how the indicator is to be constructed and calculated. The general principles are those underlying the calculation of incidence and prevalence rates, but the practice varies for each indicator, usually being reflected by the availability of data, as illustrated with life expectancy and maternal mortality.

Table 8.23 exemplifies the construction of some key health indicators. Life expectancy at birth, or at a specified age, is not based on a theoretical expectation for the individual or the actual living population but the years of life lived as calculated from the most recently available mortality rates in the population. Life expectancy is calculated from life tables (discussion of these is beyond the scope of this book). In most societies, therefore, life expectancy estimates are underestimates, because mortality rates will drop in future.

Table 8.23 Examples of the construction of some indices

Indices	Defining and operationalizing the index
Life expectancy	Years of life in a population expected on basis of current mortality rates ÷ population
Maternal mortality rate	Deaths from puerperal causes during pregnancy or within 42 days ÷ live births
Stillbirth (synonym, fetal death) rate	Stillbirths per 1000 total births
Neonatal mortality rate	Deaths in 28 days per 1000 live births
Perinatal mortality rate	Stillbirths + 1st week deaths ÷ total births
Postneonatal rate	Post 28 days to first year deaths ÷ live births
Infant mortality rate	Deaths at < 1 year ÷ live births
Birth rate	Live births ÷ population
Fertility rate	Live births ÷ women 15–44 years
Abortion rate	Number of abortions ÷ women 15–44 years
Consultation rate	Number of consultations ÷ registered population
Hospitalization rate	Discharges and deaths ÷ population
(Death rates)	As discussed earlier in Chapter 7

This, however, is not a certainty as the experience of dropping life-expectancy in some Eastern European countries and Russia (due to economic difficulties) and some African countries (due to AIDS) has shown. Knowing the life expectancy permits us to estimate the potential years of life lost by an individual (as discussed in section 8.8). The point is that a workable solution is found to estimate that which cannot be known.

The maternal mortality rate is another excellent example of how pragmatic decisions are made. We are actually interested in deaths in women associated with any aspect of childbirth. The first challenge is to define those causes of death that are associated with childbirth. Rather than create a long list of specific causes, the definition is a general one: any cause related to or aggravated by the pregnancy or its management but not from accidental or incidental causes. This leaves a judgement that is made by the health professional and the coder of the death certificate. The next question is whether there is to be a time limit. According to the WHO definition a maternal death needs to occur during pregnancy or within 42 days of the termination of pregnancy. The denominator for this rate ought to be all pregnancies. This figure cannot be estimated accurately so the definition, pragmatically, uses live births. The principle illustrated here is that definitions need to work in widely varying circumstances, to permit comparable data, say from rural China and from inner London. This requires absolute clarity (e.g. as in the time limit of 42 days) and the use of readily available data; for example, number of live births rather than, say, pregnancies or the number of women registered at antenatal clinics. The resulting fraction is multiplied to create a whole number, and is calculated for an appropriate time period. Most rates are expressed per 1000, 10 000 or 100 000 and per year.

In most rates relating to health events around birth the number of births is used rather than population size. Sometimes the denominator is all births, sometimes live births. The reader has no option but to learn the definitions, or look them up, though there is some logic behind the choices. The rate of stillbirth includes live and stillborn in the denominator, the rate of neonatal mortality does not. The numerator of stillbirth includes stillborn, so the denominator does too. The numerator for neonatal mortality excludes the stillborn, so the denominator excludes them too.

Sometimes definitions cannot be agreed internationally, either for legal or other reasons or because the availability of data differs too greatly. The WHO definition of perinatal mortality uses live births in the denominator whereas most industrialized nations use all births, dead or alive. Clearly, live births are easier to count accurately than all births.

Definitions are subject to periodic review and revision. There are, as the reader can see, intricacies and controversies behind apparently simple definitions of commonly used rates.

8.14 **Conclusion**

Clearly, epidemiological purposes, theories and study design underpin measurement, presentation, and interpretation of data. To a surprising extent, however, the capacity to measure and analyse data also alters our theories and study designs. Practical matters such as ease of analysis, and the availability of computers and computer software, also alter our choice of measures and mode of presentation. This, in turn, has a dramatic effect on the interpretation of data and the conclusions and recommendations arising. The interpretation of data, more than most aspects of epidemiology, is influenced by investigators' philosophy on the nature of knowledge (epistemology) and by the theories they hold.

Most epidemiologists adhere consciously or subconsciously to the doctrine of positivism, that is, the philosophic system that is based on facts, acquired by empirical observations, and logic. Anecdote, opinion, intuition, experience, and even observations made informally are not easily admitted as evidence. In this book, and in Chapters 3, 4, 7 and 8 specifically, I have emphasized that facts do not exist in a vacuum, but are extracted by analysis and interpretation from data that are invariably flawed. These 'facts' are contestable, and not surprisingly epidemiologists are renowned, even notorious for their capacity for critique (see Chapter 10, Sections 10.10 and 10.11).

These general points could be illustrated with many examples but let us consider just two, one reflecting a measure—the odds ratio—the other an approach—relative and absolute risk.

The odds ratio has had a profound impact on epidemiology. Its use can be traced to a paper by J. Cornfield in 1951. The appeal of the odds ratio at that time was its capacity to yield an estimate of the relative risk from case–control studies (Chapter 9). With increasing understanding of when the estimate was a good one, came a change in the design of case–control studies with an emphasis on studying incident cases and on ensuring controls were representative of the population providing the cases. The (new) mode of analysis, therefore, altered the theoretical understanding and design of case–control studies. Yet there is no imperative to analyse a case–control study using an odds ratio. Landmark case–control studies on adenocarcinoma of the vagina (Herbst *et al.*) published in 1971, and on smoking and carcinoma of the lung (Doll and Bradford Hill) published in 1950 and 1952 do not, for example, report odds ratios. Presently, the case–control study and the odds ratio are inextricably intertwined. The odds ratio has now become a dominant summary measure in a range of studies, despite its drawbacks, because its mathematical properties make analysis easy (e.g. in a logistic regression model). This is likely to change as the drawbacks are more widely debated and other models are incorporated into standard statistical computing packages.

Different ways of presenting the same data have a major impact on the perception of risk, and in particular relative and actual risks portray dramatically different priorities giving different perspectives on the health needs of populations. Usually, relative measures of risk are more useful in aetiologic enquiry while actual measures are better in health planning and policy.

The tensions inherent in the choice of whether to present data using a relative or absolute risk approach go to the core of epidemiology. What is epidemiology for? Is it a science aiming for causal understanding? If so, the 'compare and contrast' mode of analysis is the time-honoured way of generating hypotheses and the relative risk approach is right. If, however, epidemiology is equally (or even predominantly) concerned with feeding into health policy, needs assessment, clinical care and health planning, then the burden of disease as measured by absolute risk is of critical importance. In practice the relative risk approach tends to dominate. Ideally, investigators should report both relative and absolute risk, hence achieving a dual purpose. This simple advice is usually resisted because it creates extra work, makes the messages harder to convey, and takes up scarce publication space. More than that, most epidemiologists are more comfortable with the relative risk approach.

The example in Table 8.15 of the mortality of Indian subcontinent-born men illustrates the vastly different perspectives offered by relative and absolute risk. It also raises a question about how researchers see the world. Why did the original investigators not report their data in this way? Why, so often in race and ethnicity research, is the reference or standard population a 'White' one? Why is the health of the 'White' population not compared with the minority ethnic groups using the latter as the reference population? The answers are not simply technical ones. One explanation is that there is an ethnocentric approach whereby the population that is dominant in status (and possibly numbers) is automatically assigned as the standard because investigators (most of whom come from or are trained in such populations) see the world through the eyes of this population.

The measurement and portrayal of risk is a dynamic and creative aspect of epidemiology with much scope for innovation. Lee's (1998) and Gemmell et al's (2005) work described in this chapter illustrates this well. The challenges of creating simple, understandable, and valid summary measures of health states are formidable. There is the practical task, at the interphase of epidemiology and public health, of putting measures together to create a profile of the community's health, and using this to help improve it.

Epidemiological data on diseases can be combined with other information such as socio-economic circumstances, social values and attitudes to health, and behaviours relevant to health, to build up a community health profile. Combining data sets in this way helps to generate causal understanding of disease processes in populations and the means of developing interventions to improve public health. As epidemiology is a positivist discipline founded on empirical observation, mastery of quantitative data interpretation is vital to its proper practice.

Summary

Basic epidemiological data on disease occurrence and population structure can be manipulated and presented in many ways. The choice should be guided by the purposes of the research and the likely application of the findings. Data manipulation, inevitably, both sharpens the findings and distorts them. Epidemiological summary measures, broadly, estimate absolute risks (e.g. numbers, rates, life-years lost, numbers needed to treat) or relative ones (e.g. SMRs, relative risk, odds ratios).

Different ways of presenting the same data have a major impact on the perception of risk, and in particular relative and actual risks portray dramatically different perspectives on the health needs of populations. Usually, relative measures of risk are more useful in aetiologic enquiry while absolute measures are better in health planning and policy.

Epidemiological studies should indicate both relative and absolute risk. These measures allow estimation of the risk attributable to a risk factor in those exposed and in the entire population.

Avoidable mortality (and morbidity) refers to the potential to avoid death (or morbidity) from a number of specified causes if the best possible health care actions were taken. Years of life saved measures help to measure the impact of avoidable mortality in the population. Avoidable mortality helps us to focus on priorities for new research, apply epidemiological knowledge in public health, guide health care actions, and assess effectiveness of health care. The life-years lost can be adjusted for quality of life (QALY) and disability (DALY) to give a more nuanced interpretation.

Epidemiological data on diseases can be combined with other information such as socio-economic circumstances, social values and attitudes, and behaviours relevant to health, to build up a community health profile. Combining data sets in this way generates causal understanding of disease processes in populations and the means of developing rational interventions to improve public health. Advances in calculation and interpretation are vital and recent examples include the NNT and population impact numbers.

Sample examination questions

Give yourself 10 minutes for every 25% of marks.

Question 1 Define relative risk and briefly outline its value in epidemiology. (25%)
Answer Relative risk is the ratio of the incidence rate (whether measured by the cumulative incidence or person-time incidence) in those with the exposure of interest (risk factor) and those without.

Its value is in helping assess the strength of an association, part of the process of causal analysis, which in itself is important to weighing up the potential for the association arising from error, bias and confounding rather than being real.

The relative risk is key to outcome prediction models and in estimating the prospects for prevention through public health actions.

Question 2 A population register assessed the incidence of heart attacks (non-fatal and fatal events) by ethnic group in the UK population. The following data were obtained after one year of follow up:

White ethnic group

Age group	Cases of heart attack	Total number of people in study
45–54	5	7500
55–64	24	6500
65–74	37	4500
75+	71	3200
Total	**137**	**21 700**

Indian ethnic group

Age group	Cases of heart attack	Total number of people in study
45–54	3	1800
55–64	6	1500
65–74	8	800
75+	10	400
Total	**27**	**4500**

(i) Calculate the age-specific and overall (crude) incidence rates of heart attack per 1000 population for the White and Indian ethnic groups. (10 %)

Answer (i) Incidence of heart attacks by ethnic group in the UK. Age-specific and overall (crude) incidence rates.

	Age group	White	Indian
	45–54	0.66	1.6
	55–64	3.69	4.0
	65–74	8.22	10.0
	75+	22.19	25.00
Actual/Crude		6.31	6.00

(ii) Calculate the indirectly standardized rate-summarized as a standardized morbidity ratio (SMR) of heart attack for Indian ethnic groups using the White population rates as the reference population. (10%)

Answer (ii) SMR for heart attack in the Indian group; with the White population as the standard

Expected:

	45–54	1.19	Observed = 27
	55–64	5.54	Expected = 22.19
	65–74	6.58	
	75+	8.88	

Total expected   22.11 cases $SMR = \dfrac{observed}{expected} = 1.22$

(iii) Comment on the strengths and limitations of standardized and crude (actual) measures of disease incidence in (a) comparing populations and (b) planning services for one population e.g. the Indian ethnic group. (30%)

Answer (iii) The actual (crude) measures are not good for comparing populations where there are differences in other important respects e.g. age, or sex structure. Where there are large numbers of cases and people then age-specific rates are excellent. These kinds of data are, however, vital for planning services. For this we need to know the number of cases likely to be seen and their age and sex composition.

The standardized methods produce a summary that is not real world data—it is distorted by the procedure of weighting (here by age). So these summaries need to be used with care in planning health care, though they do help refine a sense of priority or need.

Standardized measures are excellent for permitting comparison where the differences in age structure (or sex or both) have been taken into account. This standardization means that age is not a confounding variable in that comparison.

Question 3 An examination of mortality data for disease A gave the following findings:

Year	Cases	Population (millions)
1961	73	4.9
1971	81	5.1
1981	87	5.2
1991	90	5.3

(i) Calculate the annual mortality rate per 100 000 population. (10%)

Answer (i)

Year	Mortality rate
1961	73/4 900 000 × 100 000 = 1.49 per 100 000
1971	81/5 100 000 × 100 000 = 1.59 per 100 000
1981	87/5 200 000 × 100 000 = 1.67 per 100 000
1991	90/5 300 000 × 100 000 = 1.70 per 100 000

(ii) Based on the 1961 rate as the standard, calculate the mortality rate ratios for the other years. (10%)

Answer (ii)

1971 rate/1961 rate	1.59/1.49 = 1.07
1981 rate/1961 rate	1.67/1.49 = 1.12
1991 rate/1961 rate	1.70/1.49 = 1.14

(iii) Describe the mortality trend. What explanations can you think of for this change? (30%)

Answer Both the actual and relative frequency measures suggest more people are dying from disease A over time although the population is also increasing. Therefore, concomitant changes in the population structure (e.g. increase in the number of old people in the population or immigration of people more susceptible to or already having disease A) are possible explanations of the increase in the mortality rate. On the other hand, it is also possible that an increase in case fatality due to changes in the disease (e.g. increased virulence if infectious in origin) or decreased resistance to the disease explains the trend, or there have been changes in diagnostic procedures or recording of deaths resulting in more deaths being attributed to disease A.

Question 4 A cohort study assessed the incidence of stroke (non-fatal and fatal events) by ethnic group in the UK population. The following data were obtained after one year of follow-up:

White ethnic group

Age group	Cases of stroke	Total number of people in study	Annual incidence rate per 1000
45–54	4	7000	0.6
55–64	19	6000	3.2
65–74	32	4500	7.1
75+	63	3500	18.0
Total	118	21 000	5.6

Indian ethnic group

Age group	Cases of stroke	Total number of people in study	Annual incidence rate per 1000
45–54	2	1700	1.2
55–64	5	1300	3.8
65–74	6	700	8.6
75+	8	400	20.0
Total	21	4100	5.1

(i) Calculate the directly standardized incidence rates of stroke for the White and Indian ethnic groups using the European standard population as the external reference population. (10%)

European standard population

Age group	European standard population
45–54	140 000
55–64	110 000
65–74	70 000
75+	40 000
Total	360 000

Answer (i)

Age group	European standard population	Expected cases of stroke: White	Expected cases of stroke: Indian
45–54	140 000	$(0.6/1000) \times 140\ 000 = 84$	168
55–64	110 000	352	418
65–74	70 000	497	602
75+	40 000	720	800
Total	360 000	$84 + 352 + 497 + 720 = 1653$	1988
Directly standardized incidence rate		$(1653/360\ 000) \times 1000 = 4.6$	5.5

(ii) Compare the results of the overall (crude) rate and the directly standardized rate in the two ethnic groups. Comment on the strengths and limitations of these two measures in (a) understanding the causes of stroke and (b) planning health services for stroke. (30%)

Answer (ii) Crude rate ratios (Indian:White) 5.1:5.6 = 0.9.

Directly standardized rate ratios (Indian:White) 5.5:4.6 = 1.2.

The data show that the incidence of stroke is higher in each age group in UK residents of Indian ethnic group than in the White population. Despite this, because the Indian population has a substantially younger age structure than the White population, and the incidence of stroke increases with age, the Indian population has a lower overall crude rate of stroke than the White population. When the differences in age structure are accounted for by age standardization, the higher risk of stroke in the Indian population is reflected in a higher directly standardized disease rate.

In general, crude disease rates provide useful information for health services planning as they reflect the actual number of cases of disease the health service will have to provide care for. Standardized rates reflect the risk of disease after accounting for differences in population structure and hence provide more useful information for understanding the causes of disease and which population subgroups are most at risk. Prioritizing health promotion interventions can be particularly challenging as a compromise between overall population health improvement and reduction in health inequalities often needs to be made (in this example most cases of stroke occur in the majority White population but disease risk is higher in the Indian population).

Question 5 What is the proportional mortality ratio? In what circumstances would you use it? What are its main limitations when comparing different populations? (25%)

Answer The proportional mortality ratio is a summary measure whereby the pattern of the causes of death in the study population is compared to a reference population. The formula is:

$$\frac{\text{Proportional mortality for disease X in study population}}{\text{Proportional mortality for disease X in reference population}}$$

The proportional mortality is the proportion of deaths from disease X, where the denominator is usually all deaths. It can, however, be deaths from another cause.

We might favour this summary measure when a mortality rate cannot be calculated for lack of a population denominator.

The proportional mortality ratio cannot, on its own, tell us whether mortality from disease X is actually different from that in the reference population. This is because differences in other diseases will also alter the ratio. For example, the proportional mortality ratio for heart disease in the study population may be high because cancer mortality is lower than in the reference population.

Question 6 In a cohort study of university students examining the association between meditation or prayer and sickness absence as a health outcome, the response rate was 70 per cent: 5700 women who responded reported they meditated or prayed, while 12 300 did not. The outcome, sickness absence, was obtained from a questionnaire to students one year later. In the meditation/prayer group, 900 students recorded having at least one day off university. In those who did not report meditating or praying, 1350 women were recorded as having at least one day off university in the same time period.
(i) Place these data in an appropriate 2 × 2 table with all appropriate labels and numbers. (10%)

Answer (i)

Relationship between meditation, prayer and sickness absence

	Sickness absence		
	Yes	No	
(a) prayed/meditated	900	4800	5700
(b) did not pray/meditate	1350	10 950	12 300
	2250	15 750	18 000

(ii) Estimate the relative risk of sickness absence in those who do not meditate or pray (use the cumulative incidence rate for your calculations with the baseline population of the denominator). (10%)

Answer (ii) $RR = \dfrac{\text{Incidence in B}}{\text{Incidence in A}} = \dfrac{1350 \div 12300}{900 \div 5700} = \dfrac{10.98}{15.78} = 0.69$

Readers may find it better to do the next part after reading Chapter 9.

(iii) Do you think this kind of study is good for showing cause and effect? What problems make it difficult to interpret the results? (30%)

Answer (iii) The cohort study is one of the classic and powerful ways of studying cause and effect. Nonetheless, the evidence arising needs to be interpreted very cautiously using frameworks for separating causal and non-causal association. One crucial issue is of timing—did the exposure truly precede the effect? Cohort studies are usually good on this matter. Nonetheless, problems arise in errors of measurement, recruitment and retention of population, confounding, and interpretation of the associations found. Studies based on incomplete data and on self-selected populations are problematic.

Appendix

Table A8.3 Population size, and cases: calculation of age-specific and actual overall (crude) rates in three populations of varying size

Age group	Population size	Cases	Rate (as %)
Population A			
21–30	1000	50	5
31–40	1000	100	10
41–50	1000	150	15
Actual overall (crude) rate	3000	300	10
Population B			
21–30	500	25	5
31–40	1500	150	10
41–50	3000	450	15
Actual overall (crude) rate	5000	625	12.5
Population C			
21–30	5000	250	5
31–40	1000	100	10
41–50	200	30	15
Actual overall (crude) rate	6200	380	6.1

Table A8.4 Standardize with the direct method: effect of young and old standard populations

Standard population	Population size	Applying age-specific rates from Table 8.3 to standard population: cases expected		
		Population A	Population B	Population C
(a) A young population (age group)				
21–30	3000	150*	150	150
31–40	1500	150	150	150
41–50	500	75	75	75
Overall	5000	375	375	375
Overall standard rate = 375/5000 =		7.5%	7.5%	7.5%
(b) An older population (age group)				
21–30	200	10	10	10
31–40	1000	100	100	100
41–50	5000	750	750	750
Overall	6200	860	860	860
Overall standardized adjusted rate = 860/6200 =		13.9%	13.9%	13.9%

*Example: from Table 8.3 we see that the rate in the age group 21–30 in populations A, B, and C is 5%. In the young standard population (a) there are 3000 people. We expect, therefore, that 5% of them will develop the disease, i.e. 150 people.

Table A8.5(b) Standardization with the indirect method

Standard population (low rates)

Age group	Population	Cases	Rate (%)
21–30	40 000	2000	5
31–40	50 000	3700	7.5
41–50	60 000	6000	10
Total	150 000	11 500	7.7

	Population A		Population B		Population C	
	Population	Cases expected	Population	Cases expected	Population	Cases expected
21–30	1000	50	500	25	5000	250
31–40	1000	75	1500	113	1000	75
41–50	1000	100	3000	300	200	20
Total	3000	225	5000	438	6200	345
Observed*/expected (standardized morbidity/ mortality ratio, SMR)	$\dfrac{300}{225} = 133\%$		$\dfrac{625}{438} = 143\%$		$\dfrac{380}{345} = 110\%$	

*Observed from Table 8.3—no. of cases in total

Chapter 9

Epidemiological study design and principles of data analysis
An integrated suite of methods

Objectives

On completion of the chapter you should understand that:

◆ understanding disease causation and/or measuring the burden of disease and/or predicting disease patterns are the three key purposes underlying all epidemiological studies;

◆ epidemiological studies are unified by their common purposes, by their utilization of the survey method and their foundation on defined populations;

◆ all study designs potentially contribute to questions of cause and effect, health policy and planning, and clinical practice;

◆ a clinical case series study is of a coherent set of cases compiled by one or a few clinicians;

◆ a population case series (or registry) study, consisting of a set of cases in a defined population and time, lays the foundation for description of disease by place, time, and characteristics of populations (sometimes erroneously described as ecological design);

◆ if a group of cases is compared with a comparison group from the same population the design is that of a case–control study, which generates and tests causal hypotheses, through the analysis of associations;

◆ a cross-sectional study measures disease and risk factor prevalence in a sample of individuals in a population in a defined time period, mainly to explore the burden of disease but also to generate associations and hence hypotheses;

◆ a cohort study consists of a sample of individuals in a population followed up over time to observe changes in health status, to measure disease incidence, and to examine associations between risk factors and health outcomes;

◆ a trial is similar in design to a cohort study except that the investigators impose an intervention on one or more of the study groups;

◆ the ecological 'design' is, usually, a mode of analysis based on variables being studied in relation to places rather than individuals—usually of a population case series (or registry study);

◆ there are conceptual and practical interrelationships between study designs.

9.1 Introduction: interdependence of study design in epidemiology, and the importance of the base population

There is a growing number of apparently disparate study designs used in epidemiology, and the labels used to describe them are numerous. There are, however, five basic designs based on individual data as listed in Box 9.1 and summarized in Table 9.1, which outlines some of their characteristics and overlapping purposes. Confusion about these five designs is common, and is accentuated by the varying use of existing terms, and continuous development and invention of new terms and designs.

There are modifications of these five study designs to suit different purposes. For example, there are retrospective and prospective cohort studies, there are case series studies based on clinical records and population-based registers, and many forms of trial design. Most textbooks and other accounts tend to consider each design as being distinct but this is taxing, particularly when a study has atypical features, or comprises a mix of designs. It is important, therefore, to understand the ideas which underlie study design, particularly in terms of purpose, form, analysis, interpretation, and basis in the concept of population. Such understanding helps to define the common ground, and relative unity, of epidemiological study design.

The common goal of epidemiological studies is understanding the frequency, pattern, and causes of disease in populations and they are usually analysed to provide one or more of the measures considered in Chapters 7 and 8. They are also united by their reliance on the survey method. This is defined by Last (2001) as an investigation in which information is systematically collected but in which the experimental method is not used (I assume, for the purposes of the discussion here, that the word experimental is used in the laboratory sense and not trials). Epidemiological studies are all rooted in the concept of population in that knowledge of the relation between the people studied and the population from which they originate is essential for interpretation, generalization, and application of data. Before reading on reflect on whether you agree with this emphasis on the population in the context of study design. Then, assuming it is correct, consider what questions arise from this perspective—questions the reader should ask, and the investigator should provide.

Box 9.1 Five basic epidemiological designs for studies based on individuals

- case series (clinical and population)
- cross-sectional
- case–control
- cohort (prospective and retrospective)
- trial

Table 9.1 Epidemiological designs and applications: an overview

Study design	Essential idea	Some research purposes
1. Case series and population case series	Count cases (numerator) and relate to population data (denominator) to produce rates and analyse patterns Look at characteristics of cases for causal hypotheses	Study signs and symptoms, and create disease definitions Surveillance of mortality/ morbidity rates Seek associations Generate/test hypotheses Source of cases or foundation for other studies
2. Cross-sectional	Study health and disease states in a population at a defined place and time Measure burden of disease and its causes	Measure prevalence (very rarely incidence) of disease and related factors Seek associations between disease and related factors Generate/test hypotheses Repeat studies (on different samples) to measure change and evaluate interventions
3. Case–control	Look for differences and similarities between a series of cases and a control group	Seek associations Generate/test hypotheses Assess strength of association (odds ratio)
4. Cohort	Follow up populations, relating information on risk factor patterns and health states at baseline, to the outcomes of interest	Study natural history of disease Measure incidence of disease Link disease outcomes to possible disease causes, i.e. seek associations Generate/test hypotheses
5. Trial	Intervene with some measure designed to improve health, then follow up people to see the effect*	Test understanding of causes Study how to influence natural history of disease Evaluate the effects (side-effects and benefits) and costs of interventions

* Measures designed to worsen health or to make no difference would be ethically unacceptable, though this may be done (with ethical or regulatory approval) on animals.

Vital epidemiological questions, therefore, include these: Where and when was the study done (as populations differ by place, and change over time)? Of which population is the study group a subset? What are the characteristics of the study and source populations? Are the findings generalizable to the whole of the population in the community, or to communities elsewhere? These questions will be reconsidered in the context of critical appraisal of epidemiological papers in Chapter 10. The underlying source population or, more technically base population, then, is the starting point of epidemiology.

All epidemiological studies permit comparisons of disease experience in terms of one or more of the triad of time, place, and person. They all contribute to measuring the burden of disease or risk factors *and*, wherever possible, study the relationship of disease and causal factors, though to a greatly varying extent. This integration is not only theoretical but is also demonstrated by the way one study design leads to another, the relatively minor modifications needed to switch the study design, and the way they complement each other, particularly in adding to the weight of evidence in causal analysis (all discussed below). One of the epidemiological criteria for causality is consistency, which requires evidence from more than one study, preferably using different study designs (Chapter 5).

Most textbooks refer to an ecological (sometimes with inverted commas as 'ecological' to reflect the author's doubts) study design, but here this is considered as a mode of analysis. This issue is briefly discussed in the section after the basic five designs are explained. First we consider the value of several dichotomous classifications of study design as these are used widely in accounts of study design, sometimes instead of more specific labels.

9.2 Classifications of study design: five dichotomies

Three commonly used dichotomies (division into two parts) distinguish between descriptive and analytic studies, retrospective and prospective studies, and observational and experimental studies (Table 9.2).

The term descriptive implies a study that provides information about the pattern of disease or risk factors but not the underlying causes. The term analytic applies to studies exploring hypotheses about causes of disease but, by inference, not primarily concerned with patterns. This is a false dichotomy because insights about hypothesis on the causation of disease are inherent in the pattern of disease and risk factors in all epidemiological studies. The pattern is used both to generate and to test hypotheses. Equally, description is

Table 9.2 Fitting study design to five dichotomous classifications

Design	Descriptive/ Analytic	Retrospective/ prospective	Observational/ Experimental	Beginning with disease/causes of disease	Specific comparison group/no such group
Case series (clinical and population)	Descriptive	Retrospective	Observational	Disease	No
Cross-sectional	Descriptive	Retrospective	Observational	Both simultaneously	Usually not, but possible
Case–control	Analytic	Retrospective	Observational	Disease	Yes
Cohort (prospective and retrospective)	Analytic	Prospective and retrospective	Observational	Usually causes	Yes (though it may be integral to the study population)
Trial	Analytic	Prospective	Experimental	Usually disease, but sometimes causes of disease	Yes

a necessary step in analysis of all studies. All epidemiological studies are simultaneously descriptive and analytic, in the sense of exploring hypotheses. One of the finest examples of causal thinking in epidemiology is the investigation by Semmelweis of childbed fever, where so-called descriptive data were the foundation for a causal hypothesis (Chapter 5, Table 5.1). Equally, cohort studies may be used to provide, in the main, descriptive data on disease incidence, and not be concerned with hypothesis testing. Table 9.2 shows the traditional view on whether the five study designs in Box 9.1 are descriptive or analytic. Readers will need to reflect on the value (if any) and limitations of this dichotomy.

Retrospective studies are said to be concerned with data in the past and prospective ones with data in the future (Table 9.2). The terms retrospective and prospective have been used synonymously with case–control and cohort studies, respectively. The distinction between retrospective and prospective studies is inaccurate, for case–control studies may enrol subjects prospectively and cohort studies may enrol subjects retrospectively (see later) and both do, of course, collect data on risk factors in the past. This classification has been (rightly) largely abandoned except to describe two forms of cohort study, prospective and retrospective. Table 9.2 shows the results of applying this classification to the five study designs.

The observational study is one where the investigator observes the natural course of events. The experimental study is one where the course of events is deliberately altered. The investigation of a natural experiment is, strictly speaking, an observational study (Table 9.2). Most epidemiology is observational, for experiments are the exception. This classification is, therefore, of little practical help. The dichotomy does, however, have value in that the biases and challenges inherent in descriptive studies are, in several respects, different from those of experimental trials, as we will see (e.g. Table 9.5). The line of critical thinking of the reader of a descriptive study will focus on matters different (e.g. confounding) to that in an experimental trial (e.g. randomization and blinding).

These three dichotomous classifications may or may not be helpful to readers, but are needed to understand epidemiological writings which use them.

Some alternative dichotomous classifications may help readers. One important distinction lies with the presence or absence of disease at the beginning of a study (Table 9.2). Studies where the disease has already occurred focus on the risk factors that led to it or influenced its course. Studies where the risk factor is present but no disease has yet occurred focus on the occurrence of disease and other outcomes.

Another division in epidemiology is between studies which incorporate a specific comparison group and those which do not (Table 9.2). Those with comparison groups are generally better for testing hypotheses about disease causation than those without, and have usually been done with this as a primary goal. In epidemiology we depend heavily on comparing and contrasting, comparing like with like, and ensuring that the principles we derive can be repeated and generalized across geographical areas and time periods. The use of a comparison population helps to achieve this. The distinctions in Table 9.2 may help understanding but they are not a classification of study design.

The five study designs are explained using the concepts of population (Chapter 2) and the natural history of disease (Chapter 6).

9.3 **Case series: clinical and population-based register studies**

9.3.1 **Overview**

Table 9.1 gives a brief summary and Table 9.2 indicates how case series fit the dichotomous classifications. As you read you may wish to reflect on the questions in Box 9.9 (page 311), but do not read the answers in Table 9.5 until later.

The clinical case series is usually a coherent and consecutive set of cases of a disease (or similar problem) from either the practice of one or more health care professionals, or a defined health care setting such as a hospital or family practice. Clinical case series are usually put together by clinicians on a topic of their interest. A case series is, effectively, a local register of cases.

The cases can be analysed to aid clinical practice and research and explored in an epidemiological way by seeking commonalities and differences in characteristics within the set of cases. The work on Legionnaires' disease, for example, described in Table 3.3 and Figure 3.7, was done by me building on a clinical case series compiled by a clinical laboratory clinician (my close collaborator the late Dr Ronald Fallon). It is not an untypical example. One of the great classics of epidemiology is the hypothesis generated by the ophthalmologist Norman McAlister Gregg after observation in 1941 of a series of 13 of his own cases of congenital cataract, and 7 of his colleagues. He devised and tested a hypothesis on why there should be so many cases of an extremely rare condition that year. The result was a new understanding of how a mild virus infection (German measles) in early pregnancy could seriously damage the fetus, and a worldwide rubella immunization programme to prevent it (see references).

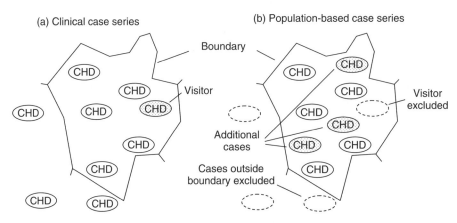

Fig. 9.1 Concept of clinical and population-based case series.

The case series is a powerful weapon in epidemiology—perhaps indispensable. Clinical case series are of value in epidemiology, at least, for studying symptoms and signs and creating case definitions, and are important for clinical education, audit, and research.

Figure 9.1(a) illustrates the concept of a clinical case series using coronary heart disease (CHD) deaths. Typically, a hospital clinician or group of clinicians would compile the case notes of all the cases seen, and analyse them to learn about the disease. As Fig. 9.1(a) illustrates, some of the cases may, indeed are likely to, live outside the defined geographical boundary and may well include patients from overseas. People living in the area, but not under the care of these particular clinicians, would not be included, and usually incidence or prevalence rates cannot be calculated because the population corresponding to the list of cases cannot be defined well.

When a clinical case series is complete for a defined geographical area for which the population is known, and people outside that area are excluded, it is, effectively, a population-based case series consisting of a population register of cases. Figure 9.1(b) illustrates a population case series. There are two main differences from Fig. 9.1(a). First, only cases within a defined geographical area are included and, second, extra cases that would not be in a clinical case series (e.g. street deaths, coroners' cases, etc.) are included. Effectively, a population case series is a collection of the cases seen by all clinicians serving a particular area, and also people living in the area but not seen by clinicians, or seen by doctors working in distant parts. Ideally, temporary migrants and visitors (and these may be overseas patients) should be excluded. In short, the list of diagnosed cases is complete for a geographical area and particular time period. To achieve this usually requires a clear and well-administered system of data collection or a rigorous case-finding study.

The biggest and epidemiologically most important sources of population case series are registers of serious diseases or deaths, and of health service utilization (e.g. hospital admissions). These registers are usually compiled for administrative and legal reasons but are used by statisticians and epidemiologists. These types of studies are sometimes called registry studies. Reflect on the questions in Box 9.2 before reading on.

Conceptually there is no difference between these two types of data sets but the clinical case series is likely to be much more detailed. The main difference between the clinical and the population case series is that in the former the list of cases is likely to be incomplete. The cases will come from an undefined area and the source or base population from which they come from may not be accurately known. The exception to this occurs

---

Box 9.2 Differences and similarities in clinical and population case series

- Is there, conceptually, a difference between a clinical case series and a population one?
- What are the differences?
- In what circumstances are clinical and population case series identical?

Box 9.3 Case series and the natural history and spectrum of disease

How does the case series (clinical and population) contribute to our understanding of the natural history and spectrum of disease?

when the clinician(s) compiling the series provides all the care to the population in a defined catchment area or has collected information on all cases diagnosed by other clinicians (including pathologists doing post-mortems) within that area. This is unlikely to occur except for rare and distinctive diseases, or for rural areas with small populations and a single healthcare provider. The difficulties of compiling a complete case series were discussed in Chapter 7 (section 4) in relation to counting the numerator for calculating incidence. Reflect on the question in Box 9.3 before reading on.

Figure 9.2 shows a case series of patients with suspected and overt coronary heart disease. Clinical case series often include the dead. The cases are, therefore, at a variety of stages in their natural history and the spectrum of symptoms, signs, and severity is likely to be broad. By delving into the past circumstances of these patients, including examination of past medical records, and by continuing to observe them to death (and necropsy as appropriate), clinicians and epidemiologists can build up a picture of the natural history and spectrum of a disease. The population case series is a systematic extension of this series which includes additional cases, such as those dying without being seen by the clinicians. Such cases will add breadth to the understanding of the spectrum and natural history of disease. For example, sudden death in the home setting from a first myocardial infarction will not appear in the hospital doctor's case series but will in the population-based case series and will be particularly valuable if linked to post-mortem data. The clinical case series might conclude that most people with myocardial infarction survive, but the population case series is likely to be contradictory—in fact about 30 per cent of all people with a first heart attack die within 30 days. The epidemiological approach seeks

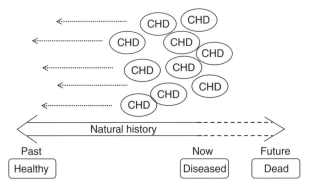

Fig. 9.2 Natural history of disease in case series.

to turn clinical case series into population-based ones—a perspective that clinicians are increasingly sharing.

Making full use of case series data needs information on the source population both to permit calculation of rates, and to develop an understanding of the context in which the disease occurs. The choice of the population at risk needs an understanding of the biology of the disease and the purpose of the analysis for calculating rates. For example, for Alzheimer's disease the population at risk might reasonably be restricted to those over 65 years of age.

The population case series is the key to understanding the distribution of disease in populations and to the study of variations over time, between places, and by population characteristics. (Readers will find this kind of work is often referred to as descriptive epidemiology or ecological studies.) Furthermore, the case series can provide the key to sound case–control and cohort studies and trials (as we shall see).

9.3.2 Design of a case series

The design of a case series is conceptually simple. The investigator defines a disease or health problem to be studied and sets up a system for capturing data on the health status of, and related factors in, consecutive cases. The database may be as simple as this: reference number, diagnosis or ICD diagnosis code, age, sex, alive or dead. In practice, however, the difficulties of developing population case series are so great that many countries have no valid large-scale data even for mortality. For example, India has a well-developed health service and service infrastructure with an established decennial census but does not have comprehensive national mortality data.

To make sense of case series data in an epidemiological sense the key requirements are:

1 the diagnosis or, for mortality, the cause of death

2 the date when the disease or death occurred (time)

3 the place where the person lived, worked, etc. (place)

4 the characteristics of the person (person)

5 the opportunity to collect additional data from medical records (possibly by electronic data linkage) or the person directly if still alive (hence reference number that gives access to personal details such as name, address etc).

6 the size and characteristics of the source population at risk.

It is important, but not immediately obvious, that the need for item 6 favours collecting data around census years or other years when population data are most accurate. Where data are collected continuously, there will be a case for analysing data around census years.

The date and time of death, for example, is recorded on the UK death certificate. The death data can thereby be analysed in relation to the time of day, day of week, month, season and, over the long term by year, decade, or even century.

When the death is not witnessed forensic methods can be used to judge the time and cause of death. Information on the main residence is also usually available on the death certificate. This can be used to find the postcode, map grid reference number, enumeration district (census tract in the USA), local government area, health authority area, region or state, and country. The home address is also vital to exclude from the analysis deaths of visitors (a procedure which may not be routinely applied). Workplace address is important for many diseases but is not usually recorded in population case series, but will be in case series of occupational medicine clinicians.

In geographical epidemiology, particularly in small area comparisons, the exact address is critical information in deciding whether the case is within the geographical area of interest. Computerized information systems usually record postcode (zip code), not address. Except in national studies, there are difficult decisions to be made on people living near the boundaries of the study area. Decisions on which small area a person lives in can be critically important, especially in investigations of rare disease, e.g. childhood leukaemia.

Population denominator data are usually only available on a grouped basis, that is, the number of people living in a particular area. In small area studies, the geographical boundary required for a study may not match that for which the denominator data are available. In this case, grid references based on the full postcode or full address may be used to assign location, but even then errors are inevitable, depending on the precision of the method of conversion.

In compiling a case series, data on some characteristics are easily obtained, such as sex and date of birth. For most other characteristics, obtaining reliable and valid information is a problem, for example, on race, ethnicity, religion, income, or socio-economic position. The problem of inaccurate information on the diagnosis was discussed in Chapter 7 (section 4). The veracity of diagnoses needs to be checked by validity studies that assess the sensitivity and specificity of diagnoses in the database (see Chapter 6). Effectively the work done in making the diagnosis, and listing the cases, is treated as for a screening test and compared to a more definitive (gold standard) data set (usually the fuller medical record). Where clinical diagnoses of death are not available 'verbal autopsies' may be done where relatives are quizzed about the circumstances of death and this information is used to code the cause of death. Extra work will be needed to supplement the basic database.

The population case series register is unlikely to hold information on the natural history of disease. However, case series data can be linked to other health data either in the past or in the future; for example, mortality data can be linked to hospital admissions including at birth and childhood, cancer registrations and other records to obtain information on both exposures and disease. The cases may also be contacted for additional information on their lifestyles, socio-economic circumstances, family history, and so on. In effect, this type of action may turn a case series design into a cohort design (described later).

9.3.3 Analysis of case series

Usually, case series data are analysed using incidence or mortality rates (Chapter 7). There are at least three circumstances, in particular, where rates are not used. First, in the study of spatial clustering of disease, techniques of point pattern analysis based on the grid reference may be preferred. The level of expected clustering may be assessed using a second case series as a control. Clearly, the chosen control disease will be one not expected to show spatial clustering. The second circumstance is when the population is stable as is usually the case for studies of short time periods, as in an examination of the number of deaths by hour of the day or day of the week. The analysis here is on the count of cases. Even if denominator data were available for such short time periods (improbable) it would be unwise to use them for the errors in measurement of the denominator would outweigh any advantage. The third case is when there is no suitable denominator, for example, in case series derived in occupational settings, where accurate information on the population at risk is unavailable, or the study is of an ethnic group which has not been identified in a census or a population register. The partial solution usually adopted is to use proportional ratios, as explained in Chapter 8 (section 2).

Rates from population case series pose serious problems of interpretation. Many clinicians are likely to be contributing to the data set. In the case of national statistics, there may be tens of thousands involved. Even for a register of a common disease in a single city there may be several dozen clinicians involved. The investigator, therefore, may have little control over the quality of numerator data, particularly in the case definitions applied and the variations in diagnostic methods. The case series may cross time periods when accurate denominator data are not available, and this is usually so, except in the census year. Awareness of the problem, training of clinicians and coders, use of agreed disease classifications such as the International Classification of Disease (ICD) and basing studies around the census year are partial solutions. Above all, however, epidemiologists' awareness and thoughtful interpretation is essential.

Population-based case series have great advantages to counter their disadvantages, for example, data sets may be complete over long periods of time, there may be huge numbers of cases, and there are likely to be comparable case series in different regions in one country and internationally. Much important epidemiology centres around such data, which are the key to health service administration, strategy development and planning, and the spur to both hypothesis generation and testing.

9.3.4 Unique insights from case series

Studies based on population case series permit two, arguably unique, forms of epidemiological analysis and insight. First, they can provide a truly national and even international population perspective on disease. Second, the disease patterns can be related to aspects of society or the environment that affect the population but have no sensible measure at the individual level (see also Chapter 2, section 5). Some indicators of the social, economic, and physical environment are not calculable at an individual level (e.g. income equality); do not exhibit individual variation within a geographical area (e.g. ozone concentration at ground level and the thickness of the ozone layer in the Earth's atmosphere); or are not available in the required accuracy in large data sets (e.g. income). For example, studies have related international rates of multiple sclerosis to the latitude of the country, mortality rates to income inequality in a region or country, and infant mortality rates to the gross national product. Reflect on the question in Box 9.4 before reading on.

Box 9.4 Making use of indicators with no valid individual measures

How might epidemiology study the potential role in disease causation of factors which vary little between individuals within a region or nation. For example, factors such as fluoride content of the water, the hardness or softness of water supplies, or weather?

Sometimes health status or exposure data are available for an aggregate population but not for each individual separately. In these cases the relations between these aggregate measures are studied. For example, we may know the fluoride content of the water in the health authority areas of a country but not the fluoride intake of individuals. We may also know the amount of expenditure on oral health, and from that the payments made for fillings, teeth extraction, and so on, but not the oral health status of each individual. These two data sets could be studied to seek associations. This type of study, based on aggregate data, is often referred to as an 'ecological' or correlation design.

The viewpoint that case series studies (whether based on individuals or aggregate data) are descriptive, observational, and epidemiologically weak is inappropriate. The ecological fallacy is commonly referred to but not the atomistic fallacy. Try the exercise in Box 9.5. These two fallacies are discussed in section 9.9. The weakness lies in the quality of data, and is not inherent in the design. These studies offer some unique opportunities and perspectives on the pattern and causes of disease in populations, and provide a solid platform from which to explore the pathways to disease causation. Sometimes, they provide the only way to explore causality in human populations when we need to integrate causes at various levels of social organization and environment. The reason for that is pragmatic, not theoretical. For this kind of work data are needed on millions of people over large geographical areas. Currently, only population case series can provide this. (This may change as the large Biobank type studies become available.) Virtually all epidemiologists will use, perhaps compile and analyse, case series data in their work. Issues relating to analysis are in section 9.11.

9.4 Cross-sectional study

9.4.1 Overview

Table 9.1 gives a brief summary and Table 9.2 shows how cross-sectional studies fit dichotomous classifications. As you read on you may wish to reflect on the questions in Box 9.9 (page 311). Do not, however, look at the answers in Table 9.5 until later. A cross-section is the shape that results from cutting an object lengthwise. In doing so we expose and study a part of it. A cross-sectional study exposes and studies disease and risk factor patterns in a representative part of the population, in a narrowly defined time period. The now rarely used synonym, prevalence study, captures the key role of cross-sectional studies in epidemiology. In addition, the cross-sectional study seeks associations between risk factors and diseases and helps generate and test hypotheses. By repetition in different

Box 9.5 Applying individual data to populations

- ◆ Reflect on whether observations on individuals are always applicable to populations.
- ◆ Can you think of an example of when this is so and when it is not?
- ◆ Why do you think this happens?

time periods, it can be used to measure change, and hence evaluate interventions or describe trends. Its focus is simultaneously on disease, population characteristics and risk factors. Comparisons between subgroups within the sample are usually made. The study can be, but is usually not, designed with comparison groups. The comparisons are usually based on differences in the prevalence of risk factors and diseases, and the association between risk factors and diseases in different populations, e.g. men versus women, or employed versus unemployed.

9.4.2 Design

An ideal cross-sectional study is of a geographically defined, representative sample of the population studied within a slice of time and space. Figures 9.3 and 9.4 illustrate the idea in relation to prevalence of CHD. A target population is defined (here, all ovals within

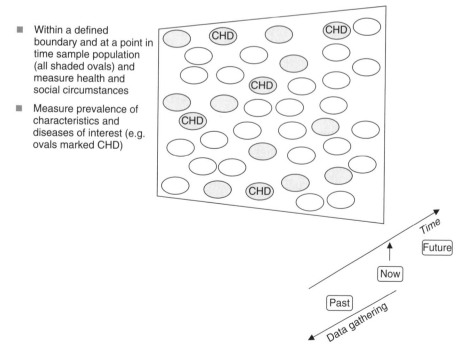

- ■ Within a defined boundary and at a point in time sample population (all shaded ovals) and measure health and social circumstances

- ■ Measure prevalence of characteristics and diseases of interest (e.g. ovals marked CHD)

Fig. 9.3 Concept of a cross-sectional study.

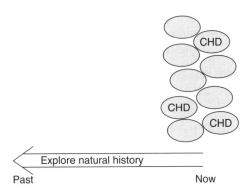

Fig. 9.4 Natural history of disease in cross-sectional studies.

the boundary in Fig. 9.3). A list is made or obtained of the target population (called a sampling frame). A sample of the population at a point in time is taken (here shaded ovals, though sometimes all people in the target population are studied). Measurements are made (preferably simultaneously) to identify people with the characteristic(s) of interest, here, coronary heart disease (marked as CHD). Assuming that the shaded ovals are representative of the population within the boundary, the findings on the sample are generalizable to the whole target population. There are, of course, limitations of random statistical variation and the method of selection of the sample, so generalization will need to be cautious.

Sometimes results are generalized beyond the target populations. For example, if the prevalence of CHD is 2 per cent in Liverpool, England, can this information be used in Newcastle, England? The answer is, probably, yes. (This result is unlikely to be valid in Newcastle, Australia). However, we would need to ensure that the characteristics of the populations of the two cities are similar and then generalize with caution. If the population in Liverpool is of a different age, sex, and ethnic structure from that in Newcastle, England the extrapolation should be avoided. The alternative to making such extrapolations is undertaking national studies, or locality-based prevalence studies, both of which are expensive and difficult endeavours. For this reason, extrapolation is done more commonly than scientific rigour would allow.

Rarely, cross-sectional studies are of the whole population. The national population census is a cross-sectional study, albeit an extremely large one, and one where the cross-section is only in time and not space. (In some countries demographic data are held in a population register. This is not a cross-section, but the demographic equivalent of the population case series.) A survey of the blood pressure of all the patients registered with a particular doctor is also one of a whole (or target) population, albeit a small and narrowly defined one. Harland *et al.* (1997) reported a study which attempted to measure the prevalence of diabetes and coronary risk factors of all Chinese people in Newcastle,

England; an example of a cross-sectional survey based on the whole target population, sometimes called a census sample. This is sometimes done when a sampling frame cannot be constructed i.e. the target population cannot be listed.

Cross-sectional surveys are sometimes thought to provide a snapshot of health. This is a simplistic but helpful analogy. The selection, compilation, and definition of the target population and the listing of the sampling frame usually conforms to the snapshot analogy, i.e. the people are present at a point in time. Measurement of risk factors and disease, however, is usually made over a period of time which varies from as little as a day to several years. A rare example of a truly snapshot study is the measurement of the prevalence of bedsores in Glasgow hospital on 21 January 1976. (Ironically, the paper's title inaccurately describes this as a study of the incidence of pressure sores [Barbenel *et al.* 1977].) This kind of snapshot is only possible in institutional settings.

In most studies the measurements are made over a relatively short period of time such as a year or two. The merit of collecting data over a year (as portrayed in Figs 7.1 and 7.2) is that seasonal differences will be evened out to give a more valid annual measure of prevalence. When the time period of data collection is long, the degree of mis-measurement of the point prevalence depends on the natural history. If the condition is permanent then the point prevalence may be overestimated because incident cases will occur and be brought to the investigator's attention during the fieldwork. Fortunately, most diseases are rare so the effect will be small.

If there is a dynamic but balanced state with new cases arising and old cases recovering in equal numbers then the mis-measure of the point prevalence is small. The mis-measurement of point prevalence is likely to be important for diseases which vary greatly by season or where the incidence is changing rapidly. The prevalence rate of a problem such as bedsores, for example, may be much higher in winter than summer. Obviously, hospitals tend to be fuller in winter so there will be more patients. The kind of patients also changes in winter with more elderly people admitted with hip and other fractures— the kind of condition that predisposes to bedsores—so the prevalence rate rises. The date on which the study was done is important. To gauge the true picture repeat cross-sectional studies at different points of the year may be advisable. Alternatively, the strategies of collecting data over a year (period prevalence) or doing surveys in parts of the population across the year might also provide the better estimate (Figs 7.1 and 7.2). For the measurement of a rapidly changing phenomenon, such as the use of different kinds of drugs in teenagers, the cross-sectional study would need to be conducted quickly (and repeated) to give useful results.

9.4.3 Value and limitations

The cross-sectional study design is excellent for measuring the population burden of disease using prevalence rates, the most reliable summary measures obtained from such surveys. Data about the past medical history and other circumstances can be, and usually are, collected. This is illustrated in Fig. 9.4 in relation to the natural history of disease. In a cross-sectional study of a sample of the general ('well') population there will be people representing virtually all stages of health and disease, and the full range of exposures of interest. They will represent a wide spectrum of disease. Cross-sectional studies can only give indirect insights on the natural history.

People with severe disease, however, may be institutionalized and either not on the sampling list from which the sample was drawn or not available for study. For example, in a study to measure the prevalence of heart failure, people with the most severe disease may be missed because they are hospitalized long term or have died since the sample list was prepared. While it is usual practice to exclude the recently dead from cross-sectional studies, there is no principle at stake here. Data on dead people could be collected from clinical records or from acquaintances and family. For pragmatic reasons the recently deceased are usually excluded. This leads to survivor bias in cross-sectional studies whereby the most severe, possibly fatal, variants of disease are missed. This imbalance can be partially corrected as discussed below.

The investigator may choose to restrict the sample, for example, by studying only people with disease. The sample may, for example, be taken from a register of people with diabetes, with the purpose of measuring, at a point in time, the prevalence of smoking in relation to diabetes and its complications. Such registers often include the recently dead and the full spectrum of disease. In doing this we have done a cross-sectional study within a case series or, even better when possible, a population case series.

9.4.4 Cross-sectional studies in relation to the iceberg, spectrum and natural history of disease

In studies of the apparently well, cross-sectional studies discover people with previously unknown disease, that is, they uncover the iceberg of disease. The full spectrum of disease can be described only by a combination of cross-sectional surveys of the apparently well population and the diseased population, the latter more often obtained from clinical case series than from cross-sectional studies. Cross-sectional studies help to piece together the natural history of disease, particularly the early stages.

9.4.5 Cross-sectional studies in relation to case series, calculating of incidence, and comparative potential

Reflect on the exercise in Box 9.6 before reading on.

A case series studies a coherent group of cases (or potential cases, i.e. those consulting) accrued over a period of time, sometimes over the entire career of a clinician or life of a clinic or service. By comparison, the cross-sectional survey studies all or a sample of the patients under care at a specified time. For example, studies of all patients ever seen at a

---

Box 9.6 Differentiating between a case series and a cross-sectional study

Reflect on the difference between a case series study and a cross-sectional study of cases, basing your thinking on a particular problem such as heart failure or diabetes.

diabetic clinic, or those seen consecutively over a year, are case series. The study of all or a sample of patients on the diabetes clinic's list at a point in time is a cross-sectional study. The distinction is subtle, and emphasizes the interrelationships between study designs.

In theory, when the data on past diseases from a cross-sectional study are accurate the disease incidence can be estimated if survivor bias can be adjusted for. In practice, collecting disease incidence using a cross-sectional design is a problem, mainly because study subjects' memory of diseases is poor and medical records may be incomplete. The possibility of estimating incidence should not, however, be dismissed, particularly for populations and topics that do not easily permit follow-up studies, for example, young people joining the workforce (18–25 years), migrants from rural to urban areas in the developing world, or ethnic minority groups in the inner city. The mobility of these groups is high and cohort studies to collect incidence data may not be possible. Some topics, such as the use of illegal drugs, experience of sexually transmitted disease, or sexual behaviour, are so sensitive that the possibility of enrolling populations for follow-up cohort studies is small and information in medical records will be incomplete. We may wish to study the incidence of gonorrhoea in young men of 18–25 years. Reliable incidence data are not available because it is treated in both primary care settings and sexually transmitted diseases clinics. In a cross-sectional study, information on whether and when in the last year the people in the sample had a diagnosis of gonorrhoea could be elicited to estimate its incidence. As clinic records are incomplete, population census denominator data are unreliable, and the possibility of long-term follow-up of a representative sample of this population is small, the cross-sectional study offers a way of measuring incidence, albeit not an absolutely ideal one, which other studies cannot achieve.

An example is shown in Table 9.3 which is from the study summarized in Table 4.8 and Box 4.6. Here the incidence of consultation for asthma with a general practitioner (physician) has been calculated as well as the prevalence of asthma. A cross-section of people was identified from the register of the population registered with general practitioners held by district health authorities. Medical case records of this sample were examined.

Table 9.3 Reasons for consultation by area in a cross-section of people registered with general practitioners in three areas of north-east England (shown here as zones CA, CB, CC)

	Zone CA	Zone CB	Zone CC
Number of people	734	724	734
Incidence rate of consultations per patient-year	3.97	4.45	3.86
Incidence rate of asthma diagnoses per patient year	0.04	0.05	0.06
Prevalence rate per thousand patients Asthma	74	97	113

Adapted from Bhopal et al., Occupational and Environmental Medicine 1998; 55, 812–22. With permission of the BMJ Publishing Group.

(Of course, we could have asked these people directly, but it is more convenient and easier to get the data from the record.) The study illustrates that cross-sectional studies can do more than measure prevalence. Later, we will reflect on the similarity between this design and a retrospective cohort study (section 9.6).

The cross-sectional study can be of populations in different places, so comparisons can be made (as in Table 9.3). Studies can also compare people with different characteristics, for example, there may be a sample of women and another of men, or one of people belonging to a Chinese origin population and another of the Indian population. Such studies are comparative cross-sectional studies. (But they are not case–control studies, which are discussed next.)

Other matters relating to analysis are in section 9.11.

9.5 Case–control study

9.5.1 Overview

Table 9.1 provides a brief summary and Table 9.2 shows how case–control studies fit the dichotomous classifications. As you read on you may wish to reflect on the questions in Box 9.9. Do not, however, look at the answers in Table 9.5 until later. The case–control study is a comparative study where people with the disease (or problem) of interest are compared with an appropriate control group. The meaning of the word case is close to its medical use to describe the characteristics and medical history of a patient. The comparison, control or reference group (all synonyms) supplies information about the expected risk factor profile in the population from which the case group is drawn. The cases are compared with controls, associations between the disease and potential risk factors are measured (usually by the odds ratio—section 8.5), and through analysis of similarities and dissimilarities hypotheses about disease causes are generated or tested.

9.5.2 Design and analysis

Once the research objectives have been set the first challenge, and usually one of the easier ones, is to find the cases. The cases can be obtained from a number of sources: a clinical case series, a population register of cases, the new cases identified in the follow-up of a cohort study, and from those identified in a cross-sectional survey. The ideal set of cases would be new (incident) and early diagnoses, and representative of all cases in the target (base) population under study. The cases from a population case series register and cohort studies usually meet this ideal the best. The cases identified in a clinical case series are usually highly selected. The exceptions will be those rare diseases where the clinicians compiling the case series see most, if not all, the cases that occur in the target (base) population. Cases from a cross-sectional study are usually prevalent ones, though there will be incident cases in a period prevalence study.

The harder challenge is to select the control group. As for all comparative work the ideal, counterfactual control group (the same people and here cases without the exposure of interest) is not achievable (see section 4.2.4). This concept, however, points to what we are looking for. Classically, the emphasis was placed on the control group being free of disease. This emphasis does not fit with the current concept of this design. The control represents the population from which the cases arise. There are three main approaches to selecting controls. First, we can define the control group at the starting point of the study. Imagine we recruit 300 children aged 5–12 years with newly diagnosed eczema between January 2008 and December 2009 from a primary case setting. We can define 300 (or more) controls in January 2008. Some of them may have, or in due course, be diagnosed with eczema but they will remain in the control group (although these cases could also be removed). Controls can, confusingly, be in the case and the control group. This case-control design is known more specifically as the case-base study.

Secondly, as cases arise, we can find appropriate controls so they are recruited over roughly the same timescale as cases, i.e. concurrent sampling of controls. This is the usual approach to selecting controls. It is normal practice to find controls without the disease, but even this is not essential, for example in a nested case–control study within a cohort study (see next section).

The third approach is to find controls at the end of the study, i.e. Dec 2009. These will exclude cases as these are already in the study.

Each of these control sampling strategies has implications for statistical methods and interpretation of the analysis. The details are outside the scope of this book but the principles given are identical. Information is obtained on the social and medical history of cases and controls and on potential causal and confounding factors. As the causal factors have already had their effect in causing disease in the case group, and the information required is recalled from the past, the case–control study is sometimes referred to as a retrospective study, but this is not a particularly helpful term (see also section 9.2).

The basic idea is shown in Fig. 9.5. Even if this is not explicit, there is an essential assumption that the source population for cases and controls is known. If not, there is no way of interpreting and generalizing the results and it creates great problems in defining the controls. Ideally, the cases are related to a defined population (all ovals in Fig. 9.5). If the aim of the study is to explore the causes of coronary heart disease (marked on Fig. 9.5 as CHD), then new cases would be identified. From the same population are drawn a set of control subjects, marked with the letter C in Fig. 9.5. These control subjects should be chosen with no selection in relation to their pattern of exposure to the postulated causes, but should otherwise be alike to the cases. If, for example, the study was on the causes of CHD (say with a focus on exercise) in post-menopausal women of about 50–75 years, then the control group should also be of women in this age group. Obviously, recruitment of men or children into the control group would be inefficient, and if they were included in the analysis, would be highly misleading. This is restriction and it is both a solution for confounding (Table 4.4) and for maximizing the efficiency of the study.

In some studies, controls are recruited to match each case; for example, if a woman of 53 years was recruited as a case, the investigator would seek a control of similar age (57 would be fine, but maybe not 72). This tight matching process is reducing the risk of confounding, here by age and sex. If a mix of ages is likely to arise anyway, the control group can be recruited without one-to-one matching, particularly in large studies. Matching cases and controls on several characteristics, such as sex, age, ethnicity, smoking status, and social

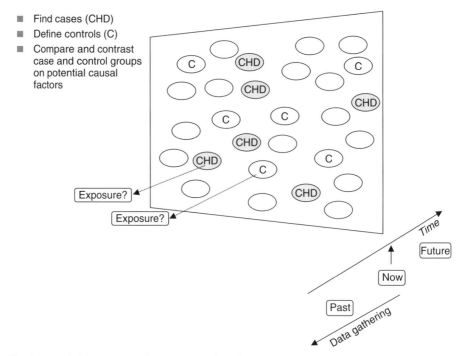

- Find cases (CHD)
- Define controls (C)
- Compare and contrast case and control groups on potential causal factors

Fig. 9.5 Population concept of a case–control study.

class, is not advisable. Such complex matching procedures create difficulties in finding controls, require more complex statistical analysis, and run the risk of 'overmatching'. Overmatching leads to missed associations because the causal factors have been inadvertently matched for. For example, in the above study, if we matched women for smoking status, social class, and income, we may find no association between CHD occurrence and exercise habits, because exercise, smoking, social class, and income are linked. The matching process has created a selection bias, such that differences between cases and controls in exercise habits have been removed or reduced.

Information is collected to confirm objectively the presence of disease in cases. In some, but not all, types of case–control study the absence of disease in controls is confirmed (though, of course, controls may be at a prediagnostic phase of the disease's natural history). Information is collected on the past exposure to factors that may have caused the disease. This is shown in relation to the natural history of disease in Fig. 9.6. Since CHD develops over years or decades (and risk factors may operate even *in utero*, or be transmitted by previous generations) the collection of information on the causal exposures will need to delve deep into the past, and inevitably will be fraught with difficulty. The concept behind the analysis is clear: to find differences in exposure to the hypothesized causes in the past lives of cases as compared with controls.

These differences can be quantified and summarized either as differences in prevalence of exposure, or more usually as the odds ratio, which in defined circumstances approximates

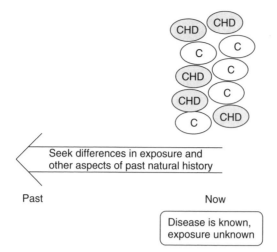

Fig. 9.6 Natural history of disease and case–control studies.

to the relative risk (Chapter 8). An exposure that may have caused disease will be more common in cases than in controls giving an odds ratio greater than one, and one that may protect against disease will be less common, giving an odds ratio less than one. For exposures that are continuous measures, e.g. mean serum cholesterol or time spent doing exercise, the average, e.g. mean, value will be compared. Here, for potential causes the mean value will be higher in cases than controls. Other matters relating to analysis are in section 9.11.

9.5.3 Population base for case–control studies

The need for a population base for a case–control study is an especially interesting issue. Of the epidemiological designs, this one is most focused on establishing aetiology and least on measuring burden of disease or risk factors, which is a by-product. So why should it be population based? Surely, it may be argued, a finding of a difference between cases and controls is informing us about fundamental differences which apply irrespective of whether the population base is known or not.

A classic study by Herbst *et al.* (1971) on the occurrence of the extremely rare disease adenocarcinoma of the vagina in girls and young women illustrates the issues. The study demonstrated an unequivocal association between the disease and use of diethylstilboestrol by mothers of cases in the first 12 weeks of pregnancy; 7 of 8 cases were treated with the drug compared with none of the 32 controls. Might it be argued that the striking findings tell an underlying biological truth independent of the population base? Do the exercise in Box 9.7 before reading on.

There are both conceptual and pragmatic reasons why this unusually clear-cut study needs, and benefits from, a population base. We must know the geographical area and the time period when the cases occurred to draw an appropriate control group. If the cases are from all over the USA, and have been admitted to one or a few hospitals because

Box 9.7 Case control studies and the source population (base): example of the study by Herbst *et al.*

◆ Why do we need an understanding of the source population (base) both to execute the study and interpret the findings?

◆ In what way would the study be impaired if the population base were unknown?

of the reputations of the local surgeons, the control group also ought to be a USA-wide sample. Taking a local control group may mislead. For example, if the local area physicians had a policy for not using diethylstilboestrol, while there was no such policy in the rest of the country, a local control group would lead to a spurious association; that is, the control group would have a low exposure to the risk factor under examination because of a local policy.

We also need to know whether the cases are typical of all cases to evaluate the public health importance of the findings. Do the findings of this study apply to this disease generally? If the selection of cases in the case–control study is not known, this question cannot be answered satisfactorily.

On a pragmatic note, the validity of the estimate of relative risk in a case–control study, the odds ratio, is based on the assumption that:

◆ the cases are incident cases drawn from a known and defined population;

◆ the controls are drawn from the same defined population and could have been in the case group;

◆ controls are selected in an unbiased way, e.g. independently of exposure status; and

◆ in some, but to emphasize not all, types of case–control studies that the disease is rare.

Case–control studies are, for these reasons, best conducted within a population framework. One source of cases and controls that meets the above criteria is the population-based cohort study as discussed next. Some authorities (see Rothman and Greenland 1998) emphasize that all case–control studies ought to be conceptualized as part of a theoretical population cohort. Issues relating to analysis are covered in section 9.11.

9.6 Cohort study

9.6.1 Overview

Table 9.1 provides a brief summary and Table 9.2 an analysis based on dichotomous classifications. As you read on you may wish to reflect on the questions in Box 9.9 (page 311). do not, however, look at the answers in Table 9.5 until later.

It is common to hear people, particularly clinicians, speak of 'their cohort', simply meaning a group, irrespective of the study design. The word cohort is derived from the Latin *cohors*, meaning an enclosure, company, or crowd. In Roman times a cohort was a body of 300–600 infantry. In modern epidemiological terms the cohort is a group of people with something in common, usually an exposure or involvement in a defined population group. Merely being associated with a doctor or health care facility does not warrant the term cohort.

The cohort study involves tracking the study population over a period of time, a feature reflected in three synonyms for this design: follow-up, longitudinal, and prospective. As with the cross-sectional survey the cohort study population may be a general one, or one with characteristics of particular interest, for example, people with a defined lifestyle or even a disease. The hallmark of this design is that health outcome or health change data are obtained on the same individuals in a population at more than one time, not just once as in the cross-sectional study or the case control study. The idea is to study part of the natural history of risk factors or diseases in individuals, and to relate one or more characteristics, exercise for example, to future outcomes such as coronary heart disease (Figs 9.7 and 9.8 illustrate this).

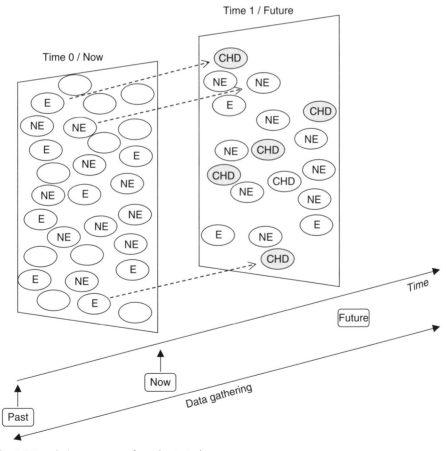

Fig. 9.7 Population concept of a cohort study.

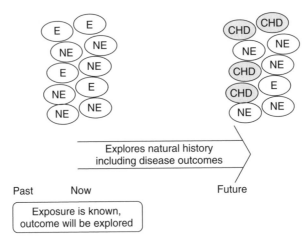

Fig. 9.8 Natural history of disease and cohort studies.

9.6.2 **Design**

In Fig. 9.7 two groups are identified in the base population (all ovals): those who exercise (ovals marked E) and those who do not (NE). These two groups are followed up to ascertain the new cases of the outcome (CHD), thereby calculating a disease incidence rate. Data are collected prospective to the construction of the sampling frame and assignment of exposure status. This applies to retrospective cohorts too (see below). Figure 9.8 shows that cohort studies are future orientated in relation to the natural history of disease.

Comparison groups are usually identified within the cohort (e.g. people who smoke or do not smoke) but sometimes separate cohorts are set up at the outset. In the latter case, the cohort study is usually exploring a specific hypothesis, which dictates the nature of the comparison group. If a particular exposure or characteristic of interest is rare then the identification of separate cohorts will be necessary. Enrichment of the study sample with people with such exposures, or so-called boosted sampling, will be necessary in these circumstances.

In causal research, cohort studies usually test the hypothesis that disease incidence differs in people with different characteristics (exposures) at baseline; that is, there is an association between exposure and outcome.

The cohort study begins by establishing baseline data, usually from a cross-sectional study, or less commonly by the extraction of baseline data from sources such as the census (for legal and ethical reasons relating to data confidentiality such cohorts are rare and will become even rarer, as discussed in Chapter 10 under ethics, section 10.10), or a routine information system such as a birth register. The cohort can either be followed up directly with repeated surveys of the same population or the baseline data can be linked to health records, so providing information on outcomes of interest, usually disease-related but potentially also on risk factors. The new cases of disease identified are incident cases and can be enrolled into a case–control study. Controls can also be identified from within the cohort, and this is often done as each case occurs. This is known as a nested case–control study. (See also section 9.5.2 on controls in case–control studies.)

Where medical records permit accurate assessment of both risk factors and disease outcomes, only possible when data are collected systematically (and preferably computerized), cohort studies may be possible without any prospective work. The label retrospective cohort study is then applied. Essentially, the cohort is identified from past records of exposure status and this is the vital step. Usually, the outcome data are also obtained from records but this information can be supplemented with direct questioning of those subjects who are alive, and can be traced. Once identified the subjects can be followed up over time (prospectively) so using both currently available and future data on outcome. Figures 9.9 and 9.10 illustrate the concept in the context of populations and the natural history of disease. The conceptual difference between this design and the prospective cohort is minimal; a retrospective cohort is assembled from historical records on exposure status, the prospective cohort on exposure status in the present. You should seek out the

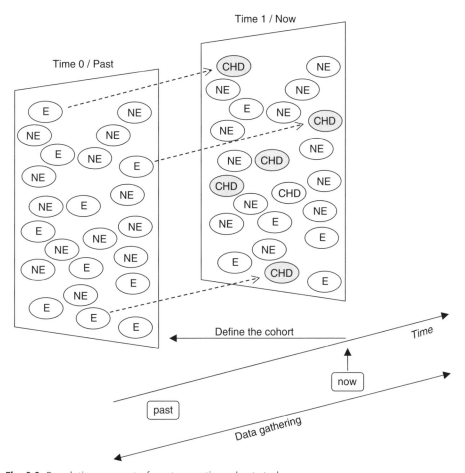

Fig. 9.9 Population concept of a retrospective cohort study.

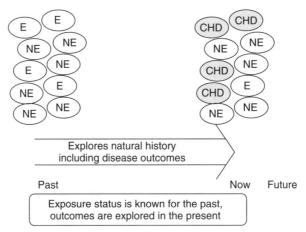

Fig. 9.10 Natural history of disease and retrospective cohort studies.

differences between figures 9.7 and 9.9. The practical work for these studies is, however, very different. Before reading on reflect on the question in Box 9.8.

The essential feature that makes the study in Table 9.3 a cross-sectional study and not a retrospective cohort is the construction of the sampling frame using a contemporary list of people living in the area of interest. The information on health is retrospective from the point at which the sampling frame was prepared in the 1990s. If the investigators had constructed a list of people living in the same areas (zones A, B and C) in, say, 1940, and looked at consultation patterns prospectively from that point, say 1941–1946, this would have been a retrospective cohort study.

Cohort studies are often described as analytic (Table 9.2) but one of their main functions is to provide information on the incidence and the natural history of disease (to describe) and not just to explore or generate hypotheses, for which they are of course extremely useful. If the cohort study is based on a defined and characterized population the incidence rates can often be extrapolated beyond the study group to similar populations elsewhere.

The most important information from a cohort study is on incidence rates. The ratio of the incidence rates in the exposed and non-exposed groups derived from the cohort

Box 9.8 Comparing a retrospective cohort with the study in Table 9.3

What is the essential feature that differentiates the cross-sectional study in Table 9.3 from a cohort study?

study is the relative risk, the primary basis for measuring the strength of an association, one of the keys to causal thinking in epidemiology. The calculation and interpretation of incidence rates was discussed in Chapter 7 and the relative risk was discussed in Chapter 8. Other matters relating to analysis are in section 9.11.

9.7 Trials—population-based experiments

9.7.1 Overview

Tables 9.1 and 9.2 provide a brief summary and description based on dichotomous classifications. As you read on you may wish to reflect on the questions in Box 9.9. Do not, however, look at the answers in Table 9.5 until later. Trials are studies where an intervention designed to improve health has been applied to a population, and the outcome assessed at follow-up. Such studies may help us to understand disease causes, assess the effectiveness of interventions to influence the natural history of disease, and weigh up the costs and benefits of interventions. Trials are experiments, and may be described by various terms including intervention studies, clinical trials, and community trials. The term 'trial' is usually reserved for experiments that are not done in the laboratory setting, and are on human or whole animal studies. The trial has, essentially, the same design as a cohort study with one vital difference, that the exposure status of the study population has been deliberately changed by the investigator to see how this alters the incidence of disease or other features of the natural history (Figs 9.11 and 9.12). This has huge implications for the ethics of research, both in terms of consent, and for ensuring safety of participants.

Clinical and public health trials are difficult and important endeavours, which usually have a practical question to answer: whether a particular intervention is sufficiently effective to be introduced into clinical or public health practice. Such trials need to be based on a study population with proper understanding of how it relates to the (target) population which will be offered the intervention should it be shown to be successful. An intervention which works in a selected population may not fulfil its goals when put into public health or clinical practice in the general population. Some trials are, however, designed solely to produce knowledge about cause and effect, the intention being to test the efficacy of the

Box 9.9 Strengths and weaknesses of the study designs

Based on the principles of study design and your knowledge of the purposes of epidemiology, consider the relative strengths and weaknesses of clinical and population case series, cross-sectional, case–control and cohort studies, and trials. Put these in a table. You may find the following key words and phrases helpful in your reflection: ease, timing, maintenance and continuity, costs, ethics, data utilization, main contributions, observer and selection bias, analytic outputs.

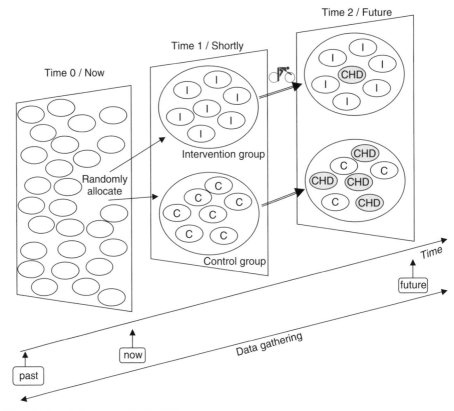

Fig. 9.11 Population concept of a trial.

intervention in actual practice at a later date. For these trials, sometimes called proof of concept trials, with their limited purpose, understanding the relationship of the study population to the target population is not so essential (but still advised). In preventive trials the intervention may be either an active intervention, say enrolment into a diet and exercise programme, or the manipulation of a natural way of life such as reducing the consumption of salt. Preventive trials are more difficult to do than trials of treatment based on drugs, for they implement complex interventions in complex circumstances.

9.7.2 Design

The first step is to define a study population suitable for answering the question, i.e. people either with disease (for clinical trials) or without (for prevention trials). Ideally, this study population will be drawn from the target population as shown in the ovals in the first box in Fig. 9.11, which is a trial of exercise in the prevention of CHD. We then divide the study population into two or more groups, the intervention group(s) and the control group(s). In the figure the intervention, symbolized by a cyclist, is an exercise programme.

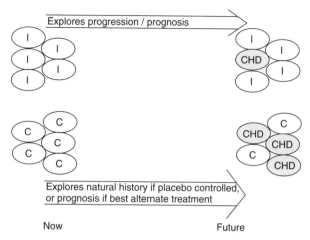

Fig. 9.12 Natural history of disease and trials.

The control group may be offered the best known alternative (e.g. meditation classes) or a placebo activity with no major expected effect on the outcome (e.g. participation in a pottery class). Trials should only be done to resolve reasonable uncertainty. There may be circumstances where the uncertainty is about the amount of an intervention that will be effective. In those circumstances different doses may be used. In the ongoing prevention of diabetes and obesity in South Asians trial (PODOSA), led by myself, the investigators agreed that the control group would be given information in a 4-visit programme that would be compared to a 15-visit intensive, interactive programme of dietary and exercise advice. This was deemed ethical and less than this unacceptable. The important thing is that, excepting the intervention, the two groups gain an equal amount of attention in the study. Otherwise, the changes seen might be attributable to differences in the amount of attention each group receives, not the intervention itself. The intervention group provides information on prognosis, the control group on the natural history (although this may be affected by the placebo or intervention offered to this group).

In the ideal trial, the study and control populations are at the same stage of the natural history of disease (Fig. 9.12), and are similar in the characteristics that affect disease outcomes, differing only in exposure to the intervention. To maximize the chances that the intervention and control groups are the same at baseline, and hence avoid confounding, the trial design should ensure that individuals in the study are assigned randomly to the groups. This process solves the problem of finding the right control group. This is the closest we get to the counterfactual comparison in epidemiology. This is a randomized, controlled trial.

Where there is no 'best known alternative', an intervention which is 'psychologically' of similar impact to the study intervention, but has no influence on the diseases process is used (a placebo, from the Latin word to please). This is a placebo-controlled randomized trial.

To prevent bias, the subject, the field investigator, and the subjects' health carer might not be told whether the subject receives the 'active' intervention or the control intervention (they are so-called 'blind'). This is a triple-blind, randomized, placebo-controlled trial (if either the subject or the health carer do not know, this is 'double-blind'). Blinding is very difficult for many complex interventions.

We now follow up the study populations and count the events of interest; in the above example, the number of cases of coronary heart disease. Analysis is by comparing incidence rates of outcome (Chapters 7 and 8), calculating relative risks (8.4) and numbers need to treat or prevent (8.11), the QALY (8.10), and other outcome measures that are beyond the scope of this book. Other matters related to analysis are in section 9.11.

9.8 Overlap in the conceptual basis of the case series, cross-sectional, case–control, cohort, and trial designs and their strengths and weaknesses

The cross-sectional study can be repeated using the same sampling methods to evaluate changes in time. The participants in the second study will be different from those studied in the first, although there may be, by the laws of chance, some overlap. This is simply a repeat cross-sectional study (and not a cohort as sometimes implied). If, however, the same sample is studied for a second time (i.e. it is followed up), the original cross-sectional study now becomes a cohort study. The cohort study can also be turned into a trial. The key difference between a cohort design and a trial is that the investigator observes the study subjects in the former but imposes an intervention in the latter. If, during a cohort study, possibly in a subgroup, the investigator imposes an intervention, a trial begins. Unfortunately, it is no longer a cohort study (unless the intervention is on a small fraction of the participants). The cohort study also gives birth to case–control studies.

When people with a particular disease are compared with a comparison group, the study is a case–control study. Ideally, the case–control study should be of new, or incident, cases. Cases that are newly discovered in a cohort study are ideal. Failing that, cases could be from a cross-sectional study (though these are mostly going to be prevalent ones) or from a case series.

Cases in a case series, particularly a population-based one, may be the starting point of a case–control study or a trial. Case series registers may also provide the data on outcomes for a cohort study or trial. A cross-sectional study of people in a case series is also possible, where people on the list are surveyed at a point in time.

These similarities and interrelations, overlooked in classifications which emphasize the distinctions in study design, integrate a series of study designs. The important thing is to understand the principles behind, and the defining features of, a particular study design.

Not every epidemiological study fits neatly into one of the basic five designs in Box 9.1. However, such atypical studies are usually variants and amalgams of the basic designs, which can be grasped with an understanding of the key features and purposes of the five designs discussed. Table 9.4 develops this point by listing a range of epidemiological studies with their general aims and then indicating the usual design options.

Table 9.4 Types, aim, and design of some epidemiological studies

Type of study	Main aims	Possible design(s)
Disease counts and description including incidence rates	Establish size of case-load; define characteristics of disease; generate hypotheses based on factors in common (similarity of cases); test hypotheses by seeing whether predicted associations occur	Case series, preferably part of a clinical or population register
Incidence rates of disease or death, in relation to risk factors	(a) Establish disease rates; assess variation over time, place, and characteristics of cases; generate or test hypotheses (b) As above plus study natural history of disease; seek associations between risk factors and disease	(a) Population case series with cases related to population usually defined by a census or other register (b) Cohort studies with populations defined by exposure
International comparisons	Explore similarities and differences in disease rates, establish the relative importance of environmental and genetic factors in disease, generate or test hypotheses	(a) Population case series, related to population census or other register (b) Multicentre cross-sectional study (c) Multicentre cohort study
Prevalence of disease or risk factors	Quantify disease and risk factor burden; seek associations between disease and risk factors; generate or test hypotheses	(a) Cross-sectional study (b) Disease or at-risk registers related to a population census or population register
Comparison of people with disease with a control group	Generate or test hypotheses by comparing similarities and dissimilarities between cases and controls	Case–control
Twin studies	Compare similarities and dissimilarities between people of similar genetic environment to give insight on the relative contribution of genetic and environmental factors in disease	Registers of monozygotic and dizygotic twins studied by cohort design (often retrospective cohort)
Migrant studies	Follow effect of environmental change, to assess relative importance of genetic and environmental factors. Measure burden of disease in immigrant populations	Analysis of population case series by country of birth or other indicator (ethnic group, race, nationality etc), and cross-sectional or cohort studies of migrants in their adopted homeland, sometimes compared with non-migrants in the land of origin
Evaluations	To assess effectiveness of interventions in decreasing disease, improving health or reducing risk factors	(a) Trial (b) Repeat cross-sectional study (c) Observations of change over time in population case series data (d) Case–control studies

Table 9.5 Some of the strengths and weaknesses of each study design

Theme	Clinical case series	Population case series	Cross-sectional	Case–control	Cohort	Trial
1 Ease	Easy to compile by clinicians or through clinicians	Difficult, as needs large number of data contributors and complex systems to ensure quality, comparable data	Difficulty depends on the study. Studies of natural living populations are hard compared with those at schools or other institutions	Usually difficult because of need for appropriate control group and problem of recall bias	Difficult because of added complexity of follow-up	Difficulty exceeds the cohort because of technical and ethical challenges of imposing an intervention
2 Timing	May be available very quickly especially if health administration systems record diagnosis	Needs much planning time. Merging of data from clinical or administrative databases, if possible, can speed up the process greatly	Usually finished within months or a few years	Usually finished within months or a few years except those on incident cases of rare diseases	Usually long-term (decades) though sometimes (e.g. studies of birth outcomes) they can be quick	Usually deliberately designed to give an answer within a few years or a decade, i.e. usually shorter than cohort studies
3 Maintenance and continuity	Possible as along as clinical commitment remains	Demands continuing effort on part of clinicians and administrators	Study is usually stopped	Study is usually stopped	Long-term continuity is essential and problematic, particularly as observations are usually on free-living people	Similar to cohort studies but when trials are in patients with diseases, the commitment to the trial may be high
4 Costs	Costs are low in compiling the series because data are at hand	Costs are high but usually hidden in the administration of the health service	Costs depend on study but lower than cohort or trial of same size	Costs are usually comparable with cross-sectional studies and, as study size is small, the overall costs may be low	Costs are high both because numbers studied are large and because costs of retaining staff and systems to collect data over many years are high	Costs are high for the same reason as the cohort study and there are additional costs of the intervention, obtaining approvals, and trial management
5 Ethics	Ethical issues such as confidentiality are not usually difficult if the investigator is the clinician	Data collection and storage systems must meet ever-stricter legal and ethical standards on consent and confidentiality	Standard ethical issues, and problem of obtaining access to a sampling frame	Standard ethical issues as in clinical case series but also those of cross-sectional studies for community controls	Confidentiality issues are acute, particularly as adverse outcomes may affect occupation and insurance premiums. Potential intrusion of repeated contact and measurement	The ethics of trials are complex and evolving, and hinge on the issues of doing no harm and informed consent

6 Data utilization	Data are likely to be used for clinical and research purposes	Data are usually under-utilized, but relevant to health care planning	Usually under-utilized, as more information is collected than needed	As analysis is straight forward, data are usually fully analysed	Data tend to be underutilized	Data concerning the central question are utilized
7 Main contribution	Contributes to clinical knowledge, health needs assessment, disease burden and may spark causal hypotheses	Contributes to understanding burden of disease, and sparking and testing causal hypotheses	Major contribution to burden of disease, substantial contribution to analysis of associations and may confirm or spark hypotheses	Major contribution to clinical knowledge, and sparking/testing causal hypotheses. Control group may supply burden of need data	Major contribution to both burden of disease (incidence) and causal analysis	Main contribution is to understanding of effectiveness of interventions, and indirectly to disease mechanisms
8 Observer bias	May be compiled by single or few observers, minimizing observer bias	Multiplicity of contributors, so vast problem of observer bias	Small studies may be done by one observer, but for most studies inter-observer bias is a problem	Small studies may be done by one observer; large studies usually need a few people so bias may be present	Usually requires multiple observers, though exceptionally, studies may be small	Usually requires multiple observers
9 Selection bias	Major problem	Minor problem as unselected cases but sometimes the diagnosis is inadequately confirmed	Selection bias arising from non-response is almost inevitable	Studies of prevalent cases have selection bias, those of incident cases minimize this although control group may have low response rates. All studies have recall bias	Selection bias due to non-response at baseline is augmented by loss to follow-up	Selection biases are particularly severe because non-participation may be high and because intervention may only be suitable for some of the target population
10 Analytic output	Case numbers, percentages, proportional morbidity/mortality ratio	Main output is disease rates, in association with census or population register data	Main output is prevalence though other measures including the odds ratio are possible (not usually the relative risk)	Proportions exposed and odds ratios	Incidence rate and the relative incidence, i.e. relative risk, and attributable risks	Incidence, survival and numbers needed to treat or prevent

Investigators usually have a choice. In general, the simpler, cheaper approaches are adopted first. Experience indicates that the order of difficulty and expense of these studies is: case series, cross-sectional, case–control, cohort, and trial. As we move along this sequence there are additional nuances; for example, the ethical and recruitment problems raised by trials add complexity to the challenge of follow-up, which is otherwise shared with cohort studies. The case–control adds the complexity of a control group to the one of establishing an unbiased case series. The cross-sectional study adds the complexity of recruitment, consent, and a community base in comparison to a case series.

Sometimes understanding the true picture requires several perspectives and, in particular cross-sectional and cohort analyses. Table 9.6 shows a classic and early example of the so-called birth cohort effect and is adapted from that of Frost. It is typical to examine age group effects, most commonly at a point in time (cross-sectional), and also standard to compare across time periods, usually using an age standardised summary (see Chapter 8) or less commonly age-specific rates. Before reading on do the exercise in Box 9.10.

In 1880 the death rate was very high in the age group 0–4, low in 5–19, and high in the others. In 1930 it was much lower in the youngest age groups than in those over 20. In every age group the rates dropped rapidly over time. For simplicity of interpretation let us assume that the data are completely accurate.

One conclusion we could reach is that the disease has changed—from one that was most common in infancy in the nineteenth century to one of older age groups by 1930. We could speculate that resistance to the infection had increased in children by 1930 as compared to 1880, and that resistance declines in older ages. This implies an age effect. If we follow those born around 1880 (0–4, 5–9) (diagonals), we see that they are the same group (cohort) that had a high rate in 1920 and 1930. In fact, all the high rate groups in 1930 come from groups (cohorts) who had very high rates in the 0–4 age group.

Box 9.10 Age trends, time trends and cohort effects in Table 9.6

- What is your assessment of the trends in tuberculosis death rates with increasing age in 1880 and 1930?
- What are the changes in these rates across time in the age groups 0–4, 30–39 and 60–69? These age groups are underlined in Table 9.6.
- What conclusion do you reach—e.g. is tuberculosis more common in the older age groups in 1930? Is this because of ageing itself?
- What alternative explanation(s) is/are there for the rising rates by age group in 1930 other than an age effect? (The column is underlined.)
- What impression is created by observing the death rates in those born in 1880 as the population grows older? This is illustrated by the diagonal line.

An alternative interpretation for the age effects in 1930 is provided by this kind of birth cohort analysis. The high rates in the older age groups in 1930 might not be a result of ageing itself, but of the high exposure to the tubercle bacillus in infancy several decades back. This is known as the generation or birth cohort effect. The age patterns at a point in time (say 1930) may reflect exposures to the causes in earlier life that are changing over time, and not necessarily the effects of ageing itself.

If there are time trends in exposure to causal agents—and there usually are—this explanation for differences by age group at a point in time needs to be at the forefront. While this is easy to remember for infections it is too readily forgotten for chronic, non-infectious diseases.

Before reading on complete the exercise in Box 9.9.

Some of the strengths and weaknesses of each study design are given in Table 9.5 (page 316). This is not a complete list. Full discussion of each point is beyond the scope of this book, and will be found in books concentrating on methods. The important point is that, contrary to a widely expressed view, each study has strengths and weaknesses and no one study design is superior. The 'hierarchy of evidence' whereby the trial is said to produce definitive evidence, and other designs weaker evidence, is a narrow idea that only applies to evaluation, particularly of drugs. Other designs are stronger for measuring the burden of disease and in generating causal ideas.

As the history of epidemiology has demonstrated repeatedly, causal understanding comes from all types of study, and above all through deep reflection on disease patterns, however generated (see Chapter 5, e.g. Table 5.9). Many of the landmark studies that have revolutionized medicine and public health would be discarded by those who apply too narrowly and unthinkingly the routines of 'evidence-based medicine'.

Table 9.6 Analysing by time, age and birth cohort, age-specific death rates per 100 000 per year from tuberculosis (all forms) among males, Massachusetts, 1880–1930

Age	Year					
	1880	1890	1900	1910	1920	1930
0–4	760	578	309	209	108	41
5–9	43	49	31	21	24	11
10–19	126	115	90	63	49	21
20–29	444	361	288	207	149	81
30–39	378	368	296	253	164	115
40–49	364	336	253	253	175	118
50–59	366	325	267	252	171	127
60–69	475	346	304	246	172	95
70+	672	396	343	163	127	95

Table adapted by me from that published by Frost. The age selection of mortality from tuberculosis in successive decades. *American Journal of Hygiene* 1939, 30, 91–96.

Understanding the concepts behind each study, however, is essential in choosing, interpreting, and evaluating reports of studies in the context of the research questions being addressed.

We now turn to so-called ecological studies, before looking at study size and analysis

9.9 Ecological studies: mode of analysis?

9.9.1 Overview

Ecology is the study of organisms in relation to their environment. As we discussed in Chapter 1 epidemiology is, in many respects, an ecological discipline and in a general sense all or most epidemiological studies are ecological. The phrase 'ecological study', however, has come to mean 'A study in which the units of analysis are populations or groups of people, rather than individuals' (Last 2001). The unit of analysis in epidemiology is always the group so all epidemiology is ecological.

Usually, though, data analysis is on aggregate measures made on individuals. Last gives as an example a study of the association between median income and cancer mortality rates in states and countries (p. 57, 4th edn). In such a study the cancer mortality rates are likely to derive from individual data from a population case series held in a database (registry) of deaths, and median income from a census or other cross-sectional studies. In this example, the investigators have chosen to analyse their data by place (rather than, say, age, sex, or social class). This choice is not an inherent design feature but a mode of analysis. This type of analysis is also sometimes called correlational, demographic, or descriptive. For example, MacMahon and Trichochopolous (1996) inform us that ecological studies are descriptive studies based on routinely collected information. In this book these studies are described as population case series or registry studies, because the label ecological is not necessary and is potentially misleading. If the label is to be used, then it should be reserved for studies where the variables measure a feature of the place and not of individuals. How, then, should we conceptualize the ecological study?

There are variables which are truly not based on individual data and that are useful in epidemiology. Such variables were discussed in Chapter 2 (Section 2.5 in particular) and in section 9.3. Sometimes such variables are merely a substitute for individualized data, which would be better but may not exist. For example, information on the duties (taxes) collected by governments on products such as alcohol and tobacco exist over long periods of time. Such data may be a partial substitute for information on consumption patterns in individuals and populations. Such data also provide additional information, for example, on government policy on the population's use of such products, the state of the economy, and the legal status of these products.

Other variables that relate to a place may have no equivalent individual level counterpart but have intrinsic importance in epidemiology (see also Chapter 2): the weather, expenditure on roads, or the type of political structure, or amount of land devoted to growing fruit and vegetables. These variables might reasonably be described as ecological, particularly those relating to the natural environment. Such variables can be studied on their own with descriptions of time trends, variation between places, and differences by the characteristics of the populations in these places. Variables can be correlated with each other, for example, the relationship between expenditure on road traffic and particulate air pollution. Assuming such a study helps to study living organisms in relation to their environment, it is an ecological study, albeit a simple one, and if it sheds light on the population pattern of disease it is also epidemiology.

There are other circumstances in which exposure data relating to a place and not to individuals (say hardness of water) are correlated with health data collected on individuals but summarized by place rather than another variable, e.g. sex. In this circumstance the boundaries are blurred. Here the study could simply be described as a population case series (or registry) study. Conceptually, the ecological component is an issue of data analysis and not study design. Cross-sectional, case–control, and cohort studies and trials (and not just population case series) could also be analysed in relation to such 'ecological' variables and such units of analysis. This thinking leads us to modify our Box 9.1 as in Table 9.7.

In Table 9.7 ecological studies are considered to be those using aggregate data on places. By this definition, the ecological design does not use aggregate information on individuals, simply because all of epidemiology does that. Studies on individuals of any design, however, can be analysed geographically using data on places. In practice, such analyses take place on population case series and large cross-sectional studies such as the census. For other studies, the numbers of people enrolled and the geographical spread is usually too small. This is reflected by placing brackets around the tick in Table 9.7. There is a worldwide movement to create large epidemiological cohort studies comprising millions of people. Those studies will be amenable to this kind of analysis. There is also a great deal of work on trials where randomization is not of individuals but places. These kinds of designs require analysis at two or more levels—known as multilevel (or mixed) modelling.

9.9.2 Some fallacies: ecological, atomistic and homogeneity

Ecological analyses are subject to the ecological fallacy (see Pearce 2000). This fallacy states that the association found with aggregate data may not apply to individuals; for

Table 9.7 Design by mode of analysis

	Aggregate data on individuals	By aggregate data on places (ecological)
Ecological	–	✓
Case series		
– clinical	✓	(✓)
– population	✓	✓
Cross-sectional	✓	(✓)
Case–control	✓	(✓)
Cohort	✓	(✓)
Trial	✓	(✓)

example, in aggregate a population with a higher risk of disease may have a higher exposure to the risk factors, but this association may not apply to individuals. Imagine a study of the rate of coronary heart disease in the capital cities of the world relating the rate to average income. Within the cities studied, coronary heart disease will be higher in the richer cities than in the poorer ones. This finding would fit the general view that coronary heart disease is a disease of affluence. We might predict from such a finding that rich people in the individual cities too have more risk of CHD than poor people. In fact, in contemporary times, in the industrialized world the opposite is the case: within cities such as London, Washington DC, and Stockholm, poor people have higher CHD rates than rich ones. The forces that cause high rates of disease at a population level are different from those at an individual level.

The ecological fallacy is usually interpreted as a major weakness of ecological analyses based on population case series. The ecological analyses, however, inform us about forces which act on whole populations which may be in conflict with those that act on individuals (see also Chapter 2). Rather than a weakness, it is a strength, for it gives us an alternative and broader perspective. Before reading on reconsider the exercise in Box 9.5.

Studies of individuals are prone to the opposite of the ecological fallacy, the so-called atomistic fallacy. Here, the fallacy is to wrongly assume from observations on the causes of disease in individuals that the same forces apply to whole populations. For example, at an individual level a high income or a marker of material success, such as employment or access to a car, is associated with a lower rate of suicide. This does not mean that populations or societies which are rich have a lower rate of suicide or better mental health. The opposite seems to be true. As in the previous example of CHD and wealth, the forces that cause or prevent disease at the individual level, for suicide factors such as family support, are different from those that work at societal level (e.g. social cohesion and expectations).

A third fallacy, which I call the fallacy of homogeneity, arises from the misinterpretation of population data from heterogeneous populations. This fallacy is most likely to arise in population case series analyses because of limitations in the detail available on the study populations. For example, studies of ethnic groups often use broad labels such as White or Asian. European origin 'White' populations in England have a lower all-cause SMR than those born in the Indian subcontinent (often called South Asians). While this is true, the highest mortality is actually within the Irish-born living in England, who are included in the White population, whose all-cause SMR is much higher than that of the South Asian population. To take a second example, the South Asian population is often described as having lower smoking prevalence than White populations. Again, while this is true, the highest recorded prevalence of smoking is actually within the South Asian population, in Bangladeshi men, as is the lowest prevalence, in Indian men and women. These examples emphasize how extrapolating from one level to another (individuals to subgroups to whole populations) is not a straightforward matter.

9.10 Size of the study

In planning a study the size of the study population is a crucial matter. Studies that are larger than they need to be are inefficient and wasteful, not only of money but also scarce epidemiological expertise, and public goodwill and time. Studies that are too small may provide misleading answers, or at least, imprecise ones.

Estimation of a desired study size is a complex issue, and one that is core to most statistics courses (and beyond this book). The principles, however, can be stated succinctly as follows:

- The sample size will be dictated by the research questions and stated study hypotheses.
- The study hypotheses need to be specified in a way that can be quantified; e.g. 'That the predicted incidence of a disease is 2% per year, and that exposure to a risk factor (say smoking) doubles the incidence'.
- The precision of the answer required needs to be stated; e.g. a study wishing to establish the incidence rate of a disease with no more than 10 per cent error, will be larger than one accepting an error of 40 per cent around the estimate.
- In studies where the hypothesis is based on a difference between groups, the size of the minimum difference that it is important to detect should be stated (alternatively, state the size of the difference expected).
- The sample size should be large enough to keep low the chances of two types of statistical error. Type 1 error is the error of rejecting a null hypothesis when it is true. In the context of most epidemiological studies a null hypothesis is one stating that there is no difference between comparison groups. In making this error one is claiming a difference when there is, in reality, none in the source (base) population, and apparent differences have occurred by chance. In most research we wish the probability of making such an error to be lower than 5 per cent.
- Type 2 error is in failing to reject a null hypothesis when it is false. In epidemiology, this usually means declaring there is no difference between comparison groups when, in the source (base) population, there is. Most studies aim to have less than 10–20 per cent probability of such an error. The power of a study is the probability that a type 2 error will not occur (so most studies aim for a power of 80 per cent or more).

With this type of information the stage is set to calculate sample size. Each study design, however, imposes its own specific requirements, and the reader will find guidance in books on statistical and epidemiological methods. Sample size calculation is not an exact discipline and requires scientific judgement. Furthermore, sample size calculations are usually based on simple outcomes and analyses where studies usually examine a range of outcomes using a range of complex multivariate methods. To specify sample size properly requires a great deal of pre-specification of data and an analysis strategy, and that may be impossible or very difficult to achieve in advance.

9.11 Data analysis and interpretation

The principles outlined in all the earlier chapters will be required to interpret data properly, particularly taking into account error, bias, and frameworks for analysis of associations (Chapters 3, 4, and 5). There is a multitude of choice in data analysis—the reader will need to consult one of many suitable textbooks—but the principles behind the basic measurements are in Chapters 7 and 8.

Box 9.11 Questions underpinning the analysis

- How do I plan the analysis?
- What is my primary focus (foci) for the analysis?
- How can I show that my data set is error free?
- How can I show my data set contains valid data?
- How can I show the potential for generalization?
- How can I demonstrate the burden of disease and the risk factors so others can use the data?
- How can I demonstrate the comparability (or otherwise) of my subpopulations that I wish to compare and contrast?
- How can I summarize these contrasts?
- How can I check whether interaction is present?
- How can I show these contrasts are not a result of error, bias or confounding?
- How can I assess the likelihood of causality?
- How do I write the findings up so they are both clear and sound?

The following simple account, nonetheless, provides a logical approach that will underpin the analysis plan, which should always be prepared in advance of beginning the analysis. Before reading on try the exercise in Box 9.11. You may wish to tackle one or a few of the questions at a time—some answers are given in sequential paragraphs.

9.11.1 Planning the analysis

Planning the analysis in advance requires, above all else, resolve to do it, steely discipline, and a great deal of foresight. Foresight comes with experience and from knowledge, particularly on the nature of the desired end point, whether in the style of a thesis, report or scientific article. While the details of the presentation differ by end product, the principles are identical. Sometimes, the analysis plan will be mandatory, and this is most likely in large scale trials where the end points are preset. Then the analysis plan will be summarized in the research proposal, expanded in the protocol, and then set out in detail prior to data analysis. This does not, of course, prevent further analysis, but this later analysis will be considered as secondary, and, therefore, not definitive. The objectives are:

1 to minimize bias
2 to minimize type 1 errors
3 to retain focus
4 to test prior hypotheses.

This same approach is rare for other kinds of studies, partly because there is more scope and need for creativity in the analysis, and partly because there is seldom an external requirement for pre-specification. Prior written specification of the analysis strategy is, nonetheless, highly recommended for the reasons above.

One effective tool for aiding this step is the creation of 'dummy' tables, or analysis of a simulation (fake) data set, or a combination of these. In dummy tables the writer thinks out the sequence of the analysis and prepares a table legend and data layout for each required table, specifying the outcome variables in relation to exposure variables (cross tabulations). The statistical tests can be stated and columns/rows to accommodate the results of the tests can be inserted. Table 8.14 is a simple example of a dummy table, but the reader can easily imagine other tables without data, e.g. Table 8.12 or Table 3.7. The approach can be extended to graphs and any other form of data output. Usually, at this stage, it is better to envisage the tabular output. Dummy tables are very hard to prepare but this approach is much preferred to diving into the analysis and hoping to turn up something interesting. The usual result of that approach, particularly for the novice, is a sense of drowning in data. This applies to primary research and systematic reviews alike. Secondary data analysers may be accused of data dredging. How are we to make the choices of which dummy tables to produce?

9.11.2 Focus

This requires you to focus on the research questions and/or aims and/or specific objectives of the work. These are the guide posts, while the proposal or protocol (including the literature review) provides the map. In doctoral and postgraduate research we aim to fill the gaps in the map, or extend it, or less commonly, in cases of doubt, to confirm the map is correct. So, there is an onus for creativity and novelty. For health service work and undergraduate/masters level work it is often enough to follow the paths set out in previous publications.

Now that you have a clear sense of the analysis plan (presumably agreed with Trial Steering Committees, Collaborators or Supervisors as appropriate) you proceed to analysis. Mostly analysis is done by computer (except for very small data sets) so let us assume this. You will need to abide by data protection principles and laws and ethical committee (review board) rulings. In so far as possible you should anonymise your data set and trim it so only those data required at this stage are in the analysis file. You may need to enter ('punch') your data onto an appropriate database. Of course, if you are analysing someone else's data, you will avoid this step. The best, though expensive, approach to data entry from paper is double entry (independently done). This minimizes the inevitable human errors that arise at entry. If the data were entered directly (i.e. not recorded on paper) such errors will probably be impossible to find.

9.11.3 Errors

The investigator's first task is to check the dataset for resolvable errors. Sometimes these will be obvious, e.g. a male is said to have a diagnostic code for cervical cancer (either the sex code or diagnostic code is wrong), or a person is said to be 174 years of age (probably the correct age is 17 years or 74 years). Sometimes errors will not be obvious, e.g. the code key for male is said to be 1, when it is 2. It is even more important for investigators to check secondary data sets, because their unfamiliarity with them will make errors hard to detect during the analysis. This checking stage is often referred to as cleaning the data. Given the structure of the data set is sound we can turn to its content.

9.11.4 Validity

Readers are probably familiar with the self-explanatory phrase 'garbage in, garbage out'. Unfortunately, garbage data are not easy to distinguish from quality data, particularly when summarized. Epidemiologists who have collected their own data have a sense of its quality, but this is not true for data they have borrowed for analysis. In Chapter 7 we considered issues around data quality, e.g. the numerator, and in Chapter 6, we covered sensitivity and specificity as indicators of validity of the screening test compared to a gold standard. The principles and methods outlined there apply here.

There is no short-cut for the investigator—information is essential on the timeliness, completeness, accuracy, or validity (i.e. the truth) and precision of measurements. For secondary data sets we need to get this information from those who collected the data. To take an example, the database says that a female of 49 years has an income between £30–40 000 per year and has diabetes. We want to know, for example, whether sex is self-reported or observed, age is self-reported or from medical records, whether income is self-reported or from an employer (or agency) database, and whether diabetes is self-reported, from medical records, or based on blood tests (if so which ones). For each of these we want to know the validity of the data. Self-report of sex and age is likely to be accurate, but self-report of income and diabetes will not be. The amount of inaccuracy needs to be estimated. To reiterate, it must not be assumed, as is often the case, that data obtained from external agencies, whether governmental or not, are accurate. It is especially important for investigators to rigorously assess the value of such data. The investigator retains the responsibility for the outcome of these secondary analyses.

9.11.5 Handling continuous data using correlation and regression: contributions to causal thinking

So far, we have concentrated on categorical data, but continuous data are important to analysis of associations, and methods of analysing such data make a large contribution to epidemiology.

Correlation is another word for association (or a link). Correlation, of course, as with association is not necessarily causation. In statistics correlation refers to a particular form of analysis of linear relationships between quantitative variables, mostly used for continuous measures. The relationship can be shown in a graph, of the type known as a scattergram (or scatter diagram) as in Figure 9.13. Here, for each person, the value for variable 1 (say height) and variable 2 (say weight) is represented by one dot. It is evident in Figure X that there is an association (Figure Y). The relationship can be calculated and summarized by a number known as a correlation coefficient (called r). The relationship can also be described by

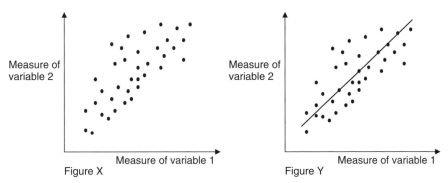

Fig. 9.13 Correlation, regression, and the scatterplot.

drawing the line that best fits the picture seen between the two variables. (The line here is drawn by eye but there are mathematical methods for doing this (least squares). If there was no association the dots would be scattered randomly but they are not. The correlation coefficient varies between 0 (no association, when the dots are random) and –1 or 1 (perfect association, when the dots form a straight line).

We do not use this measure of association as an indicator of the strength of the association in epidemiology. The reason is that we are not primarily interested in whether two variables are associated, but by the amount of increase associated with a change in one of the two. (The relative risk is the classical example of this.)

The closely aligned methods of regression analysis, however, meet this epidemiological need. The question being answered here is: by how much is a change in variable 1 associated with a change in variable 2? The scatterplot is created as above. The regression line is calculated, using the same method as for correlation (so-called least squares method), as is the summary output known as the regression coefficient (r). The regression coefficient is the statistical estimate of how much a unit of change in variable 1 is associated with variable 2. This is analogous to dose–response based on relative risks. The techniques of regression can cope with both continuous and categorical data, and permit the incorporation of numerous cofactors. The interactive and confounding effects of these cofactors can be explored. Regression methods currently dominate analysis of epidemiological data where the objective is to explore associations. Although the terminology used may imply causal inference (predict, explain, independent effects and similar terms) this is misleading. They only produce estimates of the strength of the association and extent of variation in the data explained statistically. These estimates need to be considered in the frameworks of causal reasoning in exactly the same way as any other summary measures of association, e.g. the odds ratio or relative risk. Regression techniques can be applied to categorical and quantitative variables, whether of exposure or outcome.

We are now ready to choose an appropriate statistical analysis computer package. The choices of computer packages are many and the reader will need to consult statistical and computing colleagues and other books. The important thing is that the package meets the need. There is no merit in working with a complex package like SAS® or Stata® if Microsoft Excel® will do.

9.11.6 Generalization

Virtually all epidemiological studies are designed to be generalized beyond the study population to the source population, and perhaps even beyond that. It may well be that colleagues in Osaka, Japan will be hoping to generalize from work done in Buenos Aires, Argentina, or vice versa.

Without doubt, future researchers in the same place will want to compare their results with yours. Having already stated the methods, date of fieldwork (often missing in publications) etc., you should now describe your study populations, compared with that in the source population as in the sampling frame, and if possible the target population, as in the census of that city, state or nation, as appropriate. The description should include demographic (e.g. sex, age, ethnic group), socio-economic (e.g. income, class structure etc.), behaviour (e.g. smoking etc.), and health status (e.g. BP, height, weight). This type of descriptive overview table is usually large. The investigator and reader can immediately see the kind of population recruited, and the potential selection biases that have arisen in the process. The Osakan reader can assess whether the Buenos Aires study population is similar enough to produce information of value to Osaka.

9.11.7 Burden

This kind of overview table above may well be of prime importance to assess the burden of disease or risk factors. If this is an important aim then proceed with analysis of the key variables as in Table 8.14. The analysis may be done by sex, age group, social class group, ethnic group etc. For burden of risk factors the key outputs will be absolute measures, e.g. prevalence and for disease, either incidence or prevalence. For data sets containing time of onset, diurnal, weekly, seasonal, annual and secular trends may be described. Statistical methods will help assess whether time differences are statistically significant, and to assess the precision of estimates. Where geographical variations are of interest, the data may be analysed by point pattern analysis, or by small area, region, nation or even continent. Again, spatial statistics will help evaluate the statistical significance and precision of variations. This type of analysis is of time, place and person—the epidemiological triad (Box 2.1 and Table 2.1). The prime outputs will be absolute measures (Table 7.1) including directly standardized rates. This step is vital and should not be omitted. Investigators are gaining an understanding of their population and their data, and generating new ideas that can be incorporated into the analysis strategy—potentially as secondary analysis. While the relationship between risk factors and outcomes may be analysed at this stage for the whole population, this is unlikely to be very interesting. The principles, however, will be same as in comparing subgroups, as we discuss below.

9.11.8 Comparability

Mostly, epidemiological studies are designed to compare subpopulations, and to test one or more hypotheses about difference(s). The first step is to set out your 'overview' table but for the comparison populations side-by-side. For simplicity we assume there are only two comparison populations, but there could be several—perhaps hundreds, as in international studies.

Our comparison overview table needs to include every variable that we believe is relevant to the question at hand and—here is the challenge—to make explicit those variables that we believe are relevant but we have no data on. To take an example, there is a great deal of interest in lifestyle factors such as exercise, diet, alcohol and illicit drug-taking on health. Imagine we are interested in fruit consumption and the occurrence of cancers. The comparison may be between high and low consumers of fruit. Why is an overview table by fruit-consuming category critical?

The key question is this: are there differences, other than fruit consumption, in other factors that play a role in explaining the pathway between fruit consumption and cancer? If not, which is improbable, proceed to analysis (see below). If so, as is likely, reflect on whether there may be, among the differences, some confounding or interacting factors. We may find that low fruit consumers are more likely to be male, to be older, to be smokers and to drink more alcohol. We may also find high fruit users also eat more vegetables, grains, fish and white meat. Disentangling the effects of such factors is going to be a challenge—the challenge being to isolate the independent effects. At this stage the investigators may find so many differences, and discover that many data items of relevance (e.g. exercise habits, ethnic group) have not been collected, that a sound causal analysis is not feasible, at least with the study design at hand. (It is a wonder, however, that this course of action is seldom taken, to the detriment of the science of epidemiology, through the genesis of spurious associations.) At this stage of the analysis we are still using, mainly, absolute (actual) measures.

The overview data set can be adjusted by age and sex standardization, or age/sex stratification can be used, to see if the potential confounders are now reasonable in number. If we still find numerous confounding factors (there may be 5, 10 or even more) it is possibly futile to continue the analysis as it is not going to be sound because of measurement errors and residual confounding. These numerous differences are a major and important finding and need to be published, not least to inform others of the research challenges of pursuing this line of enquiry. It is poor epidemiology—as seen in the recent past in relation to the associations between cardiovascular diseases and hormone replacement therapy, antioxidant vitamins, and alcohol use—to fail to do this analysis rigorously prior to presenting data on the strength of the association.

9.11.9 Summarizing the contrasts

Let us assume that the data set's errors are known; the extent of biases and mis-measurement errors in risk factors, outcomes and confounders are estimated; and the number of confounders is relatively small and amenable to control. We now proceed to contrast the risks in high and low fruit eaters using relative measures, preferably the relative risk (or prevalence rate ratio in cross-sectional studies and odds ratio in case–control studies).

If there are no confounding factors of note, there is no need for multivariate methods. The ratio of incidence rates (age and sex standardized if necessary) provides the relative risk, and the confidence intervals around the difference between them can be calculated to estimate the precision (and indirectly the statistical significance) of the estimate. This absence of confounding factors is unlikely except for trials.

The data are then best analysed using one or more of the many multivariate methods (e.g. multiple regression, logistic regression, Cox regression etc. depending on the kind of data). These can be used to check for interactions.

9.11.10 Interactions

Interactions were discussed in section 4.2.5. An interaction will be detected by testing whether the relative risk in one group (say high fruit-eating men), differs significantly from that in another group (say high fruit-eating women). If so, the effect of fruit on cancer is interacting with the variable, sex. If there is interaction, the groups should not be combined but analysed separately.

9.11.11 Accounting for error, bias and confounding

Multivariate methods will calculate a relative risk with (and without) adjustment for confounding factors, both individually for each risk factor and collectively, for a group of risk factors. When exposures are graded relative risks can be calculated at varying levels (doses) of the risk to give the 'dose–response' relationship. The interpretation of such analyses is problematic particularly when the data are of poor quality.

The relative risk can be corrected for measurement errors (regression dilution bias, for example see section 4.2.7).

9.11.12 Causality

The investigator is now able to apply the frameworks for assessing the association between fruit-eating and cancer. If the association is real, and not artefact, and chance is considered an unlikely player, then the causal frameworks can be applied. The analysis above only contributes to strength of the association (and dose–response), and possibly specificity. The methods may clarify temporality. A systematic review will help assess consistency, while a general review will guide us on biological plausibility. We will look for experimental confirmation from trials (if any), natural experiments and genetic studies based on Mendalian randomization.

9.11.13 Write-up

After this costly and hard work, the failure to write up and present the findings for dissemination at conferences and, more importantly, in journal articles would border on the unethical. The omission will cause publication bias (4.2.8). The partial exception is work done primarily for the education of the investigator, e.g. theses. (Doctoral theses are, however, logged on an electronic database.)

The writing up of the work is beyond this book but in the appendix to this chapter there are some hints on keeping the supervisor happy that I give my students. Your work will be assessed by peer reviewers who are experienced in critical appraisal, so write with the questions in section 10.13 in mind. Alert readers will want these questions answered.

Every study design presents choices, but the principal outputs for each study design are given in Table 9.5 (row 10 analytic output). For calculating measures of association the 2×2 table (Chapter 8, Table 8.6) provides the standard way to present data. Table 5.9 shows how different study designs contribute towards judgements of cause and effect. Chapter 10 introduces the art of critical appraisal—a skill vital to data interpretation.

9.12 Conclusion

Study design is best thought of as a system of interlinked and mutually supporting methods. The various designs have similar purposes, are rooted in population concepts of health and disease, and are conceptually overlapping. They are also subject to similar errors, biases, and problems of sampling, and similar challenges in data collection, analysis, and interpretation. In practice epidemiologists may use a mix of designs to solve a problem, and it may also be difficult to name the design of the study. Most studies can be distinguished by their focus on either disease or exposure, the relationship of the observation to calendar time and the natural history of disease, and whether there is an imposed intervention or not.

Epidemiological designs are based on the theories discussed in earlier chapters, particularly that differential exposure to the causes of disease leads to differential population patterns of disease. Only one design—the cohort study—tests this theory directly. The trial tests it indirectly by seeing whether drugs or preventive procedures that interfere with the putative causes will prevent or control diseases, thus leading to more favourable outcomes. Trials that deliberately exposed people to the causes of disease would be unethical. This is done on animals where there are animal models of human diseases. Overall, human trials help evaluate hypotheses on disease causation rather than generate them. The other designs (case series, case–control, and cross-sectional) test the theory indirectly and retrospectively. Studies of various designs, or more strictly, the data from such studies, helps to develop and refine causal theories of disease. The process of designing studies and interpreting data, and the unanswered questions arising, drive advances in methods and techniques.

This chapter only touches on the vast experience on study design and analysis; hopefully sufficient to allow the reader to understand more advanced writings and to link earlier concepts to methods. To implement a study requires a knowledge of scientific writing, winning research grants, management of staff and resources, preparation of proforma, sampling methods, measurement and other data collection, statistics, computing, and data interpretation (and other skills, all beyond the scope of this book).

The final chapter considers the art of reading and interpreting an epidemiological study, as discussed in the context of epidemiological theory, ethics, and practice. This skill, known as critical appraisal, is essential, and is best applied on a sound foundation of understanding of epidemiological concepts.

Summary

Epidemiological studies have apparently distinct designs but are unified by their common goal to understand the frequency and causes of disease, by their strategy of seeking associations between exposures (potential causes) and outcomes (disease), by their utilization of the survey method, and by their basis in defined populations. This explains why they complement each other, for example, in assessing the weight of evidence for cause and effect, and why small changes can change the design.

The population case series and the cross-sectional survey lie at the core of the epidemiological method. A case series is a coherent set of cases of a disease (or similar problem). A population case series is a register of such cases arising in a defined population and time. Cases can be analysed as rates over time, between places, and by population characteristics to generate understanding of the burden of disease and to generate associations. If such cases are compared with a control group we have a case–control study (see below). Case–control studies are analysed by comparing the odds of exposure in cases to those in controls—the odds ratio, which sometimes provides a good estimate of the relative risk.

In a population studied at a specific time and place (a cross-section), measurements can be made of disease, the factors which may cause disease, or both simultaneously. This is a cross-sectional survey and its primary output is prevalence data, though associations between risk factors and disease can be generated and tested. Such a survey might be used to identify all cases of a particular disease in a population. If the characteristics of this group of cases are compared with a control group we have, again, a case–control study (of prevalent cases). If the population in a cross-sectional survey is followed up to measure health outcomes, this study design is now a cohort study.

Cohort studies produce data on disease incidence and on associations between risk factors and disease outcomes. Cases discovered in the course of follow-up in a cohort study may be compared with a comparison group and, once again, give rise to a case–control study.

If the population of a cohort study is divided into two groups, and the investigators impose a health intervention upon one of the groups, and follows up to measure outcomes, the design is that of a trial. Trials produce data on incidence in treated populations in comparison with those untreated. They are used, primarily, to test rather than generate hypotheses, and their prime output is information on effectiveness of health interventions.

Studies based on aggregated data, usually based on geographically defined units of population, are commonly referred to as ecological studies. They represent a mode of analysis, rather than a design. All five epidemiological designs could, in theory, be analysed using 'ecologically' aggregated data. In practice, only population case series and very large cross-sectional studies such as the census lend themselves to such a form of analysis, simply because other designs usually have insufficient numbers. This is changing with the creation of massive population-based cross-sectional and cohort studies.

In all epidemiological studies interpretation and application of data are easier when the relationship between the population observed and the target population is understood. For example, case series studies need a population to construct rates; the cross-sectional study needs a case or population register to construct a sampling frame; the case–control study should, ideally, be on a defined, representative population of incident cases with a sample of controls from the same source; the cohort study should inform about risk factor–disease outcome relations in other populations; and the results of most trials are only useful if they apply outside the study population.

The principles for the analysis of all studies are similar: prepare an analysis plan based on the study research questions; check the data set for errors, mis-measurement, bias and confounding; describe your study population's characteristics in relation to the source and target populations; describe your comparison groups with particular reference to potential confounding and interacting factors; undertake the analysis, producing summary measures appropriate to the study design that take into account the effects of confounding and interacting factors; interpret the data in the light of frameworks for discriminating real and artefactual association; apply causal reasoning to associations if appropriate to the goals of the study; and write up your results for a critical audience answering the core questions underlying the appraisal of epidemiological research.

All designs contribute, though unequally, to measuring disease burden for health policy and planning, and to testing causal hypotheses. The distinction between designs which serve one function or the other is not clear-cut. The exception to this is in the evaluation of interventions, where currently the trial reigns supreme.

Sample examination questions

Give yourself 10 minutes for every 25% of marks.

Question 1 What population selection biases may arise in a cross-sectional study assessing the population burden of a disease? (25%)
Answer Population selection biases include the following:

+ an incomplete sampling frame (list of people eligible)
+ errors in the sampling frame
+ failing to invite a sample representative of the population
+ failure of the invitation to reach the person invited
+ failure of the person invited to understand the invitation
+ non-response/non-participation
+ incomplete participation, e.g. not giving blood tests.

Question 2 In a case–control study of diabetes (of type 2) in middle age and its possible link to obesity in childhood, the following data were obtained:

Of 950 people who had diabetes, 60 had demonstrable obesity in childhood. Of 900 people who did not have diabetes, 40 had had obesity in childhood.

(i) Put these data into a 2 × 2 table with all appropriate labels and numbers (10%)

Answer (i)

Relationship between DM_2 in middle aged and obesity in childhood.

		DM_2	No DM_2	
Obesity in	+	60	40	100
childhood	–	890	860	1750
		950	900	1850

(ii) Calculate the odds ratio using the no diabetes group as the control population. (10%)

Answer (ii) $OR = \dfrac{60 \times 860}{890 \times 40} = \dfrac{51\,600}{35\,600} = 1.45$

(iii) Do such data from case–control studies demonstrate cause and effect? In your answer, refer to the framework whereby associations are considered as causal or not causal (or real/artefact). (30%)

Answer Case–control studies test a hypothesis and yield an association, usually measured by the odds ratio which is in some circumstances a good estimate of the equivalent relative risk from a cohort study. The association contributes to a cause and effect analysis but is not, in itself, demonstrative of this.

The analysis of cause and effect should exclude data and study design artefacts (errors, biases, confounding) before applying a framework for causal analysis to what seems to be a real association, e.g. that of Bradford Hill/guidelines for causality. Rarely the data from case–control studies turns out to be causal and definitive. More often it makes a small contribution.

Question 3 In a cohort study of university students examining the association between meditation or prayer and sickness absence as a health outcome, the response rate was 70%.

- 5700 women who responded reported they meditated or prayed, while 12 300 did not. The outcome, sickness absence, was obtained from a questionnaire to students one year later.
- In the meditation/prayer group, 900 students recorded having at least one day off university.
- In those who did not report meditating or praying, 1350 women were recorded as having at least one day off university in the same time period.

(i) Place these data in an appropriate two-by-two table with all appropriate labels and numbers. (10%)

Answer (i) Relationship between meditation, prayer and sickness absence

	Sickness absence		
	Yes	No	
(a) Prayed/meditated	900	4800	5700
(b) Did not pray/meditate	1350	10 950	12 300
	2250	15 750	18 000

(ii) Estimate the relative risk of sickness absence in those who do not meditate or pray i.e. group (b) in the table (use the cumulative incidence rate and baseline denominators for your calculations). (10%)

Answer (ii)

$$RR = \frac{\text{Incidence in group (b)}}{\text{Incidence in group (b)}} = \frac{1350}{12300} \div \frac{900}{5700} = \frac{10.98}{15.78} = 0.69$$

(iii) Do you think this kind of study is good for showing cause and effect? What problems make it difficult to interpret the results? (30%)

Answer (iii) The cohort study is one of the classic and powerful ways of studying cause and effect. Nonetheless, the evidence arising needs to be interpreted very cautiously using frameworks for separating causal and non-causal association. One crucial issue is of timing—did the exposure truly precede the effect? Cohort studies are usually good on this matter. Nonetheless, problems arise in errors of measurement, recruitment and retention of population, confounding, and interpretation of the associations found. Studies based on incomplete data and on self-selected populations are problematic. A 70% response rate is good for such studies.

Question 4 (a) In a cross-sectional study of asthma in two cities (say city A and city B) the investigators studied children aged 10–15 years. They asked them to self-report on whether they had asthma. The study was in a classroom setting. A sample of schools was studied. They found that in city A, of 3300 children 300 reported a diagnosis of asthma while in city B of 2700 children 400 reported asthma.

   (i)   Put these data into a 2 × 2 table. (10%)

   (ii)   Calculate the prevalence rate ratio. (10%)

   (iii)   Set out, systematically, potential explanations for the higher prevalence of asthma in city B. (Note: clinical explanations are *not* required.) (30%)

Answer (i)

Place	Asthma		Totals
	Yes	No	
City A	300	3000	3300
City B	400	2300	2700
Totals	700	5300	6000

Answer (ii)

Prevalence rate in City A = 300/3300 = 0.091 = 9.1%

Prevalence rate in City B = 400/2700 = 0.148 = 14.8%

Prevalence rate ratio:

$$\frac{\text{City A rate}}{\text{City B rate}} \quad \frac{9.1\%}{14.8\%} = 0.61$$

or

$$\frac{\text{City B rate}}{\text{City A rate}} \quad \frac{14.8\%}{9.1\%} = 1.62$$

Answer (iii) The explanations are that the results are an artefact or they are real. If artefact, then it could be chance, error in study design, or data collection methods that have led to bias or confounding. For example, we may not be comparing like with like. City B schools may have access to better health care facilities that are giving the diagnosis of asthma. Or city B children may be more articulate and therefore self-report asthma more.

   Alternatively, the difference may be real and can be analysed by the epidemiological triad of host, agent and environment. City B children may be more susceptible to the disease, more exposed to agents that cause disease, or be living in environments where asthma-causing agents thrive, e.g. modern housing where ventilation is low.

Question 5 In a randomized, double-blind controlled clinical trial of the value of dietary iron supplementation in preventing sickness absence from work in women, a university department of epidemiology compared two groups. The first consisted of 4300 women who had the supplement. The trial outcome, sickness absence, was obtained from employment records one year later. 270 people were recorded as having at least one day off work.

   The control group was 4150 women who had an inactive ingredient that looked similar to the dietary supplementation, i.e. a placebo. 350 women were recorded as having at least one day off work in the same time period.

   (i)   Place these data in an appropriate 2 × 2. (10%)

   (ii) Estimate the number of people who need to be given the supplement to prevent one or more days of sickness absence. (10%)

   (iii) Do you believe this trial shows the effectiveness of dietary iron supplementation in preventing sickness absence? Write a 100 word letter to the health authority giving 3 reasons why you think the results show a benefit, and 3 reasons why the benefit might not be real. (30%)

Answer (i)

	Sickness absence (one or more day/year)		
	Yes	**No**	**Total**
Intervention group	270	4030	4300
Control group	350	3800	4150
Total	620	7830	8450

Answer (ii)

Number needed to prevent or treat:

$$= \frac{1}{(350/4150) - (270/4300)}$$

$$= \frac{1}{0.084 - 0.063}$$

$$= \frac{1}{0.021} = 47.6$$

Answer (iii)
Dear Sir or Madam,

I urge you to note the results of the iron supplementation trial carefully. First, because the trial was both randomized and double-blind, any bias in allocation to study groups (allocation bias) and ascertainment of the outcome of interest (observation bias) is unlikely to explain the findings. Second, the use of randomization also ensured comparability of the two groups, and therefore, any confounding with respect to both known and unknown factors is unlikely. Third, the use of placebo ensured that the outcome is likely to be due to the actual trial intervention rather than to any extra attention the intervention group received or their belief in the intervention.

Notwithstanding these strengths potential errors still need to be considered. Although unlikely, benefits could have arisen by chance. Bias could have occurred if the study subjects guessed whether they were on the actual treatment or a placebo. As iron has some specific effects, e.g. constipation and dark stools, recipients may have guessed the allocation. Third, there may be errors in the employment records of sickness absence.

Yours sincerely,
A. N. Epidemiologist

Question 6 In a cohort study following up 7000 people for an average of 5 years, 3000 people took a vitamin supplement and 4000 did not. There were 57 cases of cancer in the vitamin supplement group, and 43 cases of cancer in the other group.

(i)   Put these data into a 2×2 table. (10%)

(ii) Calculate the incidence rate in each group using the person-time denominator. (For simplicity, as the disease is rare you may refrain from adjusting the denominator for those developing the outcome.) (10%)

(iii) What information do these findings offer for concluding that vitamin supplementation increases the risk of cancer? (30%)

Answer (i)

Risk factor	Disease outcome		Totals
	Cancer	No cancer	
Vitamin supplement	57	2943	3000
No vitamin supplement	43	3957	4000
Totals	100	6900	7000

Answer (ii) Incidence rate (person-years) in vitamin supplement group.

$$= \frac{57}{3000 \times 5} = \frac{57}{15000} = 0.0038 = 3.8/1000$$

In no vitamin supplement group

$$= \frac{43}{20\,000} = 0.0022 = 2.2/1000$$

Note to reader: A more exact calculation would remove from the denominator 142.5 years for the vitamin group and 107.5 years for the no vitamin group as people with the outcome contribute half of the time non-cases do.

Answer (iii) The rate of cancer is about 70 per cent higher in the vitamin supplement group. This issue will need further investigation before reaching conclusions. The steps will be to consider the role of chance, bias and confounding. Among the most important questions to answer is whether the two groups were alike, other than in relation to vitamin taking. Cancers are, for example, more common in older people and those who smoke. It may be that the two groups differ in these and other important ways. If the differences cannot be explained in these ways, then there is a case for applying the epidemiological guidelines for causal reasoning.

Question 7 In a trial of the value of double glazing in preventing sickness absence from work, a housing department compared two groups. The first consisted of 3200 houses where the windows had been replaced. The head of household's sickness absence record was recorded by self-completion questionnaire—one year later. 270 people reported at least one day off work.

The control group was 20 750 homes awaiting double glazing. 2350 people reported at least one day off work in the same time period.

(i) Place these data in an appropriate 2 × 2 table. (10%)

(ii) Calculate the number of houses needed to be double glazed to prevent one or more sickness absences. (10%)

(iii) Do you believe the results of this trial? Write a 100 word letter to the health authority giving *six* reasons why the results might be unreliable.

Answer (i)

Exposure	Sickness absence		Totals
	Off work	Not off work	
Windows replaced	270	2930	3200
Windows not replaced	2350	18 400	20 750
Totals	2620	21 330	23 950

Answer (ii)

Number needed to prevent

= Inverse of: difference in incidence in control group—incidence in study group

$$= \frac{1}{(2350 \div 20\,750) - (270 \div 3200)}$$

$$= \frac{1}{0.113 - 0.084}$$

$$= \frac{1}{0.029}$$

$$= 34.5$$

Answer (iii)

Dear Sir or Madam,

I urge you to evaluate the results of the double glazing trial with caution as the results may be unreliable. First, the trial was not randomized. The people living in the two groups of houses may have been different to start with. Second, we may be seeing a placebo effect, i.e. the benefits are non-specific. Third, there is the possibility of reporting bias, i.e. the data on the sickness absence may be inaccurate. Fourth, it may be that those completing the questionnaire are more likely to report a benefit. Fifth, this might be a chance result. Finally, we have no data on the benefits in relation to the costs.

Yours sincerely,
A. N. Epidemiologist

Question 8 In a cross-sectional study of alcohol consumption and the link with acne in male teenagers aged 16 years the following data were obtained. Of 220 people who drank alcohol at least once a week, 70 had acne. Of 270 people who drank alcohol less frequently 50 had acne.

(i) Put these data into a 2×2 table. (10%)

(ii) Calculate the prevalence rate ratio using the no-alcohol group as the standard population. (10%)

(iii) Does alcohol drinking cause acne in teenagers? What are the limitations of the above research in understanding whether alcohol causes acne? Offer 5 or more non-causal explanations for the association found. (30%)

Answer (i)

Alcohol (at least once per week)	Disease (acne)		Total
	Yes	No	
Yes	70	150	220
No	50	220	270
Total	120	370	490

Answer (ii) Prevalence among drinkers: 70/220 = 31.8%; prevalence among no-alcohol group: 50/270 = 18.5%; prevalence rate ratio (drinkers/no-drinkers) = 0.318/0.185 = 1.72.
Answer (iii) A potential causal association between high alcohol consumption and acne in teenagers cannot be inferred using the cross-sectional study design. This is because it is not possible to determine which preceded which in time, the risk factor or the outcome. In this example, it may well be the case that teenagers with acne take up more drinking as a result of their condition which may impact their self-image and self-confidence. Other non-causal explanations include: error, chance, bias, quality of self-report of the frequency and amount of alcohol consumed, and confounding resulting from not comparing like with like.

Appendix I: 20 epidemiological questions

Consider which of the questions below could be answered reasonably well with a clinical case series, population case series, cross-sectional study or a truly ecological study.

Then consider which of these questions could be answered well with a case–control study, cohort study, or an experimental trial.

Overall, make your choice for each question bearing in mind the strengths and weaknesses of each study design.

Remember, most questions can be answered with a number of study designs and there is seldom a 'correct' answer.

The exercise is designed to permit you to think about the questions and study designs.
You will find possible answers in the table below this one.

Question	Potential study designs	Preferred study design with reason
1 Is leukaemia increasing in its incidence?		
2 What factors are, potentially, causes of leukaemia?		
3 What proportion of the population is exposed to virus X?		
4 Does exposure to drugs to treat epilepsy in pregnant mothers lead to congenital malformations in their offspring?		
5 Does flying on long-distance aeroplane flights increase the risk of pulmonary embolism, i.e. blood clots in the lung?		
6 What proportion of those taking long-distance aeroplane flights develop deep venous thrombosis?		
7 What are the side-effects of oral contraceptives?		
8 Are oral contraceptives more effective for the prevention of pregnancy than other methods, e.g. the condom?		
9 What are the risk factors for fatal pedestrian accidents?		
10 Does having a maximum speed limit of 30 mph reduce fatal pedestrian accidents, as compared to 40 mph?		
11 Is heart disease mortality on the rise or on the decline?		
12 Why is the incidence of heart disease mortality changing?		
13 Would doubling the amount of exercise in the population setting reduce the incidence of heart disease?		
14 What is the relationship between the wealth of the country as measured with the GNP and the consumption of illicit drugs, e.g. heroin, and legal drugs, e.g. alcohol?		
15 What proportion of school-children are obese?		

(continued)

Question	Potential study designs	Preferred study design with reason
16 Do farm subsidies to dairy farmers lead to increased consumption of dairy products in the population?		
17 What is the cause of a rare disease of your choice, e.g., phaechromocytoma, a tumour of the adrenal gland?		
18 How many cases of AIDS, or any other similar infectious disease of your choice, should the health service be planning for 5, 10 and 20 years from now?		
19 Is the amount of fruit and vegetable consumption increasing or decreasing? What is likely to happen in 10 years from now?		
20 Would screening all adults for diabetes using blood tests improve the health of the population? Would this be cost-effective?		

20 epidemiological questions—some possible answers

Question	Potential study designs	Preferred study design with reason
1 Is leukaemia increasing in its incidence?	Population and disease registers (population case series)— particularly of cancer registrations Repeat cohort studies	Cancer registration registers (analysed either with and anomalies are from a population register or census)
2 What factors are, potentially, causes of leukaemia?	Case–control studies Cohort studies/retrospective cohort studies Animal experiments Natural 'experiments' of humans (note, if the question was on factors potentially protective from leukaemia, human trials would be possible)	Case–control studies because they give the answer efficiently and quickly These may well be nested within cohorts
3 What proportion of the population is exposed to virus X?	Cross-sectional study Population registers (of people known to be infected with virus X.), with the population denominator coming from the census or a population registration scheme	Cross-sectional study

Question	Potential study designs	Preferred study design with reason
4 Does exposure to drugs to treat epilepsy in pregnant mothers lead to congenital malformations in their offspring?	Case–control study Cohort study/retrospective cohort study Analysis of data from drug side-effect schemes Case series Trials comparing different drugs	Cohort study
5 Does flying on long-distance aeroplane flights increase the risk of pulmonary embolism, i.e. blood clots in the lung?	Case–control study Cohort studies/retrospective cohort study	Case–control study followed by cohort study
6 What proportion of those taking long-distance aeroplane flights develop deep venous thrombosis?	Cohort study/retrospective cohort study	Cohort study (probably retrospective)
7 What are the side-effects of oral contraceptives?	Cohort studies/retrospective cohort studies Studies of case series/population case series/linkage of populations to long-term outcomes Studies of reported side-effects in drug surveillance schemes	Cohort study
8 Are oral contraceptives more effective for the prevention of pregnancy than other methods, e.g. the condom?	Trials Pragmatic evaluations based on analysis of case series Cohort studies	Trial
9 What are the risk factors for fatal pedestrian accidents?	Case–control study Case series/population case series	Case–control study
10 Does having a maximum speed limit of 30 mph reduce fatal pedestrian accidents, as compared to 40 mph?	Case–control studies National or international pragmatic evaluations based on case registers, i.e. population case series examining effect of changing speed limits Animal experiments Experiments using dummies simulating accidents	Pragmatic evaluations based on population case series
11 Is heart disease mortality on the rise or on the decline?	Studies of population registers of disease, i.e. population case series Repeated cohort studies	Population case series
12 Why is the incidence of heart disease mortality changing?	Modelling studies using information on risk factor–outcome relationships from cohort studies And, changing prevalence of risk factors from cross-sectional studies Repeated cohort studies	Cohort studies combined with cross-sectional studies and modelling

(continued)

Question	Potential study designs	Preferred study design with reason
13 Would doubling the amount of exercise in the population setting reduce the incidence of heart disease?	Trials, probably examining intermediate outcomes Pragmatic, before and after evaluations International, regional and local comparisons based on population case registers and information on exercise patterns based on cross-sectional studies	Trial
14 What is the relationship between the wealth of the country as measured with the GNP and the consumption of illicit drugs, e.g. heroin, and legal drugs, e.g. alcohol?	Ecological studies based on GNP and information on proxy indicators of consumption e.g. excise duties on alcohol, or amount of heroin seized at ports	Ecological study
15 What proportion of school-children are obese?	Cross-sectional study Case series	Cross-sectional study
16 Do farm subsidies to dairy farmers lead to increased consumption of dairy products in the population?	Ecological studies associating amount of subsidy to an indicator of consumption, e.g. milk produced. Cross-sectional studies measuring daily use over time, i.e. repeated Trials	Ecological studies
17 What is the cause of a rare disease of your choice e.g. phaeo-chromocytoma, a tumour of the adrenal gland?	Case–control study Case series based on clinical or population registers	Case–control study
18 How many cases of AIDS, or any other similar infectious disease of your choice, should the health service be planning for 5, 10 and 20 years from now?	Modelling based on population case registers/surveillance systems and trends in prevalence of HIV based on cross-sectional studies Expert consensus study, i.e. interview or questionnaire	Modelling based on a variety of data
19 Is the amount of fruit and vegetable consumption increasing or decreasing? What is likely to happen in 10 years from now?	Repeat cross-sectional studies Ecological studies based on farming, marketing and shopping practices Questionnaire and interview surveys to ask people about their behaviour and intentions	Repeat cross-sectional studies
20 Would screening all adults for diabetes using blood tests improve the health of the population? Would this be cost-effective?	Trials Pragmatic evaluations Modelling studies Health economics work on cost effectiveness, cost benefit and cost utility	Trials with health economic study integrated

Appendix 2

How to keep your supervisor happy; or 9 tips on research writing

1 Writing is very hard. If you are finding it easy you are probably doing it wrong. Easy writing is said to be hard reading. Expect to write 3 drafts before you release your work to others, and 6–15 drafts before you have it examined as a thesis or published.

2 Write succinctly. One sentence one point, and one paragraph one theme, are two axioms that summarize a good approach to scientific writing.

3 Dispense with adjectives!

4 Edit your word processed draft on paper with a pencil in hand. Few people seem to be able to see unnecessary words on a computer screen. Have your favourite dictionary, a thesaurus and a grammar guide by your side while you write.

5 Ensure text, tables and figures are closely integrated. Minimize the repetition of results between these three forms of presentation. On the whole tables usually work best at the earlier stages. In preparing tables work hard on legends, layout etc. Then, prepare dummy tables i.e. the table format without data. Finally, complete the table. If the table conveys the message why prepare a figure? If it does not, try a figure.

6 The accompanying text should introduce the table and point to the main findings, sometimes giving the key summary results again for special emphasis. All results that are referred to in the discussion or conclusions that are not in tables or figures need to be given in text. Ensure these extra data in the text are simple to grasp.

7 Discussions should be carefully structured. The BMJ has good guidance. Essentially comment on (a) key findings (b) strengths and limitations of the study (c) what this study adds in relation to the existing literature (d) conclusions and recommendations. Pay special attention to the abstract. Whatever the eventual layout, use the following headings: background, aims, methods, results (give the key data), conclusions.

8 Don't miss out from the acknowledgments anyone who has contributed to your success. All those meeting the accepted criteria must be participants in authorship of publications arising from the research and those who do not must be excluded (this applies to supervisors).

9 Check every reference including the layout meticulously. Use a reference management package.

Now enjoy the happy smile on the face of your supervisor.

Chapter 10

Epidemiology in the future
Theory, ethics, context, and
critical appraisal

Objectives

On completion of this chapter you should understand that:

- theory, method, and application are interrelated, therefore evolution in the one leads to change in the others;
- epidemiology serves the community in a number of ways, but predominantly through its role as one of the underpinning sciences of public health and medicine;
- ongoing vigorous debate on the future of epidemiology probably heralds a paradigm shift;
- epidemiology is both broadening and specializing;
- the context in which epidemiology is learned and practised is important in determining its nature;
- epidemiological codes of ethics and good conduct need to encompass both scientific and the medical and public health applications;
- critical appraisal of research is an essential skill for epidemiologists and requires attention to fundamental issues including the social and geographical context of research;
- epidemiologists need to study their subject's history, classical studies, and contemporary research, and to join the debates that will shape the future.

10.1 The interrelationship of theory, methods, and application: responding to criticisms of modern epidemiology

Epidemiology has entered the twenty-first century with both its exponents and critics questioning its foundations, record, and future. Modern epidemiology has been accused of being atheoretical; divorced from its source of problems, theories, and applications (public health); the source of spurious, confusing, and misleading findings; and over-dependent on the 'black box' risk factor approach. Every day the media report hugely exaggerated claims and counter-claims about epidemiological studies. Some of this research is reported by people untrained in epidemiology but the discipline's reputation is still tarnished. Almost invariably investigators (and the media) are inferring or implying cause and effect relationships from mere statistical associations. As we have discussed, such associations are rarely causal. Media publicity is, perhaps unfortunately, seen as a measure of success and is much coveted by researchers, their employers and funders of research. Guarded conclusions essential to good science do not make for exciting media reports. The result has been a profusion of unsound advice followed by the predictable and inevitable cynicism about epidemiological findings.

Even more seriously, there are questions about the relevance of epidemiology to resolving some major problems, such as the growing consumption of illegal drugs, the rising prevalence of smoking in developing countries, the obesity epidemic and the omnipresent problem of health inequalities. To participate in the resolution of such problems epidemiologists need to go beyond learning about and advancing techniques.

In 1978 Alwyn Smith criticized the atheoretical, empirical, methodological orientation of modern epidemiology and called for an integration of social, political, and biological frameworks of health and disease into epidemiology. In his 1985 review of the evolution of epidemiology in the USA, Mervyn Susser paid tribute to the methodological advances which had led to epidemiology reaching maturity as an academic discipline, but he echoed some of Smith's concerns, and emphasized that epidemiology had originated as an applied public health discipline. Nancy Krieger (1992) concluded, based partly on an examination of textbooks, that attention has been diverted from theory and concepts of epidemiology to methods and technique. These and other more recent and equally influential observations (see references), hopefully, will lead to a closer integration of theory, method, and application.

The philosophy and theory underpinning epidemiology, as in most other disciplines, is seldom made explicit and yet underpins all its work. It is a driver of change, and guides the paradigms within which epidemiology works. A full exposition of the theoretical and philosophical basis of epidemiology is not within easy grasp, and is beyond this textbook and its writer, but a more rigorous dialogue needs to be opened up. The following is a simple account that summarizes much that has been covered earlier.

Philosophically, epidemiology takes a positivist stance. The positivists' position is that problems can be solved and questions can be answered through the collection of data which are usually, but not always, quantitative. This stance has served epidemiology well. There are limitations in the quantitative approach, which is excellent for description, but insufficient for generating understanding. This book has repeatedly emphasized that great epidemiological advances may follow inspiration and insights that are not wholly based on quantitative data. A future epidemiology is likely to involve closer ties between qualitative and quantitative approaches, and a greater attention to disease mechanisms, an approach that requires closer work with social and biological scientists. These collaborators will need to understand (and respect) the theories of epidemiology so epidemiologists need to be able to communicate them.

The basic theory from which the causal contribution of epidemiology derives is that systematic variations in the pattern of health and disease exist in populations. These are a product of differences in either the prevalence of, or susceptibility to, the causal factors. The fundamental epidemiological question is why these differences in prevalence

Box 10.1 Major influences on population health and disease patterns

List five or six broad and fundamental influences on health and disease, i.e. those influences that change the population patterns of disease.

and susceptibility occur, and the challenge is to link explanations to the observed phenomena and to predict one from the other. Ultimately, such predictions could generate the 'laws' of health and disease in populations. These laws will not, however, be mathematical equations, as in physics, but principles, as in the 10 Commandments.

Epidemiological theory attributes the causes of disease to an interaction within the causal triad of host, agent, and environment. This triad works particularly well for toxic and infectious diseases, but to make it more widely applicable it needs to be developed in more detail. Development will be derived from the expanding fields described by the labels of genetic, social, life-course, and chronic disease epidemiology. This way of causal thinking was discussed in Chapters 1, 2, 3, and 5.

Epidemiologists need to think deeply about the forces that generate health and disease in populations so their specific studies are based on, and contribute to, the broader context.

Before reading on do the exercise in Box 10.1.

10.2 **Fundamental influences on health and disease in populations**

Figure 10.1 provides a simplified diagrammatic representation of the thinking below.

The fundamental influences on health and disease include natural changes in the environment; environmental changes arising from human invention, discovery, and manipulation; changes in the interaction between humans, microbes, and animals, usually for cultural reasons; changes in human circumstances, cultures, and behaviours; and the genetic evolution of microbes, animals, and humans.

These complex and interacting influences, exerting their effect over long spans of time (for human genetic effects, likely to be measured in hundreds or thousands of years), are the underlying causes of population patterns in disease. Their initial impact may be on individuals and families or small groups. Over time, due to their varying circumstances, populations begin to differ from each other, leading to the population patterns in disease and health that epidemiologists describe (symbolized in the triad of time, place, and person).

Epidemiological methods are designed to quantify variations in diseases and in their causes, to seek and quantify associations between them, and to generate and test resultant hypotheses, which are usually couched in more specific terms than above. Nonetheless, they are embedded in the above framework of influencing factors.

Variations in disease frequency give rise to hypotheses which might help to explain the patterns observed, and give insight into the natural history and causes of disease.

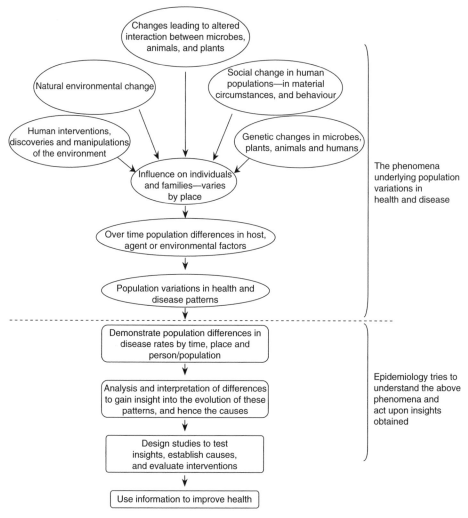

Fig. 10.1 The basis of population differences in health and disease pattern: towards a theory.

Classical epidemiological study designs (such as case–control and cohort) can be used to test such insights (Chapter 9) and, if supported, epidemiological guidelines can be applied to assess the likelihood of associations representing cause and effect (Chapter 5). Epidemiological models of cause (such as the triangle of causation) can help to conceptualize interventions for disease control (Chapter 5). Knowledge of cause and effect is essential to developing rational scientific interventions to prevent, control, and treat disease. To ensure these interventions work they need to be evaluated. Epidemiological study designs are also used for evaluating screening and diagnostic tests (Chapter 6), in evaluating preventive and other procedures, in assessing the efficacy of drugs and other interventions in curative medicine, and in studies of prognosis. While all the study designs may contribute to evaluation, the most powerful one is the trial (Chapter 9).

10.3 **Theory and practice: role of epidemiology**

As many, if not most, important advances derive from practical problems, epidemiological theory, research, and practice should intertwine. Morris, in his classic book *Uses of epidemiology* first published in 1957, and expanded in 1964, portrayed epidemiology as a discipline with multiple applications as reflected in his chapter headings: trends in disease, community diagnosis, working of health services, individual chances, completing the clinical picture, identification of syndromes, causal search, etc. In most contemporary textbooks, by comparison, the vision of epidemiology is narrower, and probably narrowing. Textbooks placing an emphasis on method, technique, and analysis wrongly imply that epidemiology is primarily about measuring disease in populations, and not primarily about how diseases develop, propagate, and are prevented in populations. Measuring disease is merely the means to the end. One vital question under current debate is whether epidemiology is primarily an applied discipline or primarily a science where methods, technique, and theory dominate over practice and applications. Whatever the outcome of the debate the fact is that epidemiology has a huge impact on health and health care. (Several recent references relating to this debate are in the reading list for this chapter.)

In measuring the frequency (incidence and prevalence) of disease in defined populations (Chapter 7), epidemiological studies almost invariably uncover morbidity, demonstrating unmet health care need, and showing the 'iceberg of disease', thus leading to expanded or new services (Chapter 6). Comparisons of disease patterns over time, between geographical areas, and by the characteristics of people within populations (e.g. by sex and age) also permit an understanding of how disease patterns are likely to change (Chapters 3 and 9), so assessing health needs and helping in health care planning. Disease trends, combined with information on demographic change and risk factor patterns, can be used to predict the future, and develop health targets. For example, epidemiological observations in the UK in the 1980s and 1990s on the trend in measles cases, with the prediction of an epidemic, gave priority to a national measles campaign targeted at school children; predictions of the HIV and AIDS epidemic in the mid-1980s gave priority to these problems; and the observations of variations in disease experience by socio-economic status have placed inequalities in health as one of the top ranking international and national priorities.

The traditional values of epidemiology are that it is concerned with the nature of health and disease in populations; that there is population group variation in disease that is worthy of scientific study; that it is important to medical and public health policy and practice; and that is it vital to prevent, control, and treat disease. There is no fundamental clash between these traditional values and modern developments in epidemiology, which emphasize measurement technique and study design and analysis. To illustrate how theory, method, and application are interdependent I have chosen two topics of personal interest: setting priorities in health care and assessing the impact on health of local polluting industries. These topics also show how epidemiological techniques continue to develop.

10.4 **Practice to theory to techniques and back**

10.4.1 **Setting priorities in health and health care: illustrative topic 1**

> Setting priorities is an issue for any organisation. The process should be sensible; it should be founded on science; it should be based on experience and research.

> Virginia Bottomley (1993)

Priority setting within health and health care is a complex mix of science and politics. Epidemiological data on disease frequency, patterns, causes, risk factors, and effectiveness stimulates the political debate on priority setting. Epidemiological criteria for priority setting (e.g. frequency and severity of disease) need to be merged with clinical, economic, and political ones to make sense of past priorities and to help determine new ones. National health policy initiatives are generally founded on epidemiology.

Priority setting cannot rest on scientific data alone. Judgements need to be made within a decision-making framework. Some of the characteristics of diseases, conditions, and problems which tend to receive high priority, in practice, are listed in Table 10.1, which is based on my judgement shaped by successive groups of postgraduate public health students who have discussed the topic. Epidemiology, alone, provides information on how common problems are. In conjunction with other clinical sciences, epidemiology has a key role in studying the outcome of disease in terms of chronicity, severity, and case-fatality and in setting out the prospects for prevention, control, and treatment. With social, laboratory and clinical sciences, epidemiology helps to define the relative importance of genetic, lifestyle, and external environmental factors in the causation of disease. The role of epidemiology is in providing background scientific information—part (a) of Table 10.1—that permits characterization of the importance of health problems.

The epidemiological principle influenced by public health, which has limitations for individual patient care, is that the most important problems are those that cause the greatest loss of life and illness, and are most amenable to prevention or effective treatment. The degree of loss can be expressed as the loss of life and the loss of life free of illness or disability (as discussed in Chapter 8).

Table 10.2 provides illustrative data on the number of deaths, the death rate, potential years of life lost (PYLL), and the standardized mortality ratios (SMR) for five health problems in an English health authority. In terms of providing diagnostic, advisory, and caring services, the data in Table 10.2, combined with basic clinical knowledge about the mode of presentation and severity of disease, show that cancers, ischaemic heart disease, and cerebrovascular disease occupy high priority. These three problems would be high priorities on the basis of the frequency data alone, but their major contributions to PYLL and the high SMR for cancer and ischaemic heart disease add to their priority status. Accidents and suicide cause relatively few deaths but the PYLL data enhance their priority status. Accidents also show a high SMR. The debate started by these data needs to be refined with information on the efficacy of treatment and preventive strategies (as discussed below in regard to risk factors), by adding the burden of disability and calculating disability-adjusted life years (DALYs), and by including economic factors, for example, by using

Table 10.1 Some characteristics of problems given high priority

A. Scientific factors
The problem is:
common
increasingly common
is commoner than expected compared with other similar populations
severe in its effects
long-lasting
communicable
epidemic
externally, or iatrogenically, acquired
one of the young
treatable
B. Social, economic and political factors
The problem is:
of high public and political interest
economically important
lobbied for by pressure groups or powerful individuals
low in stigma
socially acceptable
of interest to health professions

* Problems which do not have these characteristics, or have opposite characteristics, are given low priority. This table is similar to the one published by the author in Bhopal (1998a), Health Needs Assessment in Ethnic Minority Groups with permission (see Permissions).

Table 10.2 The number of deaths, standardized mortality ratio and potential years of life lost for selected causes of death, Newcastle upon Tyne, England, 1993

Cause of death	Number of deaths	Death rate per 100,00 population	PYLL	SMR
Cancer	943	335	6243	125
Ischaemic heart disease	884	314	3550	112
Cerebrovascular disease	348	124	1073	104
Accidents	72	26	1261	126
Suicide	26	9	870	94
All causes	3482	1236	19 264	116

SMR, standardized mortality ratio; PYLL, potential years of life lost.

I acknowledge the work of Dr Mike Lavender in helping me think through the text that describes this table and for providing this table.

quality-adjusted life years (QALYs) (Chapter 8). (The newer techniques of NNT, NEPP and PIN-ER-t may also be useful: see Chapter 8.)

Epidemiology also assesses the presence and impact of risk factors that influence mortality and morbidity. These data can be combined to estimate the risk of disease in a population that is attributable to one or more risk factors (Chapter 8). In conjunction with evaluation research these data, in turn, can be incorporated into health policy. For example, researchers have shown major variations in coronary heart disease (CHD) over time, between places, and within subgroups of populations, and have defined a number of important risk factors amenable to change (of which smoking, hypertension, and high levels of cholesterol are the best studied). Cross-sectional studies have defined the prevalence of risk factors in populations across the world, cohort and case–control studies have linked risk factors to disease, and population-based trials have assessed the efficacy of preventive strategies. Health economics has been influential in helping to define the most cost-effective interventions that address the major issues highlighted by epidemiology. The sum of this knowledge contributes to judging the priority to be given to CHD prevention, in relation to the prevention of other diseases, and in relation to 'curative' and palliative interventions.

Epidemiology provides information to use in the process of priority setting, which is, however, a political one. Some of the important political factors are given in Table 10.1 part (b). The scientific factors and social/economic/political factors are not independent. Clearly, problems which are common and severe are more likely to interest health professionals and also to be of economic and political interest. Problems which are of interest to pressure groups and politicians are more likely to be studied scientifically, and more data will become available to define the burden (and previously hidden burden) of disease and the scope for prevention or cure, thus raising its priority. The influence of politics and society on science, and vice versa, is an ethical matter (see section 10.10).

Few topics fall more clearly into the domain of applied epidemiology than priority setting. The role of epidemiology, though vast, has seldom been made explicit. Epidemiological theories, methods and data combine with other disciplines to help form difficult judgements on priorities. When the causation of a disease is known, it is easy to overlook the role of epidemiology, both in macro and micro decision-making, but historical examples make it clear. In the case of cholera, the size of the problem gave it priority (macro) but which action should take priority: cleansing the streets of filth to reduce miasma or securing water supplies uncontaminated by sewage (micro)? In the case of pellagra (disease X in Chapter 1) its importance was clear because it was common and severe (macro) but should we prioritize quarantine measures, assuming it is an infection, or supplement the diet, assuming it is a nutritional deficiency (micro)? For coronary heart disease do we prioritize cholesterol reduction or supplement the diet with folic acid or fish to reduce endothelial dysfunction (micro)? New variant CJD (Creutzfeldt-Jakob disease) in humans, arising from BSE in cattle, is a priority on epidemiological grounds because it is increasingly common, externally acquired, severe, and potentially can result in an explosive epidemic (macro consideration). Theories on causation, and predictions of the size of the epidemic, are central to prioritizing this problem but there is great uncertainty on these at present. These examples illustrate the interdependence of theory, method and data in applied epidemiology.

In conclusion, this topic illustrates how epidemiological understanding of causation is complementary to descriptive data on the burden of disease. Epidemiological theories of causation and data both help us to develop a sense of priority, and guide public health, health policy, and medical care services. The needs of policy and practice have provided the stimulus for modes of analysis (PYLL, attributable risk, etc.) that are not essential to causal epidemiology. In turn, these now classical measures are being further developed, e.g. population impact numbers (Chapter 8). The application of epidemiological knowledge spurs new questions and advancement of both method and theory; for example, the description of inequalities in health is now giving way to understanding their causes and mechanisms.

10.4.2 Impact on health of local polluting industries: Teesside study of environment and health: illustrative topic 2

Research on the impact of industrial pollution on the health of nearby populations is usually done in the midst of heavy media publicity and sometimes pending litigation. In our study of the impact of petrochemical and steel industries on the health of people in Teesside (Chapter 4, Box 4.6), my colleagues and I started with the testimony of general practitioners and with an analysis of mortality statistics. General practitioners feared, as had successive public health professionals for the last hundred years, that the pollution caused premature death, cancer, asthma, and other chest problems. Routine statistics showed appallingly high mortality in the geographical areas close to industry. This type of problem typifies applied public health's dependence on epidemiological theory and method.

The first step was to choose the theoretical framework within which to work. Ours was a positivist approach, based on epidemiological, empirical, objectively collected data.

The second step was to propose hypotheses and a study design. We had several hypotheses of which the key one was that the risk of mortality and disease, particularly for respiratory health, would be higher than expected in populations living close to industry. We defined four populations in geographical areas at varying distances from the main industrial complexes. We agreed that an association would be worthy of serious consideration as causal if there was a gradient with distance within the three areas in Teesside (called A, B, C) and if the three areas together had a higher rate than a fourth area some 20 miles distant in the city of Sunderland (called S). Our framework of causal thinking was based on the criteria (nowadays referred to as guidelines) discussed in Chapter 5. We applied a mixture of designs, including modelling of historical land use, air pollution patterns currently and in the past (truly ecological studies), analysis of population case series of mortality from routine statistics, cross-sectional analysis of primary care use (by selected diagnosis), and cross-sectional studies of self-reported health in the community using questionnaires.

The third step was to agree on how the data were to be interpreted. We agreed that if a disease or health problem was potentially causally related to living close to industry, then there would be a gradient with distance, those closest having the highest rates, and those furthest the lowest. Proximity of residence to industry, then, was the key proxy measure for exposure to industrial pollution. These decisions are based on important values, assumptions, and theories of health and disease. For example, the values and assumptions that empirical data are more reliable than the testimony of local people; and that an epidemiological approach would be better than a toxicological one where we focused on measuring the air quality, or chemicals in blood or other human tissues, rather than health status. The underlying theory of health and disease was that long-term exposure to low levels of industrial air pollution does harm, rather than good. Such important factors are seldom explicit but play a vital role in guiding the research and its interpretation. Indeed, they were not made explicit at all before, during, or after publication of the Teesside study, but in retrospect and on reflection, their importance is clear.

We found that the death rates for lung cancer in women in area A were exceptionally high and in line with the pattern predicted in our prior hypothesis. For virtually every other cause of death and cancer, while health was poor, there was no such pattern. There was no evidence in favour of our prior hypothesis for birthweight, sex ratios at birth and perinatal mortality in infants; for self-reported health; and for general practice consultation patterns.

We applied our real-artefact and causal frameworks to analyse these associations (see Chapters 4 and 5). We concluded that there was evidence that local industrial pollution had a causal role in the high rates of lung cancer in women, but that for a wide range of other health concerns alternative explanations were necessary. While there was no room for complacency some reassurance was possible. We put particular emphasis on socio-economic deprivation and environmental degradation as causes of the general poor health in Teesside. We recommended a focus on poverty, new research on lung cancer in women and new studies of air quality around industry focusing on the public's concern. Our work provided data to resolve a public health problem that had been exercising medical officers of health since the turn of the century.

The follow-up research included a case–control study of the association between proximity of residence to industry (as a proxy for long-term air pollution exposure) and lung cancer in women. Numerous studies of air pollution and lung cancer have been conducted and the pitfalls of tackling this tough topic are well documented. These pitfalls include handling the need to collect life-long data retrospectively, using recall on both residential history (the key exposure variable) and on strong confounding factors including smoking and occupational history. The study used matched controls and an innovative 'life-grid' method for data collection. Here, a person's major life-events are mapped on a time line, e.g. going to primary school, secondary school, first job, moving house, marriage, children etc. Then, the enquiry about exposures is also mapped both generally, and specifically, in relation to these life events. This life-grid approach has been developed in the social sciences but is proving useful in epidemiology. The case control study supported the earlier work, thus adding to the evidence in favour of a causal role (Edwards *et al.* 2006).

This work exemplifies how outwardly atheoretical, pragmatic, public health-orientated projects may be founded on important epidemiological theories and concepts. It also shows how epidemiology reaches out across disciplines to do the work—here toxicologists, geographers, statisticians, physicians, anthropologists, and epidemiologists worked together. When required, we went beyond epidemiology, e.g. ecological studies of land use, and the use of the life-grid method for recall.

Those readers who do not share these theories and concepts, and who are neither familiar with nor confident about the methods, will not be comfortable with the results. The public may give more credence to individual case histories of illness, and general observations on the quality of the environment, than to epidemiological data. Environmental scientists may remain unconvinced by the epidemiological findings unless the specific sources and nature of exposures can be directly linked to disease mechanisms. The crucial step, interpretation, is also dependent on theories and concepts. As epidemiologists need to communicate with both the public and other disciplines, it is important they understand how their theories and concepts compare with those of others. Indeed, epidemiologists should know and make explicit the paradigms that their work falls into.

10.5 Paradigms: the evolution of sciences, including epidemiology

> In this essay, 'normal science' means research firmly based upon one or more past scientific achievements, achievements that some particular scientific community acknowledges for a time as supplying the foundation for its further practice.
>
> Thomas Kuhn (1996, p. 10)

In 1996 Susser and Susser called for a fifth paradigm shift in epidemiology. They identified four paradigm shifts (following Kuhn) in epidemiology in the last three hundred years or so (Table 10.3) and advocated a new paradigm of multilevel eco-epidemiology, which ranges from molecule to macro environment. In doing this they struck a blow against the standard risk-factor–outcome analysis (adjusted for confounders) that characterized epidemiology in the late twentieth century. Understanding the significance of their call requires some knowledge of Kuhn's concept of scientific paradigms. Paradigms are 'shared ideas which account for relative fullness of their [i.e. scientists'] communications and their relative unanimity of judgement'. Thomas Kuhn's view is that sciences mostly work, at any one time, within a single paradigm driven by exemplars of successful work. Sciences that are maturing or changing do not have a dominant paradigm.

Table 10.3 Four paradigms in epidemiology identified by the Sussers

Exploratory description of disease (e.g. Graunt's analysis of the London Bills of Mortality in 1662, and Ramazzini and occupational exposures, 1700). In this period there was a change to sickness being seen as a result of disease entities not as humoral imbalance
Miasma theory of disease: the idea that disease arose from foul emanations from pollution (eighteenth century)
Germ theory of disease (nineteenth century)
Multiple causes as captured in the black box metaphor (twentieth century)

Table 10.4 Four components of a paradigm, or a disciplinary matrix as identified by Kuhn

Symbolic generalizations, e.g. the laws of physics as given in mathematical formulae

Beliefs in particular models, e.g. heat as kinetic energy

Values, e.g. the key goal of science being accurate predictions

Exemplars, i.e. classic examples of problems and their solutions, upon which Kuhn places special emphasis

The idea of scientific paradigms is complex, with many nuances (Table 10.4). Failure of the paradigm in solving current problems and explaining important observations inspires a search for a new paradigm that rapidly replaces the old one, which is then forgotten. This, he argues, is the foundation of scientific revolutions. Kuhn's ideas have been highly influential in the philosophy of science.

To call for a new paradigm as the Sussers did is, therefore, a severe provocation for it declares the current paradigm to be inadequate. Vigorous debate and resistance to change are identified by Kuhn as precursors to change. Current resistance to a broader role for academic epidemiology (e.g. in achieving tobacco control globally, especially in the developing world, or reducing health inequalities) might be explained as an intuition among epidemiologists that some of the dominant problems being identified lie outside the solution of current methods. Kuhn's view strikes a chord:

> .... one of the things a scientific community acquires with a paradigm is a criterion for choosing problems that, while the paradigm is taken for granted, can be assumed to have solutions. To a great extent these are the only problems that the community will admit as scientific or encourage its members to undertake.
>
> Kuhn (1966, p. 37)

This current debate in favour of new paradigms is fuelled by a combination of new patterns of disease (section 10.6), challenging new applications, a perception that the current risk factor-disease-outcome-based approach has not yielded the anticipated advances, and the availability of new techniques of data acquisition and analysis.

10.6 **Epidemiology: forces for change**

Diseases wax and wane. This has a profound effect on medical practice. Diseases that doctors saw a hundred years ago would baffle today's doctors. Diseases we now see might have baffled a doctor practising medicine a hundred years ago. What we see now is likely to be very different from what our successors will see 50–100 years from now. Some of these changes are simply reflecting new diagnostic labels but there are also remarkably rapid changes in the pattern of disease, usually for reasons that are poorly understood. The twenty-first century will rely on technology and science to resolve problems and these technologies are likely to speed up change. Before reading on do the exercise in Box 10.2.

Examples of diseases never or rarely seen in contemporary medical practice in industrialized countries include smallpox (extinct), scurvy, beriberi, rickets, and

Box 10.2 Waning of diseases

Reflect on the diseases that contemporary doctors either do not, or extremely rarely, see. Now, reflect on diseases that may not be seen by doctors in a hundred years' time.

erroneous diagnoses such as those previously attributed to masturbation, race, hysteria, and so on.

Many other massive changes, some anticipated (e.g. those due to climate change) but most not, will occur within our lifetimes. The shape of the average human body is transforming with ample nutrition causing substantial enlargement in height and, especially, bulk. Diseases that physicians in a hundred years' time may not see include mesothelioma (a cancer resulting from asbestos), tuberculosis, polio, measles, and Guinea worm infestation. With luck, even conditions such as stroke and heart disease, at least in the currently industrialized countries, may be rare. AIDS may be conquered by then. Epidemiology, and epidemiologists, need to follow and adapt to these changes, and ideally predict them, preventing adverse outcomes if possible. One adaptation that has already occurred is specialization within an expansion of the scope of epidemiology.

10.7 Scope of epidemiology and specialization

The scope of epidemiology has broadened with the discovery or invention of new applications and methods. This, and the changing pattern of diseases, has encouraged subdivisions of epidemiology, though sometimes these are artificial. There is, for example, infectious disease epidemiology and chronic disease epidemiology, health care epidemiology, public health epidemiology, life-course epidemiology, social epidemiology, clinical epidemiology, and genetic epidemiology. This list could be longer, and new forms of epidemiology could be proposed or created. The important question is whether such divisions confer benefits, and whether these benefits exceed the costs.

The benefits are those of all forms of specialization: narrowing the scope of work permits the researcher or practitioner to deepen the field, particularly by working closely with colleagues in the specialized field rather than with other epidemiologists. Concepts and methods can be refined to suit a specific application. Specific applications give rise to innovations, that are often transferable. The costs of specialization are: fragmentation of the discipline; a loss of breadth by the specialist individual or group; and a reduction in communication and cross-fertilization between epidemiologists working in the subdisciplines.

The fundamental concepts used in most subdivisions of epidemiology are similar. The same is true of the main measures of health and disease and study designs. The value of broad subdivisions such as chronic disease epidemiology is not clear, for the subdivision captures a vast territory, beyond the scope of a specialist. The similarities between infectious disease and chronic disease epidemiology far outweigh the differences. In contrast, clinical epidemiology, in the sense of epidemiology applied to patients in the clinical setting, retains a relevant distinction, and its specific needs have driven the development of new techniques of data analysis and interpretation (e.g. numbers needed to treat). The term clinical epidemiology may be used, wrongly, to distinguish medically qualified epidemiologists from others. Subspecialization is heavily influenced by the context in which epidemiology is practised.

10.8 The context of epidemiological practice: academic and service, USA and UK

Academic epidemiology in the USA is anchored in schools of public health which are mostly independent of medical schools. While there are also academic departments with epidemiologists in many medical schools their influence is much smaller. In recent decades, partly driven by the imperative to do and teach research, fewer people with a service public health background have been appointed to these schools, the posts being filled with laboratory scientists, epidemiologists, demographers, statisticians, or social scientists. The presence of clinically qualified staff (physicians and nurses) is also diminishing. In such schools of public health the vision of public health problems has become more scientific. Issues of theory, measurement, analysis, and study design receive close attention, rather than their application in disease control or prevention, so academic and service public health goals have diverged.

In contrast to the USA, British academic epidemiology and public health is mostly associated with medical schools and the public health service within the NHS (National Health Service). These medical school departments have close links to like-minded clinicians, especially in primary care and medical specialties where prevention is important, e.g. respiratory and cardiovascular medicine, and infectious diseases. These circumstances promote comparatively close links between public health and medicine, and academia and service, and generate a focus on applied work. Despite much discussion to create more, only one major university-based School of Public Health on the USA model exists in the UK—the London School of Hygiene and Tropical Medicine. This is a postgraduate school.

The US School of Public Health type of environment is large enough to offer a career path within this system for professional researchers. There, the epidemiologists see themselves, by and large, as professional epidemiologists. There are sufficient of them to form a professionalized, self-contained group and set up and sustain specialist organizations such as the Society for Epidemiological Research and the American College of Epidemiology. These are an addition to multidisciplinary societies such as the American Public Health Association. Many epidemiologists work in specialist departments of epidemiology.

In contrast to the USA, many epidemiologists in the UK perceive themselves first as statisticians, physicians, public health specialists, or social scientists. Medically qualified staff usually have a formal contract with the NHS and non-medical ones require one for research with the NHS. They mostly work in multidisciplinary departments where epidemiologists are usually a minority. Epidemiologists participate in multidisciplinary societies (Society for Social Medicine) or international epidemiological ones (IEA- the International Epidemiological Association). There are no national epidemiology societies in the UK.

These circumstances embed British epidemiologists within multidisciplinary and applied settings. They allow US epidemiologists the option of specializing and standing apart from applied public health. In mainland Europe there is a mix of systems, with most countries having major national institutes that promote epidemiological research, perhaps closer to the USA model. Service within the health care system is less common in mainland Europe than in the UK, though this is changing.

The fragmentation of American public health has been the subject of prolonged debate. A Committee for the Study of the Future of Public Health (Institute of Medicine) report stated that the 'nation has lost sight of its public health goals and has allowed the system of public health to fall into disarray'. A second report focused on the changing organization of health care, the changing role of government, the role of the community, and the need for partnership. The question for epidemiologists in such settings is: what is the role of epidemiology in such partnerships for public health? Despite much debate over 10–15 years there is no consensus. Applied public health has strengthened in the USA following investment in the infrastructure, itself spurred by the need to be prepared for terrorist attacks.

The British system of academic public health is substantially founded on applied research relevant to health policy and planning, and medical and public health practice. Epidemiology is the backbone of the applied research effort. Rigorous training in the science of epidemiology is harder to achieve than in the US and most epidemiologists are trained through the public health disciplines. The question for epidemiologists working in such settings is: what is the role of epidemiology in the world of science, and how is theoretical and methodological work to be nurtured? These questions are developed below.

10.9 **The practice of epidemiology in public health**

There is general agreement that epidemiology is a key science that underpins public health and increasingly clinical practice too. Yet the gap between academic epidemiology and public health practice may be widening. Public health, according to the definition by the Committee of Inquiry chaired by Sir Donald Acheson, is 'The science and art of preventing disease, prolonging life and promoting health through the organised efforts of society.' Public health applies science in the social and political context, inevitably creating tensions between the scientific goal of gaining knowledge and the public health goal of improving health. These tensions are being partly resolved through increasing emphasis on evidence-based policy, clinical practice and public health, with a special emphasis on evidence from clinical trials and systematic reviews/meta-analyses. This has created a common platform for academics and practitioners of medical sciences.

Epidemiology can be put into practice in many ways, including: understanding the relative impact of biology, environment, and health care on disease (e.g. the decline of tuberculosis); making the case for legislative change as was done following the London smog in 1953; setting up preventive programmes to tackle disease as done so vigorously in Finland to prevent CHD; predicting the future need for services using trends as in the field of AIDS; evaluating interventions; developing policy and clinical priorities; making clinical diagnosis in an individual patient; and providing the inspiration and methods for seeking new causal hypotheses as required for so many diseases (e.g. pancreatic cancer). So, there need not be any doubt about the role of epidemiology in public health practice. This role is not usually the focus, but a by-product, of epidemiology.

Epidemiological textbooks usually proclaim the applications of epidemiology as the foundation science of public health, but most focus on design and methods for causal research, rather than demonstrating clearly how epidemiology helps public health practice. The exemplars and classic studies used are mainly causal investigations yet much (maybe most) epidemiological effort in the public health field is on disease description and burden, prediction of trends, and evaluation of public health and clinical activity. (This book has sought a balanced perspective with equal weight to these domains.)

In a major review of epidemiology in 1985 Susser picked two studies that established the reputation of epidemiology in the modern era: the Framingham cohort study and the case–control studies on smoking as a cause of lung cancer. Susser's choices, as opposed to other triumphs such as the poliomyelitis trial of 1954 (which he discusses in detail), illustrate the dilemma. While epidemiologists may spend much of their time working on applied public health work, they still respect causal contributions most, and this is reflected in their teaching. The role of an applied science imposes on epidemiology the need for a code of ethics and good conduct that serves both its scientific and public health purposes.

10.10 Ethical basis and proper conduct of epidemiology: the need for a code

While written ethical codes for medical practice date to Hippocrates, some 2000 years ago, the idea that science in general (not just medical science, or social science) should be governed by ethical codes is recent. Discussion of such codes is currently in progress. To illustrate why applied sciences, including epidemiology, need an ethical code I have chosen to discuss three issues of interest to me: covert manipulation of scientists by the tobacco industry; the manipulation of authorship by researchers; and the purpose and direction of research on ethnicity and race (considered in some depth because of its exceptional importance to epidemiology and public health in a millennium where all societies will surely become multi-ethnic ones).

10.10.1 The tobacco industry

The pervasive and covert influence of the tobacco industry on scientific research and publication has posed mighty ethical challenges for research institutions, researchers, and journal editors. The tobacco industry puts its commercial interests before those of society. Tobacco industry archives show how the industry has manipulated research to deflect attention from tobacco's impact on health, for example, by fostering controversy about the effects of passive smoking on health; countering authoritative review articles through an international network of paid scientific 'consultants' whose activities included writing critical letters to academic journals; publishing biased 'review' articles; establishing a 'learned society' on indoor air quality; and performing research into non-tobacco causes of lung cancer (see Barnes and Bero 1998). The tobacco industry concealed or distorted evidence from its own research showing the addictive and harmful nature of smoking (see Hilts 1996). Epidemiologists working on topics such as tobacco need to be armed with an ethical code to protect them against such manipulation, and to guide them in making the right decisions in difficult circumstances, particularly when they are offered resources to pursue what are, apparently, good works. These experiences also justify policies such as declaration of conflicts of interest, sources of funding, and external influences on the research process.

10.10.2 Authorship

The authorship of scientific papers is hugely important for the status of universities and for the reputations of researchers. There is a widespread view that only work that has passed the scrutiny of peers is reliable and trustworthy (a view worthy of scrutiny, particularly as there is sparse evidence on the value of peer review). The main way for peer scrutiny is through publication in peer-reviewed journals. Publication is a key factor in academic promotion, success in competing for an academic appointment (and sometimes in service appointments too), in winning research grants, and, in the UK, determining the finances coming into universities. Not surprisingly, the pressure to publish is great, tempting individuals to accept authorship on papers to which they have not contributed sufficiently, a practice called 'gift authorship'. Richard Horton, editor of the *Lancet*, recently said, 'The mantle of authorship has become a heavy robe of fake majesty that conceals those who seek credit unworthily, priority unjustly and reward improperly' (Horton 1998).

The criteria for authorship prepared by an international committee of medical journal editors are commonly flouted (Box 10.3). Scientists, including epidemiologists, recognize that allocation of authorship is complex and raises ethical issues central to scientific integrity. (See also section 10.12 for error in scientific papers.)

10.10.3 Ethnicity and race

Ethnicity and race are among the top five or so variables in epidemiology. Their utilization, however, has put many researchers in peril of being judged as racist. Knowledge of the history of racism in science and medicine provides the essential insight into how societies may abuse data on racial differences. Some two thousand years ago Hippocrates contrasted the feebleness of the Asiatic races to the hardiness of the Europeans (see Chadwick and Mann 1950). Hippocrates' concept of race was of human groups shaped by their ancestry in different environments (especially climate). In the nineteenth century racial differences in anatomy, physiology, behaviour, and health status were avidly sought. The idea of races as distinct species, which was long and seriously debated, gave way to races as biological subspecies. On this basis race is the group a person belongs to on the basis of physique (a concept that has been hotly contested). Before reading on do the exercise in Box 10.4.

Box 10.3 The International Committee of Medical Journal Editors' criteria for authorship

Authorship should be based only on a substantial contribution to:

◆ conception and design, or analysis and interpretation of data; and

◆ drafting the article or revising it critically for important intellectual content; and

◆ final approval of the version to be published.
  Also note that:

◆ Acquisition of funding, collection of data, or general supervision of the research group, alone, does not justify authorship.

◆ All persons designated as authors should qualify for authorship, and all those who qualify should be listed.

◆ Each author should have participated sufficiently in the work to take public responsibility for appropriate portions of the content.

International Committee of Medical Journal Editors, 2007
(http://www.icmje.org/#author; accessed 22 February 2008)

In the nineteenth century, differences among races were usually assumed to be biological, interpreted to show superiority of White races, and used to justify policies which subordinated 'coloured' groups. Racism results from the belief that some races are superior to others, which is used to devise and justify actions that create inequality among racial groups.

Research focusing on problems more common in minority groups, combined with data presentation techniques designed to highlight differences in comparison with the majority population, so easily portrays the minorities as weaker. When research implies genetic factors, rather than environmental ones, as the cause of racial differences in health, racial minorities may be perceived as biologically (innately), and permanently weaker.

Science that indicated such weakness helped to justify slavery, social inequality, eugenics, immigration control, and the racist practice of medicine. Race-specific 'diseases' such as

Box 10.4 Ethnicity and race as artificial constructs

Reflect on whether there is truth to the view that races and ethnic groups are socially constructed, artificial ways of categorizing human beings. Can you think of examples of times and places when the idea of race has been used to overtly political or social ends, particularly the suppression of some groups?

drapetomania (irrational and pathological desire of slaves to run away) were invented. The Tuskegee Syphilis Study in Alabama (discussed in Chapter 4 on bias) by the US Public Health Service, which lasted from 1932 to 1972, deceived and bribed 600 Black subjects into cooperating with research which examined the progression of syphilis without treatment, even once penicillin (a cure) was available (see Jones 1993). In May 1997 President Clinton apologized on behalf of the USA to the survivors of this experiment. Osborne and Feit (1992) concluded that much American health research on race and ethnicity contributes to the idea that some human groups are inferior.

Modern genetics undermined the biological concept of race, and Nazi racism discredited both race-based science and eugenics. Race classifications are now considered to be based on a few physical features (such as colour and facial features) of small direct importance to health, which serve important social rather than biological purposes. Nonetheless, the idea of the biological basis of health differences by race (and somewhat less so for ethnicity) remains strong. This is the defining feature of the twentieth-century race concept, supported by many contemporary dictionaries and encyclopedias, and permeating biomedical thinking. The view that race is primarily a social, not primarily biological, reality is, however, emergent and slowly strengthening in the new century, despite an upsurge of interest in race in genetics.

The concept of ethnicity is that human beings identify themselves as belonging to a group because they differ culturally in fundamental ways including language, food, religion, lifestyle and, of course, their geographical origins which have shaped their genetics and physique. In epidemiological practice, perhaps unfortunately, race and ethnicity are virtually used as synonyms for overlapping underlying concepts.

Studies of ethnic and racial variations in disease pose a challenge to the maintenance of high ethical standards in epidemiology. The concepts of race and ethnicity are commonly applied in epidemiology in the hope of advancing causal understanding of disease. Contemporary race, ethnicity, and health research is mostly 'black box' epidemiology, concentrating on so-called ethnic health issues, and generating a multiplicity of interesting hypotheses. As Kiple and King (1981) discuss, the idea of a package of specific 'racial' or 'ethnic' diseases that deserve special attention and research has unfortunate echoes in history. 'Negro' susceptibility to particular diseases, such as leprosy, tetanus, pneumonia, scurvy, and sore eyes, was instrumental in 'branding blacks as an exotic breed', and the differences were explained by hypotheses on causation that can now be seen as nonsense. It may be that future generations will see current work in the same light.

Racial prejudice is fuelled by research portraying ethnic minorities as different, usually inferior to the majority. Infectious diseases, population growth, and culture are common foci for publicity. Following the release of statistics on the ethnicity of single mothers, the *Sunday Express*, an important UK newspaper, ran the headline (13 August 1996) 'The ethnic time bomb'. Researchers cannot be responsible for media reporting, but epidemiologists must be aware of the attractions of their work to the media and of the potential impact of their work on race relations.

Race and ethnicity are epidemiological variables that show, dramatically and unequivocally, the importance of historical, political, social and ethical awareness among epidemiologists.

10.11 **Ethical guidelines**

Ethical guidelines for epidemiological research have included broad statements about the duties of epidemiologists to be honest and impartial, not to distort the truth, and to uphold the public interest rather than narrow sectional interests. Other guidelines have given more specific guidance, including that epidemiologists should not accept contractual obligations contingent on reaching particular conclusions from research proposals; or accept grants or contracts in which the funder retains the right to edit or suppress results.

In 1998, the International Epidemiology Association's European Group published a code of practice for epidemiologists. This states that among other principles, some of which are given above, epidemiologists should:

- seek the truth in good faith without doing harm or jeopardizing personal integrity;
- judge their own work and ideas and those of colleagues in an impartial manner;
- disclose conflicts of interest to ethical review committees;
- publicly acknowledge all research sponsorship;
- publish all research with scientific merit;
- refuse requests to withhold findings, change, or tone down the content of reports, or delay publication unreasonably;
- ensure sponsors agree in writing that results will be published regardless of outcome and agree to the independence of the investigators;
- declare sources of funding and possible conflicts of interests in publications.

In January 2007 an updated, draft document was made available for comment by the IEA. In this revision a plea is made for a balanced approach to ethical approval with a warning that ethical rules are becoming so strict that they are undermining observational epidemiology. Bad research, however, is condemned as unethical research.

The classical medical ethics framework of autonomy (respect for individual rights), beneficence (doing good), non-maleficence (doing no harm) and justice is adopted in this document. Under autonomy the key issue for epidemiology is identified as informed consent, which is an ideal that often cannot be achieved, especially in the use of national, routinely collected databases. Linkage of databases is an especially tricky issue in relation to consent and data confidentiality.

The commonest potential problem in relation to doing no harm is avoiding disclosure of confidential data. Practical advice on how to avoid this is given by the IEA but the key point is that personal identifying data need to be removed/separated from the data set used for analysis. In making judgements on whether the data set holds personal information readers might ask this question: would a skilled investigative journalist be able to obtain private information about an individual given the data on that individual? (A full postcode/zipcode and a diagnosis might be enough.) The document supports the guidance on authorship in Box 10.3. This new guidance from the IEA will be, once finalized, core reading for the practicing epidemiologist.

The reader is encouraged to study these guidelines in more detail (the World Wide Web address is given in the references). To seek the truth and judge with impartiality (first and second bullet points above) requires, above all, a sound understanding of critical appraisal.

10.12 **Critical appraisal in epidemiology: separating fact from error and fallacy**

> Scepticism is the scalpel which frees accessible truth from the dead tissue of unfounded belief and wishful thinking.
>
> Skrabenek and McCormick (1992, p. 144)

In an era emphasizing scientific evidence as the foundation of medicine and public health, the scalpel of critical appraisal is likely to be as important to the twenty-first century doctor as the surgical scalpel was to the nineteenth century doctor. Epidemiologists have a prime role in keeping the scalpel sharp. Critical appraisal is important because much of what we know as the truth is wrong, sometimes dangerously so. Before reading on do the exercise in Box 10.5.

Historical examples of erroneous medical activities abound and include the use, for fevers and other common problems, cautery, bloodletting, purging, vomiting, and enemas. Many public health actions were equally wrong; for example, fumigation of towns to control epidemics of cholera, typhus, and yellow fever. At the time, however, these actions must have made sense to those who put them into practice.

Erroneous actions are a characteristic of modern times too. Examples of follies of the twentieth century include surgery for the floating kidney; ECT (electroconvulsive therapy) for a wide range of psychological and psychiatric disorders for which it did not work (it does work for severe depression); prolonged enforced bed rest after a heart attack when we now know that patients need to be mobilized within hours or days and not weeks or months; and treatment of heart rhythm disorders during a heart attack with the drug lignocaine. These actions were, in retrospect, dangerous.

Only with the 'retrospectoscope' can we identify follies and fallacies. At this moment life and death decisions are being made by applying uncertain knowledge about the causes, prevention, diagnosis, and management of disease. For example, is hospital birth safer than home birth for a healthy mother? Is screening for cardiovascular risk factors and cervical and breast cancer saving lives or causing unnecessary costs and anxiety?

Box 10.5 Reflection on medical and public health activities shown to be wrong

Reflect on some medical and public health activities which were widely practised but are now known to be wrong, some dangerously so. Your reflection should include both historical activities, say, before the turn of the twentieth century and more recent ones. Now, reflect on some current policies and practices that may meet the same fate.

Box 10.6 Reasons for the lack of clear answers

Reflect on and list reasons why, historically, medical and public health practice has not sought, or has not achieved, clear research-based answers to important questions.

Are drugs for moderate/mild high blood pressure, obesity, depression, and anxiety effective and safe? Why are so many antibiotics prescribed for non-bacterial illnesses? Is folate supplementation of the diet, or as a vitamin supplement, good for heart disease? What about vitamin D or probiotics for the prevention of chrome diseases? Does health education about drugs and safer sex prevent or augment problems? We often don't have clear-cut answers about the effectiveness or cost effectiveness of the activities we undertake. Before reading on do the exercise in Box 10.6.

The reasons why clear-cut answers to critically important questions do not exist include the following:

- the tendency and preference to base clinical and public health practice on personal experience and considered judgement;

- the tendency to act on good, common-sense ideas, often based on general scientific principles, in the absence of firm research evidence of effectiveness;

- the tendency to follow the ideas of distinguished colleagues;

- the difficulty and expense of doing research that gives clear-cut answers;

- the difficulty of extracting the correct interpretation of data;

- error in research.

Error in science is not rare, as the regular notification of errors in every journal shows. Several thousand errors are recorded annually in the *Index Medicus* and the prestigious journal the *Lancet* has a column called Department of Error. The popular image of the scientific process is that of steady accumulation of knowledge which is sound. The fault with science, if any, is usually said to lie in the abuse of knowledge, rather than in its accumulation and interpretation. The scientific paper, the carrier of scientific knowledge, has the authority of its authors, the elaborate peer review system, and the editorial processes of the publishing journal, and is expected to be accurate. Accuracy is a characteristic cherished and demanded by scientists. Both lay and expert readers may, however, easily overlook errors in published work, precisely because they are unexpected. Errors can then be perpetuated by quotation in secondary sources. The editorial and peer review processes are not, however, foolproof against error. The publication and continued citation of fraudulent research provides the most extreme example of the limitations of current means of detecting and excluding error in scientific literature. Fraud, however, represents an important but small proportion of errors in the scientific literature. Several studies of the use of statistics in medical journals have shown that error is a massive problem. Most errors are subtle and are made unwittingly by researchers who try hard to avoid them.

Critical appraisal is the use of the 'scalpel of scepticism' to extract truth from error in research. In evaluating research, particularly epidemiological research, researchers need to consider both technical excellence and its value in historical, political, social, and geographical context. These are heavy obligations on epidemiologists.

This book has provided the background concepts to guide the reader in critical appraisal (particularly Chapters 3, 4, and 5). In preparation for application of these concepts the reader will need to consult other books and papers (see references). Petr Skrabanek and James McCormick's (1992) book *Follies and Fallacies in Medicine* is a gold mine of examples, and the brief exposition in sections 10.12.1 to 10.12.10 is heavily based on their discussion of fallacies. (The book is available free on the Internet-see references.)

10.12.1 Some fallacies

The fallacy of association being causation

Humankind needs explanations, and this need leads us to confuse association, which is easily demonstrated, with causation, which is problematic. This matter has been discussed throughout this book (Chapters 3–5). The axiom, 'association is not causation, but it may be', is a safeguard, as is remembering that an association between factor A and disease B may be a result of:

- coincidence or chance;
- confounding (A and B share a common cause D);
- B causes A (consequenceor reverse causality);
- A causes B (cause).

This can be easily remembered as the four Cs.

The weight of evidence fallacy

The idea that pooling together weak evidence can turn it into better evidence is tempting but sometimes wrong. It is wrong to discard discordant evidence, even if it is scanty. The Popperian view of science is that progress is made by rejecting or refining hypotheses and the example of the hypothesis 'Swans are white' is memorable. More is learned about this false hypothesis by observing a single black swan (common in New Zealand) than 1000 white ones. Pooling evidence is, of course, the goal of systematic reviews and meta-analyses and is important for the causal contribution of consistency (see Chapter 5). The lesson is that critical appraisal must underpin the review process.

The fallacy of repeated citation

Is spinach a particularly good source of iron as claimed by the cartoon of Popeye the sailor man, and now widely known and cited? The answer, according to Skrabanek and McCormick, is no. In the original paper reporting these data an the iron content of spinach, the decimal point on the iron content was misplaced, giving a tenfold overestimate. (As I have not checked the original citation, this is an example of repeated citation.) The lesson is that you should check original sources and examine them with a critical eye and not rely on others' summaries. The scientific method requires replication and that is good epidemiological practice.

The fallacy of authority

Simply because an article or book is published does not make it right. Equally, the fact that it is not published because it is rejected by peer review does not make it wrong. Rejection by peers is the fate of much innovative research. The lesson is that all work, irrespective of author, needs objective examination.

The fallacy of simple explanation

Scientists and the public alike have a preference for simple explanations (usually referred to in science as elegant or parsimonious hypotheses). The emphasis in epidemiology on searching for single risk factors as causes, as opposed to ways of summarizing and studying the complex interaction of multiple risk factors, is a reflection of this preference. A quotation from H. L. Mencken summarizes Skrabanek and McCormick's view (cited on p 37 of their book) on this matter: 'for every complex problem there is a solution that is simple, direct and wrong' (see Chapter 5). Of course, sometimes there are simple explanations that are correct.

The fallacy of risk

Skrabanek and McCormick discuss a WHO study showing that women who had used oral contraceptives for 2.5 years had a relative risk of 1.5 for cervical cancer, that is, 50 per cent more than those who did not. Is this association reflecting a causal relationship, they asked? Second, does it matter and is it something for women to worry about? In terms of life expectancy, women aged 20–24 reduced, on average, their lifespan by 11 days. The principle here is: presented with a relative risk, ask yourself, what does it matter in terms of absolute risk? (See Chapters 7 and 8.)

The fallacy of inappropriate extrapolation

Just because something is unhealthy in excess (salt, milk, zinc, alcohol, weight, serum cholesterol, radiation, or water) does not mean it is unhealthy in moderation. Beware of investigators who extrapolate beyond their data, warn Skrabanek and McCormick.

The fallacy of significance tests

Any difference between two groups, no matter how small or unimportant it is, can be shown to be 'statistically significant' if the sample size is large enough. Skrabanek and McCormick ask us to (a) beware of statistically significant differences in big studies, and to (b) remember that the validity of the probability that a particular set of results has occurred by chance, shown by the significance tests (and illustrated by the p-value), depends on a prior hypothesis. They also remind us that statistically significant results are more likely to be published and that there may be unpublished studies showing no difference or the opposite (publication bias – see Chapter 4).

The fallacy of obfuscation

Beware of the use of complex language to obfuscate (to bewilder). The use of words such as 'essential', 'multifactorial', or 'functional', when describing diseases really means we don't know the causes. They are general labels to distinguish forms of disease where the causes are known, e.g. renal hypertension means kidney problems are raising the blood pressure, while essential hypertension means no specific cause is known. Such words hide ignorance yet give authority to the user.

The fallacy of covert bias

Use of language, particularly adjectives, may reflect the bias of the investigator. One writer may see a difference as important, another as insignificant. The reader needs to avoid being misled by the bias of the writer. Generally, adjectives should be minimized in scientific writing.

10.12.2 **The nature of critical appraisal**

Despite its name critical appraisal is not just about criticism and has a kinship to a book, film, or theatre review which aims to assess how good the work is in relation to expectations and what has gone before. *Citizen Kane* is an acclaimed film, but one wouldn't judge it in relation to the state of knowledge or technology of today. Similarly, in appraising a scientific paper, give credit for ideas. Do not criticize a cross-sectional study because it is not a trial (but do so if it is interpreted as if it were one!). Give a balanced view. The starting point is a mindset that is determined to examine the research painstakingly to form an independent judgement.

The next step is for the reader to attempt critical appraisal. To make this a meaningful activity engaging in the world of science the reader is advised to work on contemporary journal papers and prepare the appraisal as a letter (or rapid response electronically, if feasible) to the editor and, if it is good enough, to submit it for publication. The educational benefits of preparing a concise, critical evaluation of a scientific paper are considerable. Researchers reviewing a field should routinely search for, summarize, and cite relevant correspondence and other comments. An original scientific paper is incomplete without the accompanying published comment. Online journals now offer the ideal of electronic linkage of corrections, retractions, and correspondence to original articles. Ideally, inter-library loan requests for a paper should be for the paper together with its related commentary, whether correspondence or editorial (sadly, this is not done). The next section outlines some questions of particular relevance in epidemiological appraisal.

10.13 **Some questions relevant to the appraisal of epidemiological research**

Austin Bradford Hill posed four simple questions to guide the reading of scientific papers:

1 Why did the authors start?
2 What did they do?
3 What did they find?
4 What does it mean?

These four questions are an excellent starting point. Additional general questions include these:

- What is the importance of the research this paper describes?
- Have the authors made explicit the concepts guiding their work and defined their terms?
- What are the objectives, hypotheses, and research questions under investigation?
- Were the methods appropriate to meeting the objectives, testing the hypotheses, and answering the research questions?
- Is the sample of the right kind and size to meet the study objectives?
- What biases are inherent in the methods and what steps have been taken to minimize these?
- Do the results relate to the objectives, hypotheses and research questions addressed?
- Do the discussion and conclusions provide an objective assessment of the findings and place them correctly in relation to other scientific literature?
- What is the next step in terms of policy, practice, and research?

Such general questions can be combined with those below to produce a critical appraisal specific to epidemiological research.

- Is an epidemiological approach appropriate to the problem under study?
- What is the study design and is it suitable for the problem addressed?
- Are the dates on which the sampling frame was compiled given?
- Is the date or time period over which data were collected (fieldwork) given?
- For conditions which have a cyclical pattern, has the timing of measurements been stated? For example, for blood pressure time of day, time of week, month, and season.
- Has the target population, i.e. the one to which the findings are to be applied, been defined?
- Have the precise geographical boundaries of the study been given? If this is not a geographically defined population, can the study population be related more generally to a place?
- Have the target and study populations been defined and described in terms of their social and economic standing, and geographical and cultural origins?
- Have terms/labels used to describe populations or subpopulations been defined and justified?
- Is the study sample representative of the source and target population and, hence, are the results likely to be more widely generalizable?
- Are the sampling and measurement methods equivalent in the groups to be compared?
- Are compared populations or subgroups similar on key variables (confounding and interacting factors)?

- Where there are differences have the authors done adjustment using a weighting technique such as age standardization, or other statistical techniques such as logistic regression (see Glossary)?
- Do the statistical adjustments resolve any potential problems of confounding or might there be residual problems?
- Do the analyses provide information on both absolute and relative risks?
- If odds ratios are given, and used as an estimate of relative risk, are the required assumptions met? If not have appropriate adjustment formulae been applied?
- If the study is one exploring causality is the causal framework and model given?

The subject of critical appraisal is a large one, and the interested reader will be able to find guidance on how to critically appraise studies both in different fields of epidemiology and with different designs (see references). Some guidance adopts a checklist type approach, with an attempt to assign numerical scores to the quality of the paper. The aim of some such checklists is to exclude papers from the review. I favour the mindset that we need to extract the value from each publication, excluding mainly on irrelevance to the question at hand, but sometimes because the research is in error or is repetition. Exclusion is usually for practical reasons, saving a small amount of time or money. The research excluded, however, may have cost millions of pounds. We now turn to the need to reflect on both the past and the future, as a means of continuing one's education in epidemiology.

10.14 Building on an epidemiological education: the role of historical landmarks

One path to a solid epidemiological education is to study the classics, or in Kuhn's terminology, exemplars. Exemplars provide inspiration as well as instruction. I have chosen three examples to illustrate the value of historical studies to contemporary work.

10.14.1 James Lind and scurvy

James Lind investigated scurvy and reported his findings in 1753 (see Lind 1753). He wrote 'Scurvy alone, during the last war, proved a more destructive enemy, and cut off more valuable lives, than the united efforts of the French and Spanish wars.' He also noted that scurvy 'raged with great violence in some journeys, not at all in others'. The first observation identified the immense size of the problem, the second told him that scurvy was preventable. To prevent it he needed to create the conditions where scurvy did not rage with great violence. He generated many causal hypotheses including the role of sea climate and particularly the moist air. He chose to investigate diet and conducted his famous experiment on the ship *Salisbury* in 1747 where he 'ordered' 12 patients, divided in pairs, to take cider, elixir vitriol, vinegar, sea water, an electuary (consisting of garlic, mustard seed, radishes, balsam of Peru, gum myrrh), and oranges and lemons. He found that 'the most sudden and visible good effects were perceived from the use of the oranges and lemons'. Sadly, many lives were to be lost before his remedy was accepted and adopted about 90 years later. The British Navy then started providing limes as part of the rations, giving rise to the name limeys for

British sailors. A deficiency of vitamin C, found in fruit and vegetables, was shown in 1928 to be the cause of scurvy. Vitamin C was the first vitamin to be synthesized in 1932, nearly two hundred years after Lind's work. This story illustrates the importance of reflecting on the differing patterns of disease—here, scurvy in some journeys and not in others—and then generating a number of plausible hypotheses and testing the most likely ones. It shows that putting research into practice is a long-term endeavour. Finally, this story shows that precise mechanistic understanding, though valuable, is not crucial to put epidemiology into public health practice. The work is usually considered one of the first scientific trials (Chapter 9).

10.14.2 Edward Jenner and smallpox

Smallpox is one of history's most important diseases. The story of how Edward Jenner, a country medical practitioner in Gloucester, investigated the role of vaccination with cowpox virus is well known, but where did he get the idea? What was the observation that inspired him to take the cowpox virus from the hands of the milkmaid Sarah Nelmes and insert it into the arm of 'a lad of the name of Phipps' on 14 May 1796? The observation on which he reflected was this: that milkmaids have clear complexions and are generally free of pockmarks (a disease pattern) and that it is hard to inoculate them using smallpox virus; an observation that we would disparagingly call an old wives' tale.

Jenner investigated this tale and the local practice of exposing people to cowpox as a means of protecting against smallpox. (The farmer Benjamin Jesty had previously inoculated his family with cowpox.) He inferred that milkmaids' exposure to the cowpox protected them from smallpox. If so, he thought, why not inoculate with cowpox, rather than with smallpox, a practice that was then widespread but risky. His bold gamble was to vaccinate Phipps, and then expose him to inoculation with the smallpox virus six weeks later. Phipps did not react to the smallpox inoculation. Jenner was convinced he had demonstrated a new technique for the prevention of smallpox and, perhaps surprisingly, his contemporaries agreed (Jenner 1798). Jenner correctly forecast the elimination of smallpox.

The World Health Organization declared smallpox to be eradicated in 1980, again nearly 200 years later. I believe this is history's supreme medical advance. Smallpox is the only disease to be completely eradicated through deliberate public health endeavour. This story illustrates the need to listen to the public with an open mind, and to test a hypothesis with experiment. Finally, it shows that those making a discovery need to be champions of its dissemination and implementation. It also reinforces the long timescales between discovery, and achievement of public health goals.

10.14.3 John Snow and cholera

The classic investigation of cholera by John Snow also illustrates important principles. The pandemics of cholera in the nineteenth century sweeping from the east into Europe were causing terror, as thousands died. The description by Roy Porter gives a feel for the terror that an outbreak involving hundreds or thousands of people might cause.

> Internal disturbances, nausea and dizziness led to violent vomiting and diarrhea, with stools turning to a gray liquid (often described as 'rice water') until nothing emerged but water and fragments

of intestinal membrane. Extreme muscular cramps followed, with an insatiable desire for water, followed by a 'sinking stage' during which the pulse dropped and lethargy set in. Dehydrated and nearing death, the patient displayed the classic cholera physiognomy: puckered blue lips in a cadaverous face. There was no agreement about its cause; many treatments were tried; nothing worked.

Roy Porter (1997, p. 403)

At the time the miasma theory was favoured. Miasma was atmospheric pollution arising from decaying organic matter. John Snow investigated this disease for 20 years, culminating in his study of what he described as 'the most terrible outbreak of cholera which ever occurred in this kingdom', the epidemic of cholera in Broad Street, Soho, London (Snow 1949). On reaching the scene he immediately suspected some contamination of the water in the Broad Street pump, a conclusion he supported by his observations:

• that the dead lived or worked near the pump;

• a nearby workhouse and brewery had their own water supply and little cholera;

• people living far away but drinking Broad Street pump water were afflicted;

• the homes of people dying from cholera were clustered around the pump.

Water, not miasma in the air, he concluded, is the source of the morbid matter that causes cholera. He published in 1849 and 1855, and gave evidence to many learned committees including one in the House of Commons. He was unable to convince those in power and died in 1858 before his ideas were accepted. John Snow's book cost him two hundred pounds to publish and he sold 56 copies in three years, making 3 pounds, 12 shillings.

The lessons here are numerous. How much emphasis can we place on either peer review or indicators of research popularity such as citation practices and the judgements of committees, in assessing the importance of research? It is worth reflecting on the fact that John Snow was, primarily, an anaesthetist for whom epidemiology was a passion. All doctors, perhaps all health professionals, should see themselves as potential contributors to epidemiology. Another lesson is that confronting an established theory (miasma here) is a formidable challenge. Snow's achievement is recognized as foundational for epidemiology.

10.14.4 The emergence of epidemiology

Based on these early achievements, epidemiology and public health advanced rapidly with triumphant insights into the causes and control of diseases including puerperal fever, pellagra, typhus, beriberi, congenital rubella, adenocarcinoma of the vagina, lung cancer, coronary heart disease and, more recently, AIDS and sudden infant death syndrome. These landmarks showed how society could conquer disease.

These are the kind of examples that provide inspiration and, rightly, take pride of place in our textbooks. Kuhn identified textbooks as vehicles for perpetuating scientific paradigms and as necessary for rapid progress by the novice, including through the study of exemplars (classics). The further reading lists at the end of the book offer choices on reading exemplars, and on the wide range of epidemiological textbooks.

10.15 **A reflection on the future of epidemiology**

In industrialized countries where the economy is stable or growing the challenges for epidemiology will, increasingly, lie in the prevention and control of the diseases of older people. Paradoxically, the solutions to these problems of old age may lie in improving maternal, fetal, and infant health.

According to the fetal origins (or developmental origins) hypothesis, the environmental conditions that the fetus (or newborn) is subjected to programme metabolic adaptation, and lay the foundations for diseases of middle and later life. Relative poverty in early life, and wealth in later life, may be the basis of metabolic maladaptation, triggering diseases such as coronary heart disease and diabetes (the adaptation–dysadaptation hypothesis). The study of risk factors and disease across the life-course, indeed across generations, confronts epidemiology with immense conceptual and technical challenges. The threats to health in these countries include the fear and actuality of economic and environmental collapse, and the side-effects of wealth e.g. obesity. The impact of environmental degradation and climate change is becoming a high priority for epidemiology. This is leading epidemiology to macro-level research and scholarship, away from individuals to ecologies, governmental systems, and industrial policy.

In many developing countries the traditional public health problems of poverty (inadequate sanitation, inadequate nutrition, and the communicable disease) are combining with those of the post-industrial era including cancer, heart disease, stroke, obesity, diabetes, road traffic accidents, environmental damage and climate change, to create a public health nightmare. Disentangling the interacting effects of changing circumstances of poverty and wealth in the causation of disease (the topic of health in populations in economic transition) is a vast challenge for epidemiology. In developing countries public health information systems and infrastructures are being put in place and we can foresee an explosion of epidemiological research. This work will produce more reliable data on burden of disease e.g. causes of death on a national scale, and help judge whether risk-factor–disease-outcomes, and interventional effects, follow the pattern already demonstrated in the wealthy industrialized countries. We expect this will be the case, as already demonstrated for some diseases e.g. lung cancer and CHD

Economic and health inequalities will hold centre stage in public health as they have done for two hundred years. Modern communications increasingly exposes the injustice of gross waste in some countries, and horrendous poverty in others. The traditional 'solution' based on the moral regeneration of the poor through schooling on sobriety, frugality, and industry has proven insufficient. Poverty is now seen as a potent and direct cause of ill-health, and vice versa. Good health, therefore, will be prioritized as a drive to economic prosperity too. Epidemiology has made a vast contribution both in describing such inequalities, and in helping to understand them, given the limitations of studying a matter of such complexity.

The future holds an ethical and a technical challenge. The ethical one is whether epidemiology should be an advocate for eradication of health inequalities (i.e. participate in the policy debate) or a dispassionate observer (i.e. seek the neutral stance theoretically associated with sciences, but which is largely a myth). The technical challenge is whether epidemiology can provide insights on the mechanisms by which wealth and health interact, and whether it can design and implement efficient and solid trials of interventions. This work falls into the growing realm of social epidemiology. The other end of the spectrum is the biology and, particularly, genetics of disease (see sections 3.2 and 3.3.1).

The human genome mapping project has reignited the question of the relative importance of genetic and environmental factors as the underlying causes of disease. In assessing disease causation and prevention, even though the environment–gene interaction is all-important, the categorization of disease into 'genetic' or 'environmental' is often the first step. A few important principles will help to guide epidemiologists in the current tidal wave of genetic research.

Within populations the genetic pool changes slowly and genetic variations between populations are small; in contrast, the environment changes rapidly, and differs greatly from place to place. The frequency of occurrence of most common diseases shows massive geographical and time period variation. For instance, heart disease rates in Japan are a fraction of those in Europe. Even more strikingly, rates of many diseases, including heart disease, have been shown to vary as much as threefold between neighbouring areas within cities; areas distinguished by little more than their affluence. Variations in the incidence of cancer are also particularly striking. Geographical variations between populations appearing over short periods of time are not genetic (unless they reflect microbial genetic changes). Changes in the incidence of disease over brief timespans, say between single generations, point to the dominance of environmental causes. The causes of the current epidemic of obesity and of alcoholic liver disease, both doubling or more in about 10 years in Scotland, are not genetic as both genetics researchers and newspaper headlines sometimes claim, but environmental. This said, all biological phenomena must involve the genome to confer susceptibility.

The incidence of many diseases has changed dramatically in recent decades. In the UK, for example, stroke, gastric cancer, chronic bronchitis and, most striking of all, infections including tuberculosis, have been in decline for over 100 years. At the same time, however, asthma, AIDS, skin cancers, and hip fractures are among problems that have increased. The epidemiological pattern of coronary heart disease (CHD) exemplifies the oscillating nature of disease. While rare at the beginning of this century, CHD reached a peak in many industrialized countries in the 1960s, 1970s, or 1980s. However, the cause of this great epidemic has never been fully understood and now that it is in rapid decline the reasons are again much debated (epidemiology points to risk factor changes and medical advances both making major contributions).

Diseases fluctuate in frequency and severity, and we are left in wonder and ignorance at the pace of change in the pattern of disease. The speed of change, however, unequivocally implicates the environment rather than genetics, as the primary factor in the causative process. Studies have underlined the role of genetic inheritance in many multifactorial disorders although their interpretation is often difficult. Great advances in genetics will follow the mapping of the human genome. The genetic contribution to disease causation will be clarified and there will be a revolution in diagnostic and therapeutic medical techniques. However, the genetic revolution will not, within the next 20–30 years at least (in my view) match the revolution in public health which, based on environmental change, has within a few generations added decades to the average human lifespan. Genetic factors provide the stage in the great drama of disease causation, but the environment is the leading player. This could change in the more distant future with genetic re-engineering.

Epidemiology will need to embrace and benefit from the advances in molecular biology. While it is difficult to predict all the demands that the advances in genetics will make to epidemiology, two are clear. First, advances in genetics will undoubtedly have an impact on the diagnosis and management of disease in the future, and ultimately on population disease patterns. As a minimum genetic methods of diagnosis will change the pyramid of disease, by uncovering the iceberg, particularly raising the number of people at risk, and probably the numbers actually diagnosed. Secondly, epidemiologists will need to be trained in genetics to a much greater depth than at present. One beneficial consequence of genetic epidemiology is that studying small, interacting effects requires large studies. Shortly, we will have biobanks containing demographic, anthropometric, social, lifestyle, biochemical and genetic data on millions, perhaps tens of millions, of people. This gold mine of epidemiological research will have benefits beyond genetics.

Molecular science will deepen understanding of the interaction between the environment, lifestyle, and the gene, for example, demonstrating why some people have high serum cholesterol and how this causes atherosclerotic diseases. The public health dividend from such knowledge will come from altering the pattern of risk factors in the whole population. Reducing total serum cholesterol from the currently pathological level of 6 mmol/L and more in some populations, to a physiologically normal value of 4 mmol/L or even less, without mass medication, requires an understanding of how people and societies change. It is a remarkable indicator of the pace of change that in my 30 years since graduation I have seen professional perceptions on the level of total cholesterol requiring clinical action drop from about 7 mmol/L, to about 6 mmol/L and now to 5 mmol/L. My figure of a population average of 4 mmol/L still looks radical but it will probably be standard (or even lower) by the next edition of this book. It is not simply biochemistry that determines an individual and population's serum cholesterol level, but what and how food is grown, processed, purchased, cooked, and eaten. These factors are determined by more than personal taste. Trade agreements, agricultural policy, marketing, and economic subsidy are crucial determinants of costs, availability and consumption. Epidemiologists who wish to study the causes of raised cholesterol in individuals and populations need to study these forces.

One of the future challenges for epidemiology will be to set priorities, and to avoid being deflected from its crucial purpose, which is understanding the causes and consequences of diseases in populations, and acquiring and presenting the evidence advocating the appropriate actions to improve health. In addition to maintaining the solid middle ground of today's epidemiology, we will need to make much clearer and better observations on how diseases are generated through the interactions that people make when living in groups, in other words, the social and population determinants of disease. Epidemiologists would do well to work with social scientists who have a sounder understanding of how societies work and can be changed to promote health. Epidemiology could also potentially make a much greater contribution to clinical research, particularly that designed to improve diagnosis, treatment and prediction of disease outcome. Clinicians fully trained in epidemiology are best placed for this work.

There has been a massive increase in knowledge of methods, which has not been matched with development of theoretical frameworks. Development of theory and concepts is a pressing need. Among the priorities here are the design and analysis of mixed method studies to examine causality in its true, multilevel, ecological context. The development of graphic methods for outlining causal pathways as the basis for such work is promising. Large-scale data sets with information at various levels, powerful computer technology, and new forms of analysis are required, and are all in development. Data mining techniques using powerful computers are also available. These may be applied on linked data sets on tens of millions, perhaps hundreds of millions, of people. Epidemiologists will need political and public support to navigate through ethical and legal constraints on such approaches. The impact of such approaches on epidemiology is harder to predict but we should be fearful of being overwhelmed by the discovery of thousands of non-causal associations. An even closer collaboration between epidemiologists and researchers in other fields will be a stimulus to such advances.

Epidemiology as a discipline will grow in the next 10–20 years and will become a vital area of knowledge for all clinical and public health researchers. Epidemiology will help them to envision the causes of ill-health and diseases and the health needs of their populations. From this vision will flow the coherent global, national and local policies, laws, and health care systems to generate health from the pattern of disease.

Summary

The philosophy and theory underpinning epidemiology is seldom made explicit, and yet it underpins all work, drives change, and guides the paradigms within which it works. Epidemiology takes a positivist philosophical stance. The basic theory is that systematic variations in the pattern of health and disease exist in populations and these are a product of differences in the prevalence of, or susceptibility to, the causal factors.

Epidemiological methods are designed to quantify variations in disease patterns and their potential causes, to establish associations, and to test resultant hypotheses. Diseases arise from complex interactions of causal forces. This knowledge is applied to prevent, control, and treat disease. Philosophy, theory, method, and application are interdependent.

A vigorous ongoing debate on the future of epidemiology, and the paradigms within which it works, is being fuelled by a combination of the changing pattern of disease; new challenging applications; a perception that the current risk-factor–disease–outcome-based approach is no longer yielding the anticipated advances; and availability of new techniques of data acquisition and analysis. Major changes are anticipated. Already, epidemiology is both broadening and specializing. We can see the rise of genetic epidemiology and, at the opposite spectrum, of social epidemiology. Life course epidemiology will encompass both. Epidemiology using data on whole populations, comprising tens of millions, if not hundreds of millions of people, is on the horizon.

While epidemiology is applied in several health domains, it is a prime force in public health, whether influencing policy, strategy and planning decisions, or in disease prevention and control. It is the underpinning (but not sole) science of public health. It also has a big role in clinical medicine. This imposes on epidemiology the need for a code of ethics and good conduct that serves both its scientific and its applied purposes.

Errors in study design, data collection and interpretation may impair human health. Critical evaluation of research is, therefore, a crucial skill, and essential in the ethical conduct of epidemiology. In evaluating research, epidemiologists need to attend both to technical excellence, and to its value in the historical, political, social, and geographical context. Epidemiology is rooted in the populations it studies, and in place and time, but it seeks generalization of findings, to improve health more widely.

These obligations require epidemiologists to have an understanding of the wide determinants of health and disease. This can only be achieved by broad studies of the history and achievement of the key disciplines contributing to epidemiology, combined with a keen interest in contemporary debates on the future of epidemiology.

Sample examination question

Give yourself 10 minutes for every 25% of marks.

Question 1 Why is an ethical code important in epidemiology? (25%)
Answer Epidemiology studies human (and animal) populations, and deals with matters of life and death. The findings influence both the public directly as they are popular with the media, and indirectly via professional practice and policy. Erroneous information, and erroneous hypotheses and theories, may lead to a great deal of harm. Where information is of value, there is an obligation to bring it to the attention of those who can apply it to benefit human health.

The research process that leads to such information raises all the ethical issues of human research, e.g. informed consent, confidentiality, autonomy, respect, and equity.

For these and other related reasons an ethical code is important in epidemiology.

References and further reading (including websites)

To be effective in the science and craft of epidemiology readers of this book will need to reflect on a broad range of issues—conceptual, technical and social. An excellent starting point is a dictionary. You will probably need at least a general dictionary, an epidemiological dictionary and a medical and biological dictionary. I have drawn repeatedly upon many dictionaries but particularly:

Last, J.M. (2008) *A dictionary of epidemiology* (5th edn). Oxford University Press, New York.

Dictionary of Epidemiology, registration page; http://www.surveymonkey.com/s.asp?u= 346782009879.

The Oxford dictionary of current English. Oxford University Press, Oxford. ISBN 0 19281 91 94.

Pocket Medical Dictionary (14th edn, 1987). Roper, N. (ed.). Churchill Livingstone, Edinburgh.

Your next need is to be aware of the range of material in, and approach of, the many excellent textbooks on epidemiology and related topics. Twenty-five textbooks were formally reviewed by me in preparation for writing the first edition of this book and this may still be of use to the reader:

Bhopal, R.S. (1997) Which book? A comparative review of 25 introductory epidemiology textbooks. *J Epidemiol Community Health*, **51**, 612–622.

I am not aware of a published update, but the website http://www.epidemiolog.net/resources/ textbooks.htm maintains a list, with brief annotation, of current books. Type 'epidemiology' into the search facility of amazon.com or amazon.co.uk to get access to reviews, cost and availability of numerous epidemiology books.

Compilations of classic papers are particularly valuable. An excellent example is:

Buck, C., Llopis, A., Najera, E. and Terris, M. (1988) *The challenge of epidemiology. Issues and selected readings*. Pan American Health Organization, Washington DC.

For a historical overview of the development of epidemiology read:

Morabia, A. (ed.) (2004) *A history of epidemiologic methods and concepts*. Basel, Birkhauser.

Critical appraisal skills as applied to epidemiology are considered in depth in:

Elwood, M. (2007) *Critical appraisal of epidemiological studies and clinical trials*, 3rd edn, Oxford: Oxford University Press.

For the next step up, particularly for data analysis and interpretation, look at:

Szklo, M. and Nieto, F.J. (2007) *Epidemiology. Beyond the basics*. Sudbury, Jones and Bartlett.

The references listed below indicate the sources I have drawn upon and bring to attention others of potential interest. Many of the references are relevant to much of the book, though only a few are cited in more than one chapter.

The references are, with a few exceptions, not linked directly to the text, which means readers will need to browse the list for each chapter to find the references relevant to the text. The drawbacks are balanced by the more fluid writing style this approach permits, and by the encouragement it gives the reader to scan the reference lists.

Excellent reading lists are available in many books, including Last's *Dictionary of epidemiology* (with some websites listed) and Rothman and Greenland's book *Modern epidemiology* (see Chapter 5 reference list), a renowned, comprehensive, advanced textbook, and a new edition was published in March 2008.

I have increased the number of references associated with each chapter very substantially. It is hard to justify this when online literature searching is so easy. Nonetheless, readers may find it easier to choose from my suggestions than from the huge number of epidemiological papers that are available.

Happy reading!

Chapter 1

Alderson, P. (1998) The importance of theories in health care. *British Medical Journal*, **317**, 1007–10.

Bhopal, R.S. (1997) Which book? A comparative review of 25 introductory epidemiology textbooks. *Journal of Epidemiology and Community Health*, **51**, 612–22.

Bhopal, R.S. (1999) Paradigms in epidemiology textbooks: In the footsteps of Thomas Kuhn. *American Journal of Public Health*, **89**, 1162–5.

Chadwick, J. and Mann, W.N. (1950) *The medical works of Hippocrates*. Blackwell Scientific Publications, Oxford.

Coggon, D., Martyn, C., Palmer, K.T. and Evanoff, B. (2005) Assessing case definitions in the absence of a diagnostic gold standard. *Int J Epidemiol* **34**, 949–52.

Department of Health (1998) *Our healthier nation*. London, The Stationery Office.

Ebrahim, S. (2007) Uses of epidemiology, ways of living and dying. *Int J Epidemiol* **36**, 1159–60.

Fraser, D.W., Tsai, T.R., Orenstein, W., Parkin, W.E., Beecham, H.J., Sharrar, R.G., Harris, J., Mallison, G.F., Martin, S.M., McDade, J.E., Shepard, C.C. and Brachman, P.S. (1977) Legionnaires' disease: description of an epidemic of pneumonia. *New England Journal of Medicine*, **297**, 1189–97.

Goldberger, J. (1914) Considerations on pellagra. *Public Health Reports*, **29**, 1683–6. (Reprinted in Buck *et al.* 1988, pp. 99–102.)

Goldberger, J. (1964) *Goldberger on pellagra*. A collection of Goldberger's papers on pellagra. Edited and with an introduction by M. Terris. Louisiana State University Press, Baton Rouge.

Goldberger, J., Waring, C. and Tanner, W.F. (1923) Pellagra prevention by diet among institutional inmates. *Public Health Reports*, **38**, 2361–8. (Reprinted in Buck *et al.* 1988, pp. 726–30.)

Goldberger, J., Wheeler, G. and Sydenstricker, E. (1920) A study of the relation of family income and other economic factors to pellagra incidence in seven cotton-mill villages of South Carolina in 1916. *Public Health Reports*, **46**, 2673–714. (Reprinted in Buck *et al.* 1988, pp. 584–609.)

Krieger, N. (1994) Epidemiology and the web of causation: has anyone seen the spider? *Social Science and Medicine*, **39**, 887–903.

Kuhn, T.S. (1996) *The structure of scientific revolutions*, 3rd edn. The University of Chicago Press, Chicago.

Kuller, L.H. (1999) Invited commentary: circular epidemiology. *American Journal of Epidemiology*, **150**, 897–902.

Larson, M.G. (2006) Descriptive statistics and graphical displays. *Circulation* **114**, 76–81.

Last, J.M. (2001) *A dictionary of epidemiology*, 4th edn. Oxford University Press, New York.

Marmot, M.G., Adelstein, A.M. and Bulusu, L. (1984) *Immigrant mortality in England and Wales 1970–78*. HMSO, London.

Morris, J.N. (1964) *Uses of epidemiology*, 2nd edn. The Williams and Wilkins Company, Baltimore.

Popper, K.R. (1989) *Conjectures and refutations: the growth of scientific knowledge*, 5th edn. Routledge, London.

Roe, D. (1973) *A plague of corn: the social history of pellagra*. Cornell University Press, Ithaca.

Savitz, D.A. (1994) In defence of black box epidemiology. *Epidemiology*, **5**, 550–2.

Senior, P.A. and Bhopal, R.S. (1994) Ethnicity as a variable in epidemiological research. *British Medical Journal*, **309**, 327–30.

Shy, C.H. (1997) The failure of academic epidemiology: witness for the prosecution. *American Journal of Epidemiology*, **145**, 479–84.

Skrabanek, P. (1994) The emptiness of the black box. *Epidemiology*, 5, 553–5.

Susser, M. (1985) Epidemiology in the United States after World War II: the evolution of technique. *Epidemiologic Reviews*, 7, 147–77.

Susser, M. and Susser, E. (1996a) Choosing a future of epidemiology: I eras and paradigms. *American Journal of Public Health*, 86, 668–73.

Susser, M. and Susser, E. (1996b) Choosing a future for epidemiology: II From black box to Chinese boxes and eco-epidemiology *American Journal of Public Health*, 86, 674–7.

Taubes, G. (1995) Epidemiology faces its limits. *Science*, 269, 164–9.

Walker, A.M. (1997) Kangaroo Court: invited commentary on Shy's *The failure of academic epidemiology*: witness for the prosecution. *American Journal of Epidemiology*, 145, 485–6.

Chapter 2

Bland, J. (1990) The population mean predicts the number of deviant individuals. *British Medical Journal*, 301, 1031–4.

Christakis, N.A. and Fowler, J.H. (2007) The spread of obesity in a large social network over 32 years. *New England Journal of Medicine*, 357, 370–9.

Christakis, N. and Lamont, E. (2000) Extent and determinants of error in doctors' prognoses in terminally ill patients: prospective cohort study. *British Medical Journal*, 320, 469–74.

Diamond, J. (1998) *Guns, germs and steel—A short history of everybody for the last 13 000 years*. Vintage, London.

Durkheim, E. (1951) *Suicide: a study in sociology,* translated by J.A. Spalding and G. Simpson, edited and with an introduction by G. Simpson. Free Press, Illinois. (First published 1897.)

Herbst, A., Ulfelder, H. and Poskanzer, D. (1971) Adenocarcinoma of the vagina: Association of maternal stilbestrol therapy with tumour appearance in young women. *New England Journal of Medicine*, 284, 878–81.

Jackson, R., Lynch, J.and Harper, S. (2006) Preventing coronary heart disease. *British Medical Journal* 332, 617–18.

Kahn, R., Wise, P., Kennedy, B. and Kawachi, I. (2000) State income inequality, household income, and maternal mental and physical health; cross-sectional national survey. *British Medical Journal*, 321, 1311–15.

Kinlen, L.J., Dickson, M. and Stiller, C.A. (1995) Childhood leukaemia and non-Hodgkin's lymphoma near large rural construction sites, with a comparison with Sellafield nuclear site. *British Medical Journal*, 310, 763–8.

Kogevinas, M. (1998) The loss of the population approach puts epidemiology at risk. *Journal of Epidemiology and Community Health*, 52, 615–16.

Lind, J. (1753) *A Treatise of the Scurvy in three parts, containing an inquiry into the nature, causes, and cure of the scurvy*. Excerpted from James Lind, *A Treatise of the Scurvy in Three Parts, Containing an enquiry into the nature, causes and cure of that disease, together with a critical and chronological view of what has been published on the subject*. Sands, Murray and Cochran, Edinburgh, and reprinted in C. Buck, A. Llopis, E. Najera, and M. Terris (1988) *The challenge of epidemiology. Issues and selected readings*, pp. 20–23. Pan American Health Organization, Washington DC.

Manuel, D.G., Lim, J., Tanuseputro, P. *et al.* (2006) Revisiting Rose: strategies for reducing coronary heart disease. *British Medical Journal*, 332, 659–62.

Nusselder, W.J., Looman, C.W., Marang-van de Mheen, P.J. and Mackenbach, J.P. (2000) Smoking and the compression of morbidity. *J Epidemiol Community Health*, 54, 566–74.

Pickett, K.E. and Wilkinson, R.G. (2007) Child well-being and income inequality in rich societies: ecological cross sectional study. *British Medical Journal*, 335, 1080.

Roe, D. (1973) *A plague of corn: the social history of pellagra*. Cornell University Press, Ithaca.

Rose, G. (1985) Sick individuals and sick populations. *International Journal of Epidemiology*, 14, 32–8.

Rose, G. (1987) Environmental factors and disease: the man-made environment. *British Medical Journal*, 294, 963–5.

Rose, G. (1994) *The strategy of preventive medicine*. Oxford University Press, New York.

Rose, G. and Day, S. (1990) The population mean predicts the number of deviant individuals. *British Medical Journal*, 301, 1031–4.

US Department of Health and Human Services—Public Health Service (1990) *Healthy People 2000*. National health promotion and disease prevention objectives. Department of Health and Human Services, Washington, DC.

Walberg, P., McKee, M., Shkolnikov, V., Chenet, L. and Leon, D.A. (1998) Economic change, crime and mortality crisis in Russia: regional analysis. *British Medical Journal*, 317, 312–18.

Weitoft, G., Haglund, B. and Rosen, M. (2000) Mortality among lone mothers in Sweden: a population study. *Lancet*, 355, 1215–19.

Wilkinson, R. (1997) Health inequalities: relative or absolute material standards? *British Medical Journal*, 314, 591–5.

Chapter 3

Aidoo, M., Terlouw, D.J., Kolczak, M.S. *et al.* (2002) Protective effects of the sickle cell gene against malaria morbidity and mortality. *Lancet*, 359, 1311–12.

Antoniou, A., Pharoah, P.D., Narod, S., Risch, H.A., Eyfjord, J.E., Hopper, J.L., Loman, N., Olsson, H., Johannsson, O., Borg, A., Pasini, B., Radice, P., Manoukian, S., Eccles, D.M., Tang, N., Olah, E., Anton-Culver, H., Warner, E., Lubinski, J., Gronwald, J., Gorski, B., Tulinius, H., Thorlacius, S., Eerola, H., Nevanlinna, H., Syrjäkoski, K., Kallioniemi, O.P., Thompson, D., Evans, C., Peto, J., Lalloo, F., Evans, D.G. and Easton, D.F. (2003) Average risks of breast and ovarian cancer associated with BRCA1 or BRCA2 mutations detected in case Series unselected for family history: a combined analysis of 22 studies. *Am J Hum Genet* 72(5), 1117–30. Epub 3 April 20033.

Bhopal, R.S. (1991) A framework for investigating geographical variation in diseases, based on a study of Legionnaires' disease. *Journal of Public Health Medicine*, 13, 281–9.

Bhopal, R.S., Diggle, P. and Rowlingson, B. (1992) Pinpointing clusters of apparently sporadic Legionnaires' disease. *British Medical Journal*, 304, 1022–7.

Bhopal, R.S., Fallon, R.J., Buist, E.C., Black, R.J. and Urquart, J.D. (1991) Proximity of the home to a cooling tower and the risk of non-outbreak Legionnaires' disease. *British Medical Journal*, 302, 378–83.

Cambien, F. and Tiret, L. (2007) Genetics of cardiovascular diseases: from single mutations to the whole genome. *Circulation*, 116, 1714–24.

Cardon, L.R. and Palmer, L.J. (2003) Population stratification and spurious allelic association. *The Lancet*, 361, 598–604.

Clayton, D. and McKeigue, P.M. (2001) Epidemiological methods for studying genes and environmental factors in complex diseases. *The Lancet*, 358, 1356–60.

Davey Smith, G. and Ebrahim, S. (2005) What can Mendelian randomisation tell us about modifiable behavioural and environmental exposures? *British Medical Journal*, 330, 1076–9.

Davey Smith, G., Lawlor, D.A., Harbord, R., Timpson, N., Day, I. and Ebrahim, S. (2007) Clustered environments and randomized genes: a fundamental distinction between conventional and genetic epidemiology. *PLoS Med*, 4, e352.

Fraser, D.W., Tsai, T.R., Orenstein, W., Parkin, W.E., Beecham, H.J., Sharrar, R.G., Harris, J., Mallison, G.F., Martin, S.M., McDade, J.E., Shepard, C.C. and Brachman, P.S. (1977) Legionnaires' disease: description of an epidemic of pneumonia. *New England Journal of Medicine*, 297, 1189–97.

Gregg, N.M. (1941) Congenital cataract following German measles in the mother. *Transactions of the Ophthalmological Society of Australia*, 3, 35–46. Reprinted in Buck *et al.* 1988, pp. 426–34.

Ioannidis, J.P., Boffetta, P., Little, J. *et al.* (2008) Assessment of cumulative evidence on genetic associations: interim guidelines. *Int J Epidemiol*, 37, 120–32.

Janssens, A.C., Moonesinghe, R., Yang, Q., Steyerberg, E.W., van Duijn, C.M. and Khoury, M.J. (2007) The impact of genotype frequencies on the clinical validity of genomic profiling for predicting common chronic diseases. *Genet Med*, 9(8), 528–35.

Khoury, M.J., Davis, R., Gwinn, M., Lindegren, M.L. and Yoon, P. (2005) Do we need genomic research for the prevention of common diseases with environmental causes? *Am J Epidemiol*, 161, 799–805.

Khoury, M.J., Little, J., Gwinn, M. and Ioannidis, J.P. (2007) On the synthesis and interpretation of consistent but weak gene-disease associations in the era of genome-wide association studies. *Int J Epidemiol*, 36, 439–45.

Loscalzo, J. (2007) Association studies in an era of too much information: clinical analysis of new biomarker and genetic data. *Circulation*, 116, 1866–70.

Olsen, S.F., Martuzzi, M. and Elliott, P. (1996) Cluster analysis and disease mapping—why, when, and how? A step by step guide. *British Medical Journal*, 313, 863–6.

Openshaw, S. and Blake, M. (1995) Geodemographic segmentation systems for screening health data. *Journal of Epidemiology and Community Health*, 49(suppl 2), S34–8.

Pennisi, E. (2007) Breakthrough of the year. Human genetic variation. *Science*, 318, 1842–3.

The Wellcome Trust Case Control Consortium (2007) Genome-wide association study of 14,000 cases of seven common diseases and 3,000 shared controls. *Nature*, 447, 661–78.

World Health Organisation (1992) *ICD-10: International statistical classification of diseases and related health problems*. World Health Organisation, Geneva.

Wright, A., Charlesworth, B., Rudan, I., Carothers, A. and Campbell, H. (2003) A polygenic basis for late-onset disease. *Trends Genet*, 19, 97–106.

Chapter 4

Barnett, A.G., van der Pols, J.C. and Dobson, A.J. (2005) Regression to the mean: what it is and how to deal with it. *Int J Epidemiol*, 34, 215–20.

Bhopal, R. (1997) Is research into ethnicity and health racist, unsound, or important science? *British Medical Journal*, 314, 1751–6.

Bhopal, R.S., Moffatt, S., Pless-Mulloli, T., Phillimore, P.R., Foy, C., Dunn, C.E., and Tate, J. (1998) Does living near a constellation of petrochemical, steel, and other industries impair health? *Occupational and Environmental Medicine*, 55, 812–22.

Bhopal, R.S., Phillimore, P., Moffatt, S., and Foy, C. (1994) Is living near a coking works harmful to health? *Journal of Epidemiology and Community Health*, 48, 237–47.

Bhopal, R.S., Tate, J.A., Foy, C., Moffatt, S., and Phillimore, PR. (1999) Residential proximity to industry and adverse birth outcomes. *Lancet*, 354, 920.

Boccia, S., La Torre, G., Persiani, R., D'Ugo, D., van Duijn, C.M. and Ricciardi, G. (2007) A critical appraisal of epidemiological studies comes from basic knowledge: a reader's guide to assess potential for biases. *World Journal of Emergency Surgery*, 2, Published online 15 March 2007, doi: 10.1186/1749–7922–2–7.

Brenner, H. (1998) A potential pitfall in control of covariates in epidemiologic studies. *Epidemiology*, 9, 68–71.

Brusin, S. (1999) The communicable disease surveillance system in the Kosovar refugee camps in the former Yugoslav Republic of Macedonia April–August 1999. *Journal of Epidemiology and Community Health*, 54, 52–7.

Davey Smith, G. and Phillips, A.N. (1992) Confounding in epidemiological studies: why 'independent' effects may not be all they seem. *British Medical Journal*, **305**, 757–59.

Davey Smith, G. and Phillips, A.N. (1996) Inflation in epidemiology: 'the proof and measurement of association between two things' revisited. *British Medical Journal*, **312**, 1659–61.

Duffy, S.W., Warwick, J., Williams, A.R. *et al.* (2004) A simple model for potential use with a misclassified binary outcome in epidemiology. *J Epidemiol Community Health*, **58**, 712–17.

Ecob, R. and Williams, R. (1991) Sampling Asian minorities to assess health and welfare. *Journal of Epidemiology and Community Health*, **45**, 93–101.

Fewell, Z., Davey, S.G. and Sterne, J.A. (2007) The impact of residual and unmeasured confounding in epidemiologic studies: a simulation study. *Am J Epidemiol*, **166**, 646–55.

Frost, C. and White, I.R. (2005) The effect of measurement error in risk factors that change over time in cohort studies: do simple methods overcorrect for 'regression dilution'? *Int J Epidemiol*, **34**,1359–68.

Gould, S.J. (1984) *The mismeasure of man*. Pelican, London.

Greenland, S. (1980) The effect of misclassification in the presence of covariates. *American Journal of Epidemiology*, **112**, 564–9.

Grimes, D.A. and Schulz, K.F. (2002) Bias and causal associations in observational research. *Lancet*, **359**, 248–52.

Hammond, E.C., Selikoff, I.J., Seidman, H. Asbestos exposure, cigarette smoking and death rates. Ann N Y Acad Sci 1979; 330: 473–90.

Health Education Authority (1994) *Health and lifestyles: Black and minority ethnic groups in England*. HEA, London.

Hozawa, A., Okamura, T., Kadowaki, T. *et al.* (2007) Is weak association between cigarette smoking and cardiovascular disease mortality observed in Japan explained by low total cholesterol? NIPPON DATA80. *Int J Epidemiol*, **36**, 1060–7.

Jones, J.H. (1993) *Bad blood. The Tuskegee Syphilis Experiment*, 2nd edn. Free Press, New York.

Jousilahti, P., Salomaa, V., Kuulasmaa, K., Niemela, M. and Vartiainen E. (2005) Total and cause specific mortality among participants and non-participants of population based health surveys: a comprehensive follow up of 54 72 Finnish men and women. *J Epidemiol Community Health*, **59**, 310–15.

Jurek, A.M., Greenland, S., Maldonado, G. and Church T.R. (2005) Proper interpretation of non-differential misclassification effects: expectations vs observations. *Int J Epidemiol*, **34**, 680–7.

Kaptchuk, T.J. (2003) Effect of interpretive bias on research evidence. *British Medical Journal* **326**, 1453–5.

Key, T.J., Fraser, G.E., Thorogood, M., Appleby, P.N., Beral, V., Reeves, G., Burr, M.L., Chang-Claude, J., Frentzel-Beyme, R., Kuzma, J.W., Mann, J., and McPherson, K. (1999) Mortality in vegetarians and nonvegetarians: detailed findings from a collaborative analysis of 5 prospective studies. *American Journal of Clinical Nutrition*, **70** (suppl 3), 516S–24S.

Knol, M.J., van D.T., Grobbee, D.E., Numans, M.E. and Geerlings, M.I. (2007) Estimating interaction on an additive scale between continuous determinants in a logistic regression model. *Int J Epidemiol*, **36**, 1111–18.

Kuhn, T.S. (1996) *The structure of scientific revolutions*, 3rd edn. The University of Chicago Press, Chicago.

Lillie-Blanton, M., Anthony, J.C., and Schuster, C.R. (1993) Probing the meaning of racial/ethnic group comparisons in crack smoking. *Journal of the American Medical Association*, **269**, 993–7.

Loannidis, J.P.A. (2008) Why most published research findings are false. *PLos Medicine*, **2**, e124, doi:10.1371/journal.pmed.0020124.

Mamdani, M., Sykora, K., Li, P. *et al.* (2005) Reader's guide to critical appraisal of cohort studies: 2. Assessing potential for confounding. *British Medical Journal*, **330**, 960–2.

Moffatt, S., Mulloli, T.P., Bhopal, R., Foy, C. and Phillimore, P. (2000, a) An exploration of awareness bias in two environmental epidemiology studies. *Epidemiology*, **11**, 199–208.

Moffatt, S., Phillimore, P., Hudson, E., and Downey, D. (2000, b) 'Impact? What impact?' Epidemiological research findings in the public domain: a case study from North-East England. *Social Science and Medicine*, **51**, 1755–69.

Morton, L.M., Cahill, J. and Hartge, P. (2006) Reporting participation in epidemiologic studies: a survey of practice. *Am J Epidemiol*, **163**, 197–203.

Phillips, A.N. and Davey, S.G. (1993) Confounding in epidemiological studies. *British Medical Journal*, **306**,142.

Popper, K.R. (1989) *Conjectures and refutations: the growth of scientific knowledge*, 5th edn. Routledge, London.

Rose, G. (1985) Sick individuals and sick populations. *International Journal of Epidemiology*, **14**, 32–8.

Schilling, L.M., Kozak, K., Lundahl, K. and Dellavalle, R.P. (2006) Inaccessible novel questionnaires in published medical research: hidden methods, hidden costs. *Am J Epidemiol*, **164**,1141–4.

Schwartz,S. and Carpenter, K.M. (1999) The right answer for the wrong question: consequences of type III error for public health research. *Am J Public Health*, **89**, 1175–80.

Tu, Y., Gunnell, D.J. and Gilthorpe, M.S. (2008) Simpsons Paradox, Lord's Paradox, and Suppression Effects are the same phenomenon – the reversal paradox. *Emerging Themes in Epidemiology*, **5**, doi:10.1186/1742–7622–5–2.

Yank, V., Rennie, D. and Bero, L.A. (2007) Financial ties and concordance between results and conclusions in meta-analyses: retrospective cohort study. *British Medical Journal*, **335**, 1202–5.

Chapter 5

Beiser, C. (1997) Recent advances: HIV infection–II. *British Medical Journal*, **314**, 579.

Bhopal, R.S. (1992) Smoking and suicide. *Lancet*, **304**, 1095.

Bhopal, R.S., Phillimore, P., Moffatt, S. and Foy, C. (1994) Is living near a coking works harmful to health? *Journal of Epidemiology and Community Health*, **48**, 237–47.

Bradford Hill, A. (1965) The environment and disease: association or causation? *Occupational Medicine*, 295–300.

Chadwick, J. and Mann, W.N. (1950) *The medical works of Hippocrates*. Blackwell Scientific, Oxford.

Charemza, W.W. and Deadman, D.F. (1997) *New directions in econometric practice: general to specific modelling, cointegration, and vector autoregression*, 2nd edn. Elgar, Cheltenham.

Cleophas, T.J. and Zwinderman, A.H. (2007) Meta-analysis. *Circulation*, **115**, 2870–5.

Cottingham, J. (1996) *Western philosophy—an anthology*. Blackwell, Oxford.

Doll, R. (1998) Uncovering the effects of smoking: historical perspective. *Statistical Methods in Medical Research*, **7**, 87–117.

Doll, R. and Bradford Hill, A. (1956) Lung cancer and other causes of death in relation to smoking. *British Medical Journal*, **2**, 1071–81.

Elwood, M. (2007) *Critical appraisal of epidemiological studies and clinical trials*, 3rd edn, Oxford, Oxford University Press.

Evans, A. (1978) Causation and disease: a chronological journey. *American Journal of Epidemiology*, **108**, 249–58.

Gilbert, R., Salanti, G., Harden, M. and See S. (2005) Infant sleeping position and the sudden infant death syndrome: systematic review of observational studies and historical review of recommendations from 1940 to 2002. *Int J Epidemiol*, **34**, 874–7.

Gould, S.J. (1984) *The mismeasure of man*. Pelican, London.

Greenland, S. and Brumback, B. (2002) An overview of relations among causal modelling methods. *Int J Epidemiol*, **31**, 1030–7.

Herbst, A., Ulfelder, H. and Poskanzer, D. (1971) Adenocarcinoma of the vagina: Association of maternal stilbestrol therapy with tumour appearance in young women. *New England Journal of Medicine*, **284**, 878–81. (Reprinted in Buck *et al.* 1988, pp. 446–50.)

Hernan, M.A. (2004) A definition of causal effect for epidemiological research. *J Epidemiol Community Health*, **58**, 265–71.

Hicks, J. (1979) *Causality in economics*. Blackwell, Oxford.

Hofler, M. (2005) The Bradford Hill considerations on causality: a counterfactual perspective. *Emerg Themes Epidemiol*, **2**, 11.

Kaufman, J.S., Kaufman, S. and Poole C. (2003) Causal inference from randomized trials in social epidemiology. *Soc Sci Med* **57**, 2397–409.

Kaufman, J.S. and Cooper, R.S. (1999) Seeking causal explanations in social epidemiology. *American Journal of Epidemiology*, **150**, 113–20.

Krieger, N. (1994) Epidemiology and the web of causation: has anyone seen the spider? *Social Science and Medicine*, **39**, 887–903.

Kuhn, T.S. (1996) *The structure of scientific revolutions*, 3rd edn. The University of Chicago Press, Chicago.

Lewontin, R.C. (2006) The analysis of variance and the analysis of causes. *Int J Epidemiol*, **35**, 520–5.

Lilford, R.J. and Braunholtz, D. (2000) Who's afraid of Thomas Bayes? *J Epidemiol Community Health*, **54**, 731–9.

Maldonado, G. and Greenland, S. (2002) Estimating causal effects. *Int J Epidemiol*, **31**, 422–9.

Mausner, J.S. and Kramer, S. (1985) *Epidemiology*, 2nd edn. W.B. Saunders, Philadelphia.

McPherson, K. (1998) Wider 'causal thinking in the health sciences'. *Journal of Epidemiology and Community Health*, **52**, 612–13.

Ogilvie, D., Fayter, D., Petticrew, M. *et al.* (2008) The harvest plot: a method for synthesising evidence about the differential effects of interventions. *BMC Med Res Methodol*, **8**, 8.

Olsen, J. (2003) What characterises a useful concept of causation in epidemiology? *J Epidemiol Community Health*, **57**, 86–88.

Onyebuchi, A. (2008) The role of causal reasoning in understanding Simpson's paradox, Lord's paradox, and the suppression effect: covariate selection in the analysis of observational studies. *Emerging Themes in Epidemiology*, **5**, DOI: 10.1186/1742–7622–5–5.

Oswald, A.J. (2007) Commentary: human well-being and causality in social epidemiology. *Int J Epidemiol*, **36**, 1253–4.

Phillips, C.V. and Goodman, K.J. (2006) Causal criteria and counterfactuals; nothing more (or less) than scientific common sense. *Emerg Themes Epidemiol*, **3**, 5.

Renton, A. (1994) Epidemiology and causation: a realist view. *Journal of Epidemiology and Community Health*, **48**, 79–85.

Rigas, J., Feretis, C., and Papavassiliou, E.D. (1999) John Lykoudis: an unappreciated discoverer of the cause and treatment of peptic ulcer disease. *Lancet*, **354**, 1634–5.

Rothman, K.J. and Greenland, S. (2005) Causation and causal inference in epidemiology. *Am J Public Health*, **95**(Suppl 1), S144–S150.

Rothman, K.J. (1986) *Modern epidemiology*, 1st edn. Little, Brown, Boston.

Rothman, K.J. (1988) *Causal inference*. Epidemiology Resources Inc., Chestnut Hill, Massachusetts.

Rothman, K.J. and Greenland, S. (1998) *Modern epidemiology*. Lippincott-Raven, Philadelphia.

Semmelweis, I. (1983) *The etiology, concept and prophylaxis of childbed fever*, translated by K. Codell Carter. University of Wisconsin, Madison. Excerpted and reprinted in Buck *et al.* 1988, pp. 46–59.

Shrier, I., Boivin, J.F., Steele, R.J. *et al.* (2007) Should meta-analyses of interventions include observational studies in addition to randomized controlled trials? A critical examination of underlying principles. *American Journal of Epidemiology*, **166**, 1203–9.

Skrabanek, P. (1994) The emptiness of the black box. *Epidemiology*, **5**, 553–5.

Smith, G.D., Phillips, A.N. and Neaton, J.D. (1992) Smoking as 'independent' risk factor for suicide: illustration of an artifact from observational epidemiology? *Lancet*, **340**, 709–12.

Susser M. (2001) Glossary: causality in public health science. *J Epidemiol Comm Health*, **55**, 376–8.

Susser, M. (1977) *Causal thinking in the health sciences*, 2nd edn. Oxford University Press, New York.

Tesh, S.N. (1988) *Hidden arguments*. Rutgers University Press, New Brunswick.

Thygesen, L.C., Andersen, G.S. and Andersen, H. (2005) A philosophical analysis of the Hill criteria. *J Epidemiol Community Health*, **59**, 512–16.

Vineis, P. and Kriebel, D. (2006) Causal models in epidemiology: past inheritance and genetic future. *Environ Health*, **5**, 21.

Vineis, P. (1997) Proof in observational medicine. *Journal of Epidemiology and Community Health*, **51**, 9–13.

Wade, D.T. and Halligan, P.W. (2004) Do biomedical models of illness make for good healthcare systems? *British Medical Journal*, **329**, 1398–401.

Wald, N.J. and Morris, J.K. (2003) Teleoanalysis: combining data from different types of study. *British Medical Journal*, **327**, 616–18.

Weed, D. (1997) On the use of causal criteria. *International Journal of Epidemiology*, **26**, 1137–41.

Chapter 6

Fowkes, F. (1986) Diagnostic vigilance. *Lancet*, **i**, 493–4.

Grimes, D.A. and Schulz, K.F. (2002) Uses and abuses of screening tests. *Lancet*, **359**, 881–4.

Holland, W. and Stewart, S. (1990) *Screening in health care*. Nuffield Provincial Hospitals Trust, London.

Jones, J.H. (1993) *Bad blood. The Tuskegee Syphilis Experiment*, 2nd edn. Free Press, New York.

Khoury, M.J., McCabe, L.L. and McCabe, E.R. (2003) Population screening in the age of genomic medicine. *New England Journal of Medicine*, **348**, 50–8.

Last, J. (1963) The iceberg 'completing the clinical picture' in general practice. *Lancet*, **ii**, 28–31.

Last, J.M. (2001) *A dictionary of epidemiology*, 4th edn. Oxford University Press, New York.

Low N. (2007) Screening programmes for chlamydial infection: when will we ever learn? *British Medical Journal*, **334**, 725–8.

Marijon, E., Ou, P., Celermajer, D.S. *et al.* (2007) Prevalence of rheumatic heart disease detected by echocardiographic screening. *New England Journal of Medicine*, **357**, 470–6.

Raffle, A.E. (2000) Honesty about new screening programmes is best policy. *British Medical Journal*, **320**, 872.

Rothman, K.J. and Greenland, S. (1998) *Modern epidemiology*. Lippincott-Raven, Philadelphia.

Vernooij, M.W., Ikram, M.A., Tanghe, H.L. *et al.* (2007) Incidental findings on brain MRI in the general population. *New England Journal of Medicine*, **357**, 1821–8.

Wilson, J.M.G. and Jungner, G. (1968) *Principles and practice of screening for disease*. World Health Organization, Geneva.

Zimmern, R.L. and Kroese, M. (2007) The evaluation of genetic tests. *J Public Health (Oxf)*, **29**, 246–50.

Chapter 7

Barros, A.J. and Hirakata, V.N. (2003) Alternatives for logistic regression in cross-sectional studies: an empirical comparison of models that directly estimate the prevalence ratio. *BMC Med Res Methodol*, **3**, 21.

Berlin, A., Bhopal, R.S., Spencer, J.A., and van Zwanenberg, T.D. (1993) Creating a death register for general practice. *British Journal of General Practice*, **43**, 70–2.

Bodansky, H.J., Airey, CM., Chell, S.M., Unwin, N. and Williams, D.R.R. (1997) The incidence of lower limb amputation in Leeds, UK: setting a baseline for St Vincent. International Diabetes Federation Meeting. *Diabetologia*, A1850.

Calman, K. (1996) Cancer: science and society and the communication of risk. *British Medical Journal*, 313, 799–802.

Calman, K. and Royston, G. (1997) Risk language and dialects. *British Medical Journal*, 315, 939–42.

Choi, B., de Guia, N. and Walsh, P. (1998) Look before you leap, stratify before you standardize. *American Journal of Epidemiology*, 149, 1087–96.

Department of Health (1997) *Communicating about risks to public health: Pointers to good practice*, pp. 1–35. Department of Health, London.

Edwards, A., Elwyn, G. and Mulley, A. (2002) Explaining risks: turning numerical data into meaningful pictures. *British Medical Journal*, 324, 827–30.

Elandt-Johnson, R. (1975) Definition of rates: Some remarks on their use and misuse. *American Journal of Epidemiology*, 102, 267–71.

Gottlieb, S. (1999) Updates for US heart disease death rates. *British Medical Journal*, 318, 79.

International Working Group for Disease Monitoring and Forecasting (1995a) Capture–recapture and multiple-record systems estimation I: History and theoretical development. *American Journal of Epidemiology*, 142, 1047–58.

International Working Group for Disease Monitoring and Forecasting (1995b) Capture–recapture and multiple-record systems estimation II: Applications in human diseases. *American Journal of Epidemiology*, 142, 1059–68.

Last, J.M. (2001) *A dictionary of epidemiology*, 4th edn. Oxford University Press, New York.

Law, M.R. and Wald, N.J. (2002) Risk factor thresholds: their existence under scrutiny. *British Medical Journal*, 324, 1570–76.

Maudsley, G. and Williams, E. (1996) 'Inaccuracy' in death certification—where are we now? *Journal of Public Health Medicine*, 18, 59–66.

Paling, J. (2003) Strategies to help patients understand risks. *British Medical Journal*, 327, 745–8.

Pickles, W.N. (1939) *Epidemiology in country practice*. Wright, Bristol.

Rothman, K.J. and Greenland, S. (1998) *Modern epidemiology*. Lippincott-Raven, Philadelphia.

Sonderegger-Iseli, K., Burger, S., Muntwyler, J. and Salomon, F. (2000) Diagnostic errors in three medical eras: a necropsy study. *Lancet*, 355, 2027–32.

Tapia Granados, J.A. (1997) On the terminology and dimensions of incidence. *J Clin Epidemiol*, 50, 891–87.

The Global Lower Extremity Amputation Study Group (2000) Epidemiology of lower extremity amputation in centres in Europe, North America and East Asia. *British Journal of Surgery*, 87, 328–37.

Unwin, N., Alberti, K.G.M.M., Bhopal, R., Harland, J., Watson, W. and White, M. (1998) Comparison of the current WHO and the new ADA criteria for the diagnosis of diabetes in three ethnic groups in the UK. *Diabetic Medicine*, 15, 554–7.

World Health Organisation (1992) *ICD-10: International statistical classification of diseases and related health problems*. World Health Organisation, Geneva.

Chapter 8

Arnesen, T. and Nord, E. (1999) The value of DALY life: problems with ethics and validity of disability-adjusted life years. *British Medical Journal*, 319, 1423–6.

Bartlett, C.J. and Coles, E.C. (1998) Psychological health and well-being: why and how should public health specialists measure it? Part 1: rationale and methods of the investigation, and review of psychiatric epidemiology. *Journal of Public Health Medicine*, 20, 281–94.

Bland, J. and Altman, D. (2000) The odds ratio. *British Medical Journal*, 320, 1468.

Charlton, J.V.R. (1986) Some international comparisons of mortality amenable to medical intervention. *British Medical Journal*, **292**, 295–301.

Cook, R. and Sackett, D. (1995) The number needed to treat: a clinically useful measurement of treatment effect. *British Medical Journal*, **310**, 452–6.

Cornfield, J. (1951) A method of estimating comparative rates from clinical data. Applications to cancer of the lung, breast and cervix. *Journal of the National Cancer Institute*, **11**, 1269–75.

Cornfield, J. and Haenszel, W (1960) Some aspects of retrospective studies. *Journal of Chronic Disease*, **11**, 523–34.

Doll, R. and Bradford Hill, A. (1956) Lung cancer and other causes of death in relation to smoking. *British Medical Journal*, **2**, 1071–81.

Doll, R. and Hill, A.B. (1950) Smoking and carcinoma of the lung: preliminary report. *British Medical Journal*, **2**, 739–48.

Etches, V., Frank, J., Di, R.E. and Manuel, D. (2006) Measuring population health: a review of indicators. *Annu Rev Public Health* **27**, 29–55.

Gemmell, I., Heller, R.F., McElduff, P., Payne, K., Butler, G., Edwards, R., *et al.* (2005) Population impact of stricter adherence to recommendations for pharmacological and lifestyle interventions over one year in patients with coronary heart disease. *J Epidemiol Community Health*, **59**,1041–6.

Gemmell, I., Heller, R.F., Payne, K., Edwards, R., Roland, M. and Durrington, P. (2006) Potential population impact of the UK government strategy for reducing the burden of coronary heart disease in England: comparing primary and secondary prevention strategies. *Qual Saf Health Care*, **1**, 339–43.

Herbst, A., Ulfelder, H. and Poskanzer, D. (1971) Adenocarcinoma of the vagina: Association of maternal stilbestrol therapy with tumour appearance in young women. *New England Journal of Medicine*, **284**, 878–81.

Julious, S.A. and George, S. (2007) Are hospital league tables calculated correctly? *Public Health*, **121**, 902–4.

Julious, S., Nicholl, J. and George, S. (2000) Why do we continue to use standardized mortality ratios for small area comparisons? *Journal of Public Health Medicine*, **23**, 39–46.

Lee, W. (1998) The meaning and use of the cumulative rate of potential life lost. *International Journal ofEpidemiology*, **27**, 1053–6.

Li, W., Stanek, E.J., III and Bertone-Johnson, E.R. (2008) Should adjustment for covariates be used in prevalence estimations? *Epidemiol Perspect Innov*, **5**, 2.

Lopez, A.D., Mathers, C.D., Ezzati, M., Jamison, D.T. and Murray, C.J. (2006) Global and regional burden of disease and risk factors, 2001: systematic analysis of population health data. *Lancet*, **367**, 1747–57.

Low, A, and Low, A. (2006) Importance of relative measures in policy on health inequalities. *British Medical Journal*, **332**, 967–9.

Mackenbach, J.P., Bouvier-Colle, M.H. and Jougla, E. (1990) 'Avoidable' mortality and health services: a review of aggregate data studies. *Journal of Epidemiological and Community Health*, **44**, 106–11.

Mackintosh, J., Bhopal, R.S., Unwin, N. and Ahmad, N. (1998) *Step-by-step guide to epidemiological health needs assessment for ethnic minority groups*. Department of Epidemiology and Public Health, University of Newcastle upon Tyne, Newcastle upon Tyne. Available at www.minorityhealth.gov.uk/docs/step_by_step.doc.

Marmot, M.G., Adelstein, A.M. and Bulusu, L. (1984) *Immigrant mortality in England and Wales 1970–78*. HMSO, London.

Mausner, J.S. and Kramer, S. (1985) *Epidemiology*, 2nd edn. W.B. Saunders, Philadelphia.

Morrato, E.H., Elias, M. and Gericke, C.A. (2007) Using population-based routine data for evidence-based health policy decisions: lessons from three examples of setting and evaluating national health policy in Australia, the UK and the USA. *J Public Health (Oxf)*, **29**, 463–71.

Moser, K., Frost, C. and Leon, D.A. (2007) Comparing health inequalities across time and place—rate ratios and rate differences lead to different conclusions: analysis of cross-sectional data from 22 countries 1991–2001. *Int J Epidemiol*, **36**, 1285–91.

Murray, C.J.L. and Lopez, A.D. (1997) Mortality by cause for eight regions of the world: Global burden of disease study. *Lancet*, **349**, 1269–76.

Nolte, E. and McKee, M. (2003) Measuring the health of nations: analysis of mortality amenable to health care. *British Medical Journal*, **327**, 1129.

Pless-Mulloli T., Phillimore, P., Moffatt, S., Bhopal, R., Foy, C., Dunn, C. and Tate, J. (1998) Lung cancer, proximity to industry, and poverty in northeast England. *Environ Health Perspect*, **106**, 189–96.

Rockhill, B., Newman, B. and Weinberg, C. (1998) Use and misuse of population-attributable fractions. *American Journal of Public Health*, **88**, 15–19.

Roman, E., Beral, V., Inskip, H., McDowall, M. and Adelstein, A.A. (1984) Comparison of standardised proportional mortality ratios. *Statistics in Medicine*, **3**, 7–14.

Schwartz, L.M., Woloshin, S., Dvorin, E.L. and Welch, H.G. (2006) Ratio measures in leading medical journals: structured review of accessibility of underlying absolute risks. *British Medical Journal*, **333**, 1248.

Schwartz, L., Woloshin, S. and Welch, H. (1999) Misunderstandings about the effects of race and sex on physicians; referrals for cardiac catherization. *New England Journal of Medicine*, **341**, 279–85.

Silcocks, P.B.S., Jenner, D.A. and Reza, R. (2000) Life expectancy as a summary of mortality in a population: statistical considerations and suitability for use by health authorities. *Journal of Epidemiology and Community Health*, **55**, 38–43.

Singh, S.P. (1997) Ethnicity in psychiatric epidemiology: need for precision. *Br J Psychiatry*, **171**, 305–8.

Vandenbroucke, J. (1989) Statistical modelling: the old standardisation problem in disguise? *Journal of Epidemiology and Community Health*, **43**, 207–8.

Wyatt, J. (1999) Same information, different decisions: format counts. *British Medical Journal*, **318**, 1501–2.

Wilson, D. and Bhopal, R.S. (1998) Impact of infection on mortality and hospitalisation: a study in the North East of England. *Journal of Public Health Medicine*, **106**, 189–96.

Chapter 9

Barbenel, J., Jordan, M., Nicol, S. and Clark, M.O. (1977) Incidence of pressure-sores in the Greater Glasgow Health Board area. *Lancet*, **2**, 548–50.

Ben-Shlomo, Y. (2005) Real epidemiologists don't do ecological studies? *Int J Epidemiol* **34**, 1181–2.

Benson, K. and Hartz, A.J. (2000) A comparison of observational studies and randomized, controlled trials. *New England Journal of Medicine*, **342**, 1878–86.

Bhopal, R.S., Moffatt, S. and Pless-Mulloli, T. *et al.* (1998) Does living near a constellation of petro-chemical, steel, and other industries impair health? *Occupational and Environmental Medicine*, **55**, 812–22.

Bhopal, R.S., Unwin, N., White, M., Yallop, J., Walker, L. and Alberti, K.G.M.M. *et al.* (1999) Heterogeneity of coronary heart disease risk factors in Indian, Pakistani, Bangladeshi and European origin populations: cross sectional study. *British Medical Journal*, **319**, 215–20.

Cockings, S., Dunn, C., Bhopal, R. and Walker, D. (2004) Users' perspectives on epidemiological, GIS and point pattern approaches to analysing environment and health data. *Health and Place*, **10**, 169–82.

Coker, W.J., Bhatt, B.M., Blatchley, N.F. and Graham, J.T. (1999) Clinical findings for the first 1000 Gulf war veterans in the Ministry of Defence's medical assessment programme. *British Medical Journal*, **318**, 290–4.

Concato, J., Shah, N. and Horwitz, R.I. (2000) Randomized, controlled trials, observational studies, and the hierarchy of research designs. *New England Journal of Medicine*, **342**, 1887–92.

Cornfield, J. and Haenszel, W. (1960) Some aspects of retrospective studies. *Journal of Chronic Disease*, **11**, 523–34.

Dawber, T., Kannel, W. and Lyell, L. (1963) An approach to longitudinal studies in a community: The Framingham Study. *Annals New York Academy of Sciences*, **107**, 539–56. (Reprinted in Buck *et al.* 1988, pp. 619–630).

De Stavola, B.L., Nitsch, D., dos Santos Silva, I. *et al.* (2006) Statistical issues in life course epidemiology. *Am J Epidemiol*, **163**, 84–96.

Diez-Roux, A. (1998) Bringing context back into epidemiology: variables and fallacies in multilevel analysis. *American Journal of Public Health*, **88**, 1–13.

Dunn, C.E., Bhopal, R.S., Cockings, S., Walker, D., Rowlingson, B. and Diggle, P. (2007) Advancing insights into methods for studying environment-health relationships: a multidisciplinary approach to understanding Legionnaires' disease. *Health and Place*, **13**, 677–90.

Editorial (1990) Should we case-control? *The Lancet*, **335**, 1128.

Edwards, R., Pless-Mulloli, T., Howel, D., Chadwick, T., Bhopal, R., Harrison, R., *et al.* Does living near heavy industry cause lung cancer in women? A case-control study using life grid interviews. *Thorax*, 2006 Dec; 61(12): 1076–82.

Fletcher, J. (2007) Subgroup analyses: how to avoid being misled. *British Medical Journal*, **335**, 96–97.

Gatto, N.M., Campbell, U.B., Rundle, A.G. and Ahsan H. (2004) Further development of the case-only design for assessing gene-environment interaction: evaluation of and adjustment for bias. *Int J Epidemiol*, **33**, 1014–24.

Gregg, N.M. (1941) Congenital cataract following German measles in the mother. *Transactions of the Opthalmological Society of Australia*, **3**, 35–46. Reprinted in Buch *et al.* 1988, pp. 426–34.

Harland, J., Unwin, N., Bhopal, R.S., White, M., Watson, B., Laker, M. and Alberti, K.G.M.M. (1997) Low levels of cardiovascular risk factors and coronary heart disease in a UK Chinese population. *Journal of Epidemiology and Community Health*, **51**, 636–42.

Herbst, A., Ulfelder, H. and Poskanzer, D. (1971) Adenocarcinoma of the vagina: Association of maternal stilbestrol therapy with tumour appearance in young women. *New England Journal of Medicine*, **284**, 878–81.

Hopewell, S., Clarke, M., Moher, D. *et al.* (2008) CONSORT for reporting randomised controlled trials in journal and conference abstracts: explanation and elaboration. *PLoS Med*, **5**, 0048–0056.

Jha, P., Gajalakshmi, V., Gupta, P.C. *et al.* (2006) Prospective study of one million deaths in India: rationale, design, and validation results. *PLoS Med*, **3**, e18.

Keavney, B., Danesh, J., Parish, S. *et al.* (2006) Fibrinogen and coronary heart disease: test of causality by 'Mendelian randomization'. *Int J Epidemiol*, **35**, 935–43.

Kermack, W.O., McKendrick, A.G. and McKinlay, P.L. (2001) Death-rates in Great Britain and Sweden. Some general regularities and their significance. *Int J Epidemiol*, **30**, 678–83.

Krieger, N., Lowy, I., Aronowitz, R. *et al.* (2005) Hormone replacement therapy, cancer, controversies, and women's health: historical, epidemiological, biological, clinical, and advocacy perspectives. *J Epidemiol Community Health*, **59**, 740–8.

Magnusson, P.K., Rasmussen, F., Lawlor, D.A., Tynelius, P. and Gunnell, D. (2006) Association of body mass index with suicide mortality: a prospective cohort study of more than one million men. *Am J Epidemiol*, **163**, 1–8.

McMahon, B. and Trichopoulos, D. (1996) *Epidemiology*, 2nd edn. Little, Brown, Boston.

Mencken, H. L. (1928). Prejudices. 6th series. Jonathan Cape, London, p. 237.

Miettinen, O. (1976) Estimability and estimation in case-referent studies. *Am J Epidemiol* **103**, 226–35.

Nitsch, D., Molokhia, M., Smeeth, L., DeStavola, B.L., Whittaker, J.C. and Leon D.A. (2006) Limits to causal inference based on Mendelian randomization: a comparison with randomized controlled trials. *Am J Epidemiol*, **163**, 397–403.

Pearce, N. (2000) The ecological fallacy strikes back. *Journal of Epidemiology and Community, Health*, **54**, 326–7.

Perera, R., Heneghan, C. and Yudkin, P. (2007) Graphical method for depicting randomised trials of complex interventions. *British Medical Journal*, **334**, 127–9.

Poole, C. (1999) Controls who experienced hypothetical causal intermediates should not be excluded from case-control studies. *Am J Epidemiol*, **150**, 547–51.

Rich, A.R. (2007) On the frequency of occurrence of occult carcinoma of the prostrate. *Int J Epidemiol*, **36**, 274–7. (Reprinted from *J Urology* 1934; 33: 15–23)

Rose, K., Morgan, I., Smity, W., Burlutsky, G., Mitchell, P. and Saw, S. (2008) Myopia, lifestyle and schooling in students of Chinese ethnicity in Singapore and Sydney – an ecological approach. Archives of Ophthalmology, 126, 527–530.

Rothman, K.J. and Greenland, S. (1998) *Modern epidemiology*. Lippincott-Raven, Philadelphia.

Uusitalo, U., Feskens, E., Tuomilehto, J., Dowse, G., Haw, U. and Fareed, D. *et al.* (1996) Fall in total cholesterol concentration over five years in association with changes in fatty acid composition of cooking oil in Mauritius: cross-sectional survey. *British Medical Journal*, **313**, 1044–6.

Wen, S.W., Demissie, K., August, D. and Rhoads, G.G. (2001) Level of aggregation for optimal epidemiological analysis: the case of time to surgery and unnecessary removal of the normal appendix. *J Epidemiol Community Health*, **55**, 198–203.

Yusuf, S., Hawken, S., Ounpuu, S. *et al.* (2004) Effect of potentially modifiable risk factors associated with myocardial infarction in 52 countries (the INTERHEART study): case–control study. *Lancet*, **364**, 937–52.

Chapter 10

Action on Smoking and Health UK. Philip Morris Scandal documents show how Philip Morris and its lawyers, Covington and Burling invented and orchestrated controversy around passive smoking by infiltrating highly respected science and policy institution and by buying up scientists. Available at http://www.ash.org.uk/.

Alper, J.S. and Natowicz, M.R. (1992) The allure of genetic explanations. *British Medical Journal*, **305**, 666.

Armstrong, R., Waters, E., Moore, L. *et al.* (2008) Improving the reporting of public health intervention research: advancing TREND and CONSORT. *J Public Health (Oxf)*, **30**, 103–9.

Ashton, J. (ed.) (1994) *The epidemiological imagination. A reader*. Open University Press, Philadelphia.

Barkan, E. (1992) *The retreat of scientific racism*. Cambridge University Press, London.

Barnes, D.E. and Bero, L.A. (1998) Why review articles on the health effects of passive smoking reach different conclusions. *Journal of the American Medical Association*, **279**, 1566–70.

Beauchamp, T.L. Cook, R.R. Fayerweather, W.E., Raabe, G.K., Thar, W.E., Cowles, S.R., *et al.* (1991) Ethical guidelines for epidemiologists. *Journal of Clinical Epidemiology*, **44**, 151S–169S.

Bholal R. S. Challenges of collecting and interpreting data using the concepts of ethnicity and race. Ethnicity, race, and health in multicultural societies. Oxford: Oxford University Press; 2007. p. 29–59.

Bhopal, R. (1997) Is research into ethnicity and health racist, unsound, or important science? *British Medical Journal*, **314**, 1751–6.

Bhopal, R.S. (1998a) Setting priorities for health care in ethnic minority groups. In S. Rawaf and V. Bahl (eds) *Health needs assessment in ethnic minority groups*, pp.. Royal College of Physicians, London pp 57–64.

Bhopal, R.S. (1998b) The context and role of the American School of Public Health: Implications for the UK. *Journal of Public Health Medicine*, **20**, 144–8.

Bhopal, R.S. (1999) Paradigms in epidemiology textbooks: in the footsteps of Thomas Kuhn. *American Journal of Public Health*, **89**, 1162–5.

Bhopal, R.S. (2000) Race and ethnicity as epidemiological variables. In H. Macbeth (ed.) *Ethnicity and health*, pp. 21–40. Taylor and Francis, London.

Bhopal, R.S. (2001) Generating health from the pattern of disease. *Proceedings of the Royal College of Physicians of Edinburgh*, **31**, 293–8.

Bhopal, R.S. and Thomson, R.A. (1991) Form to help learn and teach about the assessment of medical audit papers. *British Medical Journal*, **303**, 1520–2.

Bhopal, R.S. and Tonks, A. (1994) The role of letters in reviewing research. *British Medical Journal*, **308**, 1582–3.

Bhopal, R.S., Rankin, J., McColl, E., Thomas, L., Kaner, E., Stacy, R., Pearson, P., Vernon, B. and Rodgers, H. (1997) The vexed question of authorship: views of researchers in a British medical faculty. *British Medical Journal*, **314**, 1009–12.

Bhopal, R.S. (2007) *Ethnicity, race, and health in multicultural societies; foundations for better epidemiology, public health, and health care*. Oxford, Oxford University Press, 2007, pp 357. http://www.oup.com/uk/catalogue/?ci=9780198568179

Blettner, M., Heuer, C. and Reeder, R.C. (2000) Critical reading of epidemiological papers. *European Journal of Public Health*, **11**, 97–101.

Blettner, M., Sauerbrei, W., Schlehofer, B. and Scheuchenpflug, T. (1999) Traditional reviews, meta-analyses and pooled analyses in epidemiology. *International Journal of Epidemiology*, **28**, 1–9.

Bobrow, M. and Grimbaldeston, A. (2000) Medical genetics, the human genome project and public health. *Journal of Epidemiology and Community Health*, **54**, 645–9.

Bonneux, L., Barendregt, J. and Van der Maas, P. (1998) The expiry date of man: a synthesis of evolutionary biology and public health. *Journal of Epidemiology and Community Health*, **52**, 619–23.

Bottomley, V. (1993) Priority setting in the NHS. Ch 3 in *Rationing in Action*, p. 25–32. London, BMJ Publishing Group.

Brown, P. (1992) Popular epidemiology and toxic waste contamination: Lay and professional ways of knowing. *Journal of Health and Social Behaviour*, **33**, 267–81.

Buckley, B., Murphy, A.W., Byrne, M. and Glynn, L. (2007) Selection bias resulting from the requirement for prior consent in observational research: a community cohort of people with ischaemic heart disease. *Heart*, **93**, 1116–20.

Carlson, R.V., Boyd, K.M. and Webb, D.J. (2004) The revision of the Declaration of Helsinki: past, present and future. *Br J Clin Pharmacol*, **57**, 695–713.

Carpiano, R.M. and Daley, D.M. (2006) A guide and glossary on post-positivist theory building for population health. *J Epidemiol Community Health*, **60**, 564–70.

Chadwick, J. and Mann, W.N. (1950) *The medical works of Hippocrates*. Blackwell Scientific, Oxford.

Colditz, G. (1997) Epidemiology—future directions. *International Journal of Epidemiology*, **26**, 693–7.

Committee for the Study of the Future of Public Health (Institute of Medicine) (1988) *The future of public health*. National Academy Press, Washington, DC.

Committee of Inquiry (1988) *Public health in England*. HMSO, London.

Cooper, R. (1984) A note on the biological concept of race and its application in epidemiological research. *American Heart Journal*, **108**, 715–23.

Day, R.A. (1994) *How to write and publish a scientific paper*, 4th edn. Oryx, Phoenix.

Department for Business Enterprise and Regulatory Reform (BERR) (2007) Rigour, respect and responsibility: A universal ethical code for scientists. 1. Available at (http://www.berr.gov.uk/dius/science/science-and-society/public_engagement/code/page28030.html).

Diez Roux, A.V. (2002) A glossary for multilevel analysis. *J Epidemiol Community Health*, **56**, 588–94.

Down, J.L.H. (1995) Observations on an ethnic classification of idiots (reprinted from *Journal of Mental Science*, 1867). *Mental Retardation*, **3**, 54–6.

Edwards, R. and Bhopal, R. (1999) The covert influence of the tobacco industry on research and publication: a call to arms. *Journal of Epidemiology and Community Health*, **53**, 261–2.

Edwards, R., Pless-Mulloli, T., Howel, D., Chadwick, T., Bhopal, R., Harrison, R., et al. Does living near heavy industry cause lung cancer in women? A case-control study using life grid interviews. Thorax 2006 Dec; 61(12): 1076–82.

Gamble, V. (1993) A legacy of distrust: African Americans and medical research. *American Journal of Preventive Medicine*, **9**, 35–7.

Gotzsche, P.C. (2006) Believability of relative risks and odds ratios in abstracts: cross sectional study. *British Medical Journal*, **333**, 231–4.

Greenland, S. (ed.) (1987) *Evolution of epidemiologic ideas: Annotated readings on concepts and methods.* Epidemiology Resources Inc, Massachusetts.

Herbst, A., Ulfelder, H. and Poskanzer, D. (1971) Adenocarcinoma of the vagina: Association of maternal stilbestrol therapy with tumour appearance in young women. *New England Journal of Medicine*, **284**, 878–1.

Hilts, P.J. (1996) *Smokescreen: the truth behind the tobacco industry cover-up.* Addison-Wesley, Massachusetts.

Hopewell, S., Clarke, M., Moher, D. *et al.* (2008) CONSORT for reporting randomised trials in journal and conference abstracts. *The Lancet*, **371**, 281–3.

Horton, R. (1998) The unmasked carnival of science. *Lancet*, **351**, 688–9.

Huth, E.J. (1990) *How to write and publish papers in the medical sciences*, 2nd edn. Williams and Wilkins, Baltimore.

Ingelfinger, J.R. and Drazen, J.M. (2204) Registry research and medical privacy. *New England Journal of Medicine*, **350**, 1452–3.

International Committee of Medical Journal Editors (1997) Uniform requirements for manuscripts submitted to biomedical journals. *Journal of the American Medical Association*, **277**, 927–34. (See http://www.icmje.org/ for update).

Iversen, A., Liddell, K., Fear, N., Hotopf, M. and Wessely, S. (2006) Consent, confidentiality, and the Data Protection Act. *British Medical Journal*, **332**, 165–9.

Jenner, E. (1798) An inquiry in to the causes and effects of the variolae vaccine. Excerpt in Buck *et al.* 1988, pp. 31–2.

Jones, J.H. (1993) *Bad blood. The Tuskegee Syphilis Experiment*, 2nd edn. Free Press, New York.

Kalra, D., Gertz, R., Singleton, P. and Inskip, H.M. (2006) Confidentiality of personal health information used for research. *British Medical Journal*, **333**, 196–8.

Kavvoura, F.K., Liberopoulos, G. and Ioannidis, J.P. (2007) Selection in reported epidemiological risks: an empirical assessment. *PLoS Med*, **4**, e79.

Kiple, K.F. and King, V.H. (1981) *Another dimension to the black diaspora.* Cambridge University Press, London.

Krieger, N. (1992) The making of public health data: paradigms, politics, and policy. *Journal of Public Health Policy*, **65**, 412–27.

Krieger, N.D., Rowley, D.L. and Herman, A. (1993) Racism, sexism and social class: implications for studies of health, disease, and wellbeing. *American Journal of Preventive Medicine*, **9**, 82–122.

Kuhn, T.S. (1996) *The structure of scientific revolutions*, 3rd edn. The University of Chicago Press, Chicago.

Last, J.M. (1990) Guidelines on ethics for epidemiologists. *International Journal of Epidemiology*, **19**, 226–9.

Lawlor, D.A. (2007) Quality in epidemiological research: should we be submitting papers before we have the results and submitting more hypothesis-generating research? *Int J Epidemiol* **36**, 940–3.

Lilienfeld, D.E. (2007) The general epidemiologist: is there a place in today's epidemiology? *Am J Epidemiol*, 166, 1–4.

Lilienfeld, D.E. and Stolley, P.D. (1994) *Foundations of epidemiology*, 3rd edn. Oxford University Press, New York.

Lillie-Blanton, M., Anthony, J.C. and Schuster, C.R. (1993) Probing the meaning of racial/ethnic group comparisons in crack smoking. *Journal of the American Medical Association*, 269, 993–7.

Lind, J. (1753) *A Treatise of the Scurvy in three parts, containing an inquiry into the nature, causes, and cure of the scurvy*. Excerpted from James Lind, *A Treatise of the Scurvy in Three Parts, Containing an enquiry into the nature, causes and cure of that disease, together with a critical and chronological view of what has been published on the subject*. Sands Murray and Cochran, Edinburgh, and reprinted in Buck *et al.* 1988, pp 20–23.

Mackenbach, J.P. (2004) Streets of Paris, sunflower seeds, and Nobel prizes. Reflections on the quantitative paradigm of public health. *J Epidemiol Community Health*, 58, 734–7.

Mackenbach, J.P. (2006) The origins of human disease: a short story on 'where diseases come from'. *J Epidemiol Community Health*, 60, 81–6.

MacMahon, B., Pugh, T.F. and Ipsen, J. (1960) *Epidemiological methods*. J and A Churchill, London.

March, D. and Susser, E. (2006) The eco- in eco-epidemiology. *Int J Epidemiol*, 35, 1379–83.

Marmot, M.G., Adelstein, A.M. and Bulusu, L. (1984) *Immigrant mortality in England and Wales 1970–78*. HMSO, London.

Mausner, J.S. and Kramer, S. (1985) *Epidemiology*, 2nd edn. W. B. Saunders Company, Philadelphia.

Merlo, J., Chaix, B., Yang, M., Lynch, J. and Rastam L. (2005) A brief conceptual tutorial of multilevel analysis in social epidemiology: linking the statistical concept of clustering to the idea of contextual phenomenon. *J Epidemiol Community Health*, 59, 443–9.

Merlo, J., Yang, M., Chaix, B., Lynch, J. and Rastam, L. (2005) A brief conceptual tutorial on multilevel analysis in social epidemiology: investigating contextual phenomena in different groups of people. *J Epidemiol Community Health*, 59, 729–36.

Moher, D., Tetzlaff, J., Tricco, A.C., Sampson, M. and Altman, D.G. 92007) Epidemiology and reporting characteristics of systematic reviews. *PLoS Med*, 4, e78.

Morabia, A. (2007) Epidemiologic interactions, complexity, and the lonesome death of Max von Pettenkofer. *American Journal of Epidemiology*, 166, 1233–8.

Morabia A. (2007) Morabia responds to 'The context and challenge of von Pettenkofer's contributions to epidemiology'. *American Journal of Epidemiology*, 166, 1242–3.

Morris, J.N. (1964) *Uses of epidemiology*, 2nd edn. The Williams and Wilkins Company, Baltimore.

Morrison, T. (1993) *Beloved*. Chatto and Windus, London.

Olsen, J. (2007) Good epidemiological practice (GEP) proper conduct in epidemiologic research. See http://www.dundee.ac.uk/iea/GEP07.htm, for update.

Oppenheimer, G.M. and Susser, E. (2007) Invited commentary: the context and challenge of von Pettenkofer's contributions to epidemiology. *American Journal of Epidemiology*, 166, 1239–41.

Osborne, N.G. and Feit, M.D. (1992) The use of race in medical research. *Journal of the American Medical Association*, 267, 275–9.

Pearce, N. (2008) Corporate influences on epidemiology. *Int J Epidemiol*, 37, 46–53.

Pearce, N. and Merletti, F. (2006) Complexity, simplicity, and epidemiology. *Int J Epidemiol*, 35, 515–19.

Pearce, N. (1996) Traditional epidemiology, modern epidemiology, and public health. *American Journal of Public Health*, 86, 678–83.

Popay, J. (2006) Whose theory is it anyway? *J Epidemiol Community Health*, 60, 571–2.

Porta, M. and Alvarez-Dardet, C. (1998) Epidemiology: bridges over (and across) roaring levels. *Journal of Epidemiology and Community Health*, 52, 605.

Porter, R. (1997) *The greatest benefit to mankind: A medical history of humanity from antiquity to the present*. Harper Collins, London.

Potter, J.D. (2005) Epidemiology informing clinical practice: from bills of mortality to population laboratories. *Nat Clin Pract Oncol*, **2**, 625–34.

Reynolds, G. (1993) Foreword. *Annals of Epidemiology*, **3**, 119.

Rothman, K.J. (2007) The rise and fall of epidemiology, 1950–2000 A.D. *Int J Epidemiol*, **36**, 708–10. Reprinted from NEJM 1981; 304: 600–602.

Rothman, K., Adami, H. and Trichopoulos, D. (1998) Should the mission of epidemiology include the eradication of poverty? *Lancet*, **352**, 810–13.

Rothman, K. J. Measuring Disease Occurence and Causal Effects. Epidemiology An Introduction. New York: Oxford University Press; 2002. p. 24–56.

Rothman, K. J. Types of Epidemiologic Study. Epidemiology An Introduction. New York: Oxford University Press; 2002. p. 57–93.

Sanderson, S., Tatt, I.D. and Higgins, J.P. (2007) Tools for assessing quality and susceptibility to bias in observational studies in epidemiology: a systematic review and annotated bibliography. *Int J Epidemiol*, **36**, 666–76.

Saracci, R. (1997) The World Health Organization needs to reconsider its definition of health. *British Medical Journal*, **314**, 1409–10.

Saracci, R. (2007) Epidemiology: a science for justice in health. *Int J Epidemiol*, **36**, 265–8.

Semmelweis, I. (1983) *The etiology, concept and prophylaxis of childbed fever*, translated by K. Codell Carter. University of Wisconsin, Madison. Excerpted and reprinted in Buck *et al.* 1988, pp. 46–59.

Singer, E. and Bossarte, R.M. (2006) Incentives for survey participation when are they 'coercive'? *Am J Prev Med*, **31**, 411–18.

Skrabanek, P. and McCormick, J. (1992) *Follies and fallacies in medicine*, 2nd edn. Tarragon Press, Chippenham, UK. (Download from: www.medicine, tcd.ie/public_health_primary_care/skrabanek/publications.phf

Smith, A. (1978) The epidemiological basis of community medicine. In A.E. Bennett (ed.) *Recent advances in community medicine*, pp. 1–10. Longman, Edinburgh.

Snow, J. (1949) *The Cholera near Golden Square* (extracted from *Snow on Cholera*, Cambridge, Hybrid University Press.) Reprinted in Buck *et al.* 1988, pp. 415–418. *The challenge of epidemiology. Issues and selected readings*, pp. 415–18. Pan American Health Organization, Washington DC.

Stepan, N. (1982) *The idea of race in science*. MacMillan Press, London.

Stoto, M., Abel, C. and Dievler, A. (1996) *Healthy communities: New partnerships for the future of public health* (Institute of Medicine). National Academy Press, Washington DC.

Stroup, D.F., Berlin, J.A., Morton, S.C. *et al.* (2000) Meta-analysis of observational studies in epidemiology: a proposal for reporting. Meta-analysis Of Observational Studies in Epidemiology (MOOSE) group. *JAMA*, **283**, 2008–12.

Susser, M. (1985) Epidemiology in the United States after World War II: the evolution of technique. *Epidemiologic Reviews*, **7**, 147–7.

Susser, M. (1998) Does risk factor epidemiology put epidemiology at risk? Peering into the future. *Journal of Epidemiology and Community Health*, **52**, 608–11.

Terris, M. (1978) Epidemiology as a basic science in the education of health professionals. *International Journal of Epidemiology*, **7**, 294–6.

US Department of Health and Human Services—Public Health Service (1990) *Healthy People 2000*. National health promotion and disease prevention objectives. Department of Health and Human Services, Washington, DC.

Vandenbroucke, J.P., von Elm, E., Altman, D.G. *et al.* (2007) Strengthening the Reporting of Observational Studies in Epidemiology (STROBE): explanation and elaboration. *PLoS Med*, **4**, e297.

Ward, H.J., Cousens, S.N., Smith-Bathgate, B. *et al.* (2004) Obstacles to conducting epidemiological research in the UK general population. *British Medical Journal*, **329**, 277–279.

Weed, D.L. and McKeown, R.E. (1998) Epidemiology and virtue ethics. *International Journal of Epidemiology*, **27**, 343–9.

Winkelstein, W. (1996) Editorial: Eras, paradigms, and the future of epidemiology. *American Journal of Public Health*, **86**, 621–2.

Wright, J., Williams, R. and Wilkinson, J. (1998) Development and importance of health needs assessment. *British Medical Journal*, **316**, 1310–14.

Websites

The task of compiling a comprehensive list of relevant websites would be futile, because there are so many and the pace of change is so rapid. Obviously, an Internet search program will bring thousands of websites to your attention. So, here is a small selection that will provide a valuable return for your time and links to many others.

American College of Epidemiology
http://www.acepidemiology2.org/policystmts/EthicsGuide.asp

CDC (Centres for Disease Control and Prevention)
http://www.cdc.gov/

Epi monitor
http://www.epimonitor.net/index.htm

Epidemiology.net Epidemiology learning materials
http://www.epidemiolog.net/

Equator network. Guidelines for reporting systematic reviews and meta-analyses.
http://www.equator-network.org:80/?o=1073

EUPHA (European Public Health Association)
http://www.eupha.org/

History of Epidemiology and its concepts
http://www.epidemiology.ch/index3.htm

International Classification of Diseases
ftp://ftp.cdc.gov/pub/Health_Statistics/NCHS/Publications/ICD10/each10.txt

International Epidemiological Association (IEA)
http://www.dundee.ac.uk/iea/

Medicine and Health: Epidemiology http://www.epibiostat.ucsf.edu/epidem/epi-dem.html

PAHO (Pan American Health Organisation)
http://www.paho.org/

Research Process Flow Chart
http://www.rdinfo.org.uk/flowchart/Flowchart.html

Supercourse. Epidemiology, the Internet and Global Health
http://www.pitt.edu/~super1/index1.htm

Society for Social Medicine (SSM)
http://www.socsocmed.org.uk/

WHO (World Health Organisation)
http://www.who.int/en/

Appendix

Curriculum for teaching in taught courses: suggestions

The key objective for Master's level postgraduate students is a thorough but broad grasp of the strengths and weaknesses of the epidemiological approach and the principles of sound data interpretation. They can build on such a foundation in doctoral and postdoctoral work.

Undergraduate students need to see the scope of the subject and its potential relevance to their own studies. Above all the undergraduate's interest must be captured and held. Techniques are unlikely to be important for most such students (until they are doing their own projects, when they need to know sources of highly specific advice).

Policy-makers and managers need to see the grand scope of the subject and its potential relevance to the solution of their health and health service challenges. The route to this will usually lie with examples of the application of epidemiology and not causal research.

These suggestions for a course curriculum assume literacy and numeracy at the level expected in a 16–17-year-old person who studies maths, English and science. No exposure to medicine or medical sciences is necessary, though it is helpful. This book is designed for postgraduate and continuing professional education but has proven itself useful in a wider arena. I base these ideas on my courses for managers (half-day), professionals and students.

To teach on virtually the entire content of the book is feasible (in my experience based on the 1st edition) in about 12 lectures (50 minutes each) with 12 practical sessions of the same length. This suits courses based on 15-week semesters as these usually have 12 or 13 teaching weeks. Teachers running shorter courses will need to make choices on material to be left out, or to be identified as for private study. Examples of examination questions are given in each chapter.

These suggestions follow the section headings and numbers by chapter. If an item is in parenthesis I consider it as optional – this applies to the first two columns.

Chapter and section heading/number	Postgraduate or CPD (12–13 weeks with about 25 contact hours)	Postgraduate or CPD (10 weeks with 20 contact hours)	Undergraduate medical or health sciences students (5 weeks with 10 contact hours)	Policy-makers and managers (4 contact hours)
1 What is epidemiology? The nature and scope of a biological, clinical, social, and ecological science and of its variables				
1.1 The individual and the population	✓	✓	✓	✓

Chapter and section heading/number	Postgraduate or CPD (12–13 weeks with about 25 contact hours)	Postgraduate or CPD (10 weeks with 20 contact hours)	Undergraduate medical or health sciences students (5 weeks with 10 contact hours)	Policy-makers and managers (4 contact hours)
1.2 Definition of epidemiology and statement of its central paradigm	✓	✓	✓	✓
1.3 Directions in epidemiology and its uses	✓	✓	✓	✓
1.4 Epidemiology as a science, practice, and craft	✓	(✓)		
1.5 The nature of epidemiological variables	✓	✓	✓	
1.6 Definition and diagnosis of disease: an illustration of the interdependence of clinical medicine and epidemiology	✓	✓		
1.7 The basic tools of epidemiology: measuring disease frequency and study design	See chapters 7–9			
1.8 Seeking the theoretical foundations of epidemiology	✓	(✓)		
Summary				
2 The epidemiological concept of population				
2.1 The individual and the population	✓	✓	✓	✓
2.2 Harnessing variety in dividual and group level disease and risk factor patterns	✓	✓		
2.3 Disease patterns as an outcome of individuals living in changing social groups	✓	✓	✓	
2.4 Sick populations and sick individuals	✓	✓	✓	✓
2.5 Individual and population level epidemiological variables	(✓)			
2.6 Epidemiology and demography: interdependent population sciences	✓	✓		
2.7 The dynamic nature of human population	✓			
2.8 Applications of the epidemiological population concept	✓	✓		✓
2.9 Conclusion	✓			
Summary				

Chapter and section heading/number	Postgraduate or CPD (12–13 weeks with about 25 contact hours)	Postgraduate or CPD (10 weeks with 20 contact hours)	Undergraduate medical or health sciences students (5 weeks with 10 contact hours)	Policy-makers and managers (4 contact hours)
3 Variation in disease by time, place, and person:				
A framework for analysis				
3.1 Introduction	✓	✓	✓	✓
3.2 Reasons for analysing disease variations	✓	✓	✓	✓
3.3 Introducing human genetic variation and genetic epidemiology	✓	✓	✓	
3.3.1 The human genome	✓			
3.3.2 Genomic variation as the basis of human disease and population variation	✓			
3.3.3 Susceptibility to diseases, chronic diseases and genetics	✓	(✓)		
3.3.4 Tools of genetic epidemiology	✓	(✓)		
3.3.5 Population level differences in disease and genetics: the example of race	✓	✓		
3.4 Variations and associations: real or artefact?	✓	✓	✓	
3.5 Applying the real-artefact framework	✓	✓	✓	
3.6 Disease clustering and clusters in epidemiology	✓	(✓)		
3.7 Applications of observations of disease variation	✓	✓	✓	✓
3.8 Epidemiological theory underpinning or arising from this chapter	✓			
3.9 Conclusion	✓	✓		
Summary				
4 Error, bias, confounding and risk modification/interaction in epidemiology				
4.1 Introduction	✓	✓	✓	✓
4.2 A classification of error and bias	✓	✓		
4.2.1 Bias in the research question, theme or hypothesis	✓	✓	✓	✓
4.2.2 Choice of population—selection bias	✓	✓		
4.2.3 Non-participation: non-response bias	✓	✓		

Chapter and section heading/number	Postgraduate or CPD (12–13 weeks with about 25 contact hours)	Postgraduate or CPD (10 weeks with 20 contact hours)	Undergraduate medical or health sciences students (5 weeks with 10 contact hours)	Policy-makers and managers (4 contact hours)
4.2.4 Comparing disease patterns and risk factor-disease-outcome relationships in populations which differ (context for confounding)	✓	✓	✓	
4.2.5 Risk/effect modification, susceptibility and interaction	✓	(✓)		
4.2.6 Measurement errors: differential and non-differential	✓	✓		
4.2.7 Misclassification bias: non-differential measurement errors, and regression to the mean	✓	✓		
4.2.8 Analysis and interpretation	✓	✓		✓
4.2.9 Publication	✓	✓		✓
4.2.10 Judgement and action				
4.3 A practical application of the research chronology schema of bias and error	✓	✓		
4.4 Conclusion	✓	✓	✓	✓
Summary				
5 Cause and effect: The epidemiological approach				
5.1 Introduction: causality in science and philosophy	✓	✓	✓	✓
5.2 Epidemiological causal strategy and reasoning: the example of Semmelweiss	✓	✓	✓	✓
5.3 Models of cause in epidemiology	✓	✓		
5.3.1 Interplay of host, agent, and environment	✓	✓	✓	
5.3.2 Necessary and sufficient cause, proximal and distal cause and the interacting component causes, models	✓	✓		
5.4 Guidelines (elsewhere criteria) for epidemiological reasoning on cause and effect	✓	✓		
5.4.1 Comparison of epidemiological and other concepts of causal reasoning	✓	(✓)		
5.4.2 Application of causal guidelines to associations	✓	✓	✓	

Chapter and section heading/number	Postgraduate or CPD (12–13 weeks with about 25 contact hours)	Postgraduate or CPD (10 weeks with 20 contact hours)	Undergraduate medical or health sciences students (5 weeks with 10 contact hours)	Policy-makers and managers (4 contact hours)
5.4.3 Judging the causal basis of the association	✓	✓		
5.4.4 Reviews, systematic reviews and meta-analysis	✓	(✓)	✓	
5.4.5 Interpretation of data, paradigms, study design, and causal criteria	✓	✓		
5.5 Epidemiological theory illustrated by this chapter	✓	✓		
5.6 Conclusion	✓	✓	✓	✓
Summary				
6 Interrelated concepts in the epidemiology of disease: natural history, spectrum, iceberg, population patterns, and screening				
6.1 Natural history of disease, the incubation period and acute/chronic diseases	✓	✓	✓	✓
6.2 The population pattern of disease: changes over time (secular trends)	✓	✓		
6.3 Spectrum of disease: a clinical concept fundamental to epidemiology	✓	✓	✓	
6.4 The unmeasured burden of disease: the metaphors of the iceberg and the pyramid	✓	✓	✓	✓
6.5 Screening: picking up disease or disease susceptibility early	✓	✓	✓	
6.5.1 Introduction: definition, purposes, and ethics	✓	✓	✓	✓
6.5.2 Choosing what to screen for: criteria of Wilson and Jungner	✓	(✓)		
6.5.3 Sensitivity, specificity, and predictive powers of screening tests	✓	✓	✓	
6.5.4 Setting the cut-off point for a positive screening test: introducing the relation between sensitivity and specificity and the ROC curve	✓			
6.5.5 Distributions of the factors we are screening for – explaining the relations between sensitivity and specificity	✓			

Chapter and section heading/number	Postgraduate or CPD (12–13 weeks with about 25 contact hours)	Postgraduate or CPD (10 weeks with 20 contact hours)	Undergraduate medical or health sciences students (5 weeks with 10 contact hours)	Policy-makers and managers (4 contact hours)
6.6 Applications of the concepts of natural history, spectrum, population pattern and screening	✓	✓		✓
6.7 Epidemiological theory: symbiosis with clinical medicine and social sciences	✓	✓		
6.8 Conclusion	✓	✓		
Summary				
7 The concept of risk and fundamental measures of disease frequency: incidence and prevalence				
7.1 Introduction: risks, risk factors, and causes	✓	✓	✓	✓
7.2 Quantifying disease frequency, risk factors, and their relationships: issues of terminology	✓	✓		
7.3 Numerator: defining, diagnosing, coding disease accurately	✓	✓	✓	
7.4 Incidence and incidence rate: the concepts of person-time incidence and cumulative incidence	✓	✓	✓	
7.5 Denominator	✓	✓	✓	
7.6 Prevalence and prevalence rate	✓	✓	✓	
7.7 Relationship of incidence and prevalence	✓			
7.8 Choice of incidence or prevalence measures	✓	✓		
7.9 Presenting rates: overall and specific	✓	✓	✓	✓
7.10 Conclusion	✓	✓		
Summary				
8 Presentation and interpretation of epidemiological data on risk				
8.1 Introduction	✓	✓	✓	✓
8.2 Proportional morbidity or mortality ratio	✓	✓		
8.3 Adjusted overall rates: standardization and the calculation of the SMR (standardized mortality ratio)	✓	✓		
8.3.1 Direct standardization	✓	✓		
8.3.2 Indirect standardization	✓	✓		

Chapter and section heading/number	Postgraduate or CPD (12–13 weeks with about 25 contact hours)	Postgraduate or CPD (10 weeks with 20 contact hours)	Undergraduate medical or health sciences students (5 weeks with 10 contact hours)	Policy-makers and managers (4 contact hours)
8.4 Relative measure: relative risk	✓	✓	✓	✓
8.5 The odds ratio (OR)	✓	✓		
8.6 Measurements to assess the impact of a risk factor in groups and populations: attributable risk and related measures	✓	✓	✓	✓
8.6.1 Attributable risk/exposed group: estimating benefits of changing exposure in the at risk group	✓	✓		
8.6.2 Population attributable risk and population impact number: estimating the benefits of reducing exposure in the population as a whole	✓	(✓)		
8.7 Presentation and interpretation of epidemiological data in applied settings	✓	✓	✓	✓
8.8 Avoidable morbidity and mortality and life-years lost	✓	(✓)	✓	✓
8.9 Comparison of summary measures of health status	✓			
8.10 Disability-adjusted life years and quality-adjusted life years	✓		✓	✓
8.11 Numbers needed to treat (NNT) or to prevent (NNP); and the number of events prevented in your population (NEPP)	✓	✓ (NNT only)	✓ (NNT only)	✓ (NNT only)
8.12 Describing the health status of a population	✓	(✓)		✓
8.13 The construction and development of health status indicators	✓			
8.14 Conclusion	✓	✓		
Summary				
9 Epidemiological study design: an integrated suite of methods				
9.1 Introduction: interdependence of study design in epidemiology, and the importance of the base population	✓	✓	✓	✓
9.2 Classifications of study design: five dichotomies	✓	(✓)		
9.3 Case-series: clinical and population based register studies	✓	✓		
9.3.1 Overview	✓	✓	✓	✓

Chapter and section heading/number	Postgraduate or CPD (12–13 weeks with about 25 contact hours)	Postgraduate or CPD (10 weeks with 20 contact hours)	Undergraduate medical or health sciences students (5 weeks with 10 contact hours)	Policy-makers and managers (4 contact hours)
9.3.2 Design of a case series	✓	✓		
9.3.3 Analysis of case series	✓	✓		
9.3.4 Unique insights from case series	✓	✓		
9.4 Cross-sectional study				
9.4.1 Overview	✓	✓	✓	✓
9.4.2 Design	✓	✓		
9.4.3 Value and limitations	✓	✓		
9.4.4 Cross-sectional studies in relation to the iceberg, spectrum and natural history of disease	✓	✓		
9.4.5 Cross-sectional studies in relation to case series, calculating of incidence, and comparative potential	✓	(✓)		
9.5 Case–control study				
9.5.1 Overview	✓	✓	✓	✓
9.5.2 Design and analysis	✓	✓		
9.5.3 Population base for case–control studies	✓	(✓)		
9.6 Cohort study				
9.6.1 Overview	✓	✓	✓	✓
9.6.2 Design	✓	✓		
9.7 Trials—population-based experiments				
9.7.1 Overview	✓	✓	✓	✓
9.7.2 Design	✓	✓	✓	
9.8 Overlap in the conceptual basis of the case-series, cross-sectional, case–control, cohort, and trial designs; and strengths and weaknesses	✓	✓		
9.9 Ecological studies: mode of analysis?				
9.9.1 Overview	✓	(✓)		
9.9.2 Some fallacies: ecological, atomistic and homogeneity	✓	(✓)		
9.10 Size of the study	✓	(✓)	(✓)	
9.11 Data analysis and interpretation	✓	(✓)		
9.11.1 Planning the analysis	✓	✓		

Chapter and section heading/number	Postgraduate or CPD (12–13 weeks with about 25 contact hours)	Postgraduate or CPD (10 weeks with 20 contact hours)	Undergraduate medical or health sciences students (5 weeks with 10 contact hours)	Policy-makers and managers (4 contact hours)
9.11.2 Focus	✓	(✓)		
9.11.3 Errors	✓	(✓)		
9.11.4 Validity	✓	(✓)		
9.11.5 Handling continuous data using correlation and regression: contributions to causal thinking	✓	(✓)		
9.11.6 Generalization	✓	(✓)		
9.11.7 Burden	✓	(✓)		
9.11.8 Comparability	✓	(✓)		
9.11.9 Summarizing the contrasts	✓	(✓)		
9.11.10 Interactions	✓	(✓)		
9.11.11 Accounting for error, bias and confounding	✓	(✓)		
9.11.12 Causality	✓	(✓)		
9.11.13 Write-up	✓	(✓)		
9.12 Conclusion	✓	✓		
Summary				
10 Epidemiology in the future: Theory, ethics, context, and critical appraisal				
10.1 The interrelationship of theory, methods, and application: responding to criticisms of modern epidemiology	✓	✓		
10.2 Fundamental influences on health and disease in populations	✓	✓	✓	✓
10.3 Theory and practice: role of epidemiology	✓	✓		
10.4 Practice to theory to techniques and back	✓			
10.4.1 Setting priorities in health and health care	(✓)			✓
10.4.2 Impact on health of local polluting industries: Teesside study of environment and health	✓	✓		
10.5 Paradigms: the evolution of sciences, including epidemiology	✓	✓		
10.6 Epidemiology: forces for change	✓	✓	✓	✓

Chapter and section heading/number	Postgraduate or CPD (12–13 weeks with about 25 contact hours)	Postgraduate or CPD (10 weeks with 20 contact hours)	Undergraduate medical or health sciences students (5 weeks with 10 contact hours)	Policy-makers and managers (4 contact hours)
10.7 Scope of epidemiology and specialization	(✓)			
10.8 The context of epidemiological practice—academic and service, USA and UK	(✓)			
10.9 The practice of epidemiology in public health	✓	✓		✓
10.10 Ethical basis and proper conduct of epidemiology: the need for a code	✓	✓	✓	
10.10.1 The tobacco industry	✓	(✓)	✓	✓
10.10.2 Authorship	✓			
10.10.3 Ethnicity and race	✓			
10.11 Ethical guidelines	✓	✓		
10.12 Critical appraisal in epidemiology: separating fact from error and fallacy	✓	✓	✓	
10.12.1 Some fallacies	✓	✓	✓	
10.12.2 The nature of critical appraisal	✓	✓	✓	
10.13 Some questions relevant to the appraisal of epidemiological research	✓	✓	(✓)	
10.14 Building on an epidemiological education: role of historical landmarks				
10.14.1 James Lind and scurvy	✓	✓	✓	✓
10.14.2 Edward Jenner and smallpox	✓			
10.14.3 John Snow and cholera	✓			
10.14.4 The emergence of epidemiology	✓	✓		
10.15 A reflection on the future of epidemiology	✓	✓	✓	✓
Summary				

Index

Page numbers in **bold** refer to figures and tables